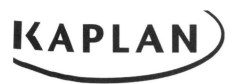

MCAT® 528

Advanced Prep

2021–2022

Published by Kaplan Publishing, a division of Kaplan, Inc.
750 Third Avenue
New York, NY 10017

10 9 8 7 6 5 4 3 2

ISBN: 978-1-5062-6405-9

Kaplan Publishing print books are available at special quantity discounts to use for sales promotions, employee premiums, or educational purposes. For more information or to purchase books, please call the Simon & Schuster special sales department at 866-506-1949.

TABLE OF CONTENTS

GO ONLINE

*www.kaptest.com/
mcatbookresources*

The *Kaplan MCAT 528* Team

Deeangelee Pooran-Kublall, MD/MPH
Editor-in-Chief

Christopher Durland
Kaplan Content Manager

Laura Ambler
Kaplan MCAT Faculty, Author

Elizabeth Flagge
Kaplan Content Manager

Brandon Deason, MD
Kaplan MCAT Faculty, Author/Editor

Lauren White
Kaplan Content Manager

Samer T. Ismail
Kaplan MCAT Faculty, Author/Editor

Matthew Dominick Eggert
Kaplan MCAT Faculty, Author

Thomas C. C. Sargent II
Kaplan MCAT Faculty, Author

Laura Krivicich
Kaplan MCAT Faculty, Author/Editor

MCAT faculty writers/contributors: Marilyn Engel, Aeri Kim, PhD, Brandon McKenzie, Jason Selzer, Uneeb Qureshi, Neha Rao, Charles Richards, Noah Silva, and Rebecca Stover.

Countless thanks to Kim Bowers; Eric Chiu; Samantha Fallon; Owen Farcy; Dan Frey; Chris Gage; Robin Garmise; Rita Garthaffner; Joanna Graham; Adam Grey; Allison Harm; Alex Macnow, MD; Aaron Lemon-Strauss; Keith Lubeley; Petros Minasi; John Polstein; Rochelle Rothstein, MD; Larry Rudman; Sylvia Tidwell Scheuring; Carly Schnur; Lee Weiss; and many others who made this project possible.

How This Book Was Created

The *Kaplan MCAT 528* book was created to give advanced Medical College Admission Test (MCAT) students an edge on the MCAT. This book summarizes the required content for Test Day. Through careful analysis, we identified the content topics for which even the most advanced students might need extra instruction. Then we had our most qualified item writers create challenging, test-like passages. Additionally, the *Kaplan MCAT 528* book contains strategic callouts derived from Kaplan's experience in test taking. Tips are provided to help students work through the tough passages and get the academic boost that will allow them to get the highest score possible (528) on the MCAT.

A team of highly dedicated writers worked very long hours to create this resource. This book was submitted for publication in June 2018. For any updates after this date, please visit **www.kaptest.com/retail-book-corrections-and-updates**.

If you have any questions about the content presented here, email **KaplanMCATfeedback@kaplan.com**. For other questions not related to content, email **booksupport@kaplan.com**.

This book has seen at least five rounds of review. To that end, the information presented is true and accurate to the best of our knowledge. Still, your feedback helps us improve our prep materials. Please notify us of any inaccuracies or errors in the books by sending an email to **KaplanMCATfeedback@kaplan.com**.

Using This Book

Kaplan's *MCAT 528* brings the best of Kaplan's classroom experience to you—right in your home, at your convenience. This book offers the same Kaplan strategies and practice that make Kaplan the #1 choice for MCAT prep.

This book is designed to help you approach the most challenging topics covered on the MCAT in a strategic way. It represents just one of the practice resources available to you as part of your purchase. Additional resources are available in your Online Center, including more practice questions, video science review, and full-length practice. Register for your Online Center at **kaptest.com/booksonline**.

This book summarizes the content necessary for Test Day success and should be viewed as a supplement to your pre-med courses and other MCAT resources. For more thorough content, review Kaplan's *Complete 7-Book Subject Review*.

No matter how confident you are in the content for the MCAT, please understand that content review—no matter how thorough—is not sufficient preparation for the MCAT! The MCAT tests not only your science knowledge but also your critical reading, reasoning, and problem-solving skills. Do not assume that simply memorizing the content will earn you high scores on Test Day; to maximize your score, you must also improve your reading and test-taking skills through MCAT-style questions and practice tests.

That is precisely what this book strives to offer: challenging, MCAT-style worked examples and practice targeting the most high-yield and high-difficulty topics on the exam.

STRATEGIC OVERVIEW

This book simplifies the skills tested by the Association of American Medical Colleges (AAMC) and Kaplan's methods for applying those skills in the different content areas by answering three main questions:

1. What are the skills/strategies/content you need to know?
2. How are the skills/strategies/content presented on the exam?
3. How can you get the edge in that particular skill/strategy/content area?

MCAT PRACTICE

In this book, MCAT practice is provided in two forms:

1. The first type of practice is in the form of worked examples. These passages and question sets were designed for you to try on your own and/or see how an expert would work through them using Kaplan's methods, thereby giving you the tools you need to succeed on Test Day.
2. The second type of practice is in the form of practice passages/sections (in the book and online) that help you apply the strategies and tips that were demonstrated in the worked examples so that you gain mastery and can use them seamlessly on Test Day.

The following is a list of the four types of sidebars you'll find in *MCAT 528*:

- **Key Concept:** These sidebars draw attention to the most important takeaways in a given topic and sometimes offer synopses or overviews of complex information. If you understand nothing else, make sure you understand the Key Concepts for any given subject.
- **MCAT Expertise:** These sidebars point out how information may be tested on the MCAT or offer key strategy points and test-taking tips that you should apply on Test Day.
- **Things to Watch Out For:** These sidebars warn you of common traps students fall into when answering a specific question type.
- **Takeaways:** These sidebars help you understand the point of a question so you won't just walk away from it bogged down with details.

HIGH-YIELD BADGES

Beginning with the 2019–2020 edition of this book, we introduced High-Yield badges. You'll see these badges in the "Preparing for the MCAT" sections. They are designed to be a guide to the number of test-worthy facts that are likely to be derived from a given topic.

These High-Yield badges were created based on material released by the AAMC. In other words, according to the test maker and all our experience with their resources, a badge means more questions on Test Day.

In the end, this is your book. So write in the margins, draw diagrams, highlight the key points—do whatever is necessary to help you get that higher score. We look forward to working with you as you achieve your dreams and become the doctor you deserve to be!

PART ONE

MCAT Basics and Test Strategy

CHAPTER 1

The Path to Medical School

The Medical College Admission Test (MCAT) is a standardized, multiple-choice test administered by the American Association of Medical Colleges (AAMC). It is the entrance exam for medical school.

The MCAT is offered only on specific days of the year (usually about 30 days a year). Test dates range from January to September with only a handful of dates in January and none in February. Every exam begins at 8 a.m. and is administered on a computer. Typically the AAMC opens registration for the earlier exams in October of the previous year and for the later exams in February of the same year. The cost to register varies depending upon when registration is complete, and fees increase as the registration date approaches the test date.

The AAMC does make exceptions to the standard testing experience. Requests for accommodations should be applied for and approved well in advance.

KEY CONCEPT

In response to the COVID-19 pandemic, the AAMC has modified their testing schedule (dates and times) and the length of the MCAT (each section has been shortened to 48 questions). As of the printing of this book it is unknown how long those changes will last.

1.1 The MCAT

Three of the four sections on the MCAT test your basic science knowledge by requiring you to use information critically rather than just provide individual scientific facts. Therefore, you should know how to integrate and analyze information in different contexts using various skills and content databases.

The second section on Test Day, Critical Analysis and Reasoning Skills (CARS), is a unique part of the exam in that it is a pure test of critical thinking. Passages on topics within the social sciences and humanities are presented. Then a series of questions asks you to reason about the material presented—just as you would be expected to do in medical school and in your medical careers.

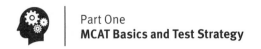
CHEMICAL AND PHYSICAL FOUNDATIONS OF BIOLOGICAL SYSTEMS

In this section, you are required to combine your knowledge of the basic physical sciences with that of the biological sciences. Therefore, understanding the basic chemical and physical principles that underlie the mechanisms operating in the human body and applying these general principles to living systems will be essential.

CRITICAL ANALYSIS AND REASONING SKILLS

This section asks you to analyze passages rooted in the social sciences and humanities. Unlike the other sections, specific knowledge is not required for this section because all of the information is presented in the passages. Some of the subject areas from which content is drawn include ethics and philosophy, cultural studies, and population health.

BIOLOGICAL AND BIOCHEMICAL FOUNDATIONS OF LIVING SYSTEMS

In this section of the MCAT, you have to demonstrate an understanding of the basic processes that foster life, such as growing, reproducing, acquiring energy, etc. Equally important in the study of medicine is your knowledge of how cells and organ systems within an organism act both independently and in concert to accomplish these processes.

PSYCHOLOGICAL, SOCIAL, AND BIOLOGICAL FOUNDATIONS OF BEHAVIOR

This section assesses your ability to implement research and statistical principles within the realm of behavioral and sociocultural determinants of health and health outcomes. Basically, you are required to integrate psychological, sociological, and biological bases of behaviors and relationships.

PASSAGES

Passages on the MCAT are written to test science concepts *in the context of living systems*. In other words, it is unlikely that you will see a passage describing a roller coaster car descending a track at an angle θ, with a given height h and coefficient of kinetic friction μ_k, that is accompanied by questions asking for plug-and-chug application of these principles. Rather, solution chemistry could be tested as an underlying theme in our understanding of urolithiasis (the formation of kidney and bladder stones), organic oxidation and reduction mechanisms as a component of the metabolism of toxins such as ethanol, and atomic absorption and emission spectrometry as it relates to bioluminescence.

QUESTIONS AND SKILLS

A full-length MCAT contains science questions divided into four Scientific Inquiry and Reasoning Skills (SIRS). Although these skills are further explained in Part Two, it is worthwhile to note the increased number of questions focusing on experimental and research design (Skill 3) as well as on data and statistical analysis (Skill 4). These previously made a minimal appearance on the MCAT. However, they now constitute a significant proportion of the questions—perhaps about 20 percent, combined between the two skills.

BIOLOGICALLY BASED PASSAGES

How often have you wondered to yourself—while cramming for that organic chemistry or physics final—"Why do I need to know this as a doctor?" Many pre-medical students question the relevance of some of the material on the MCAT.

How information is presented on the MCAT has changed over time, thereby changing the answer to this question of relevance. Rather than testing thermodynamics through a gas-piston system, which fails to demonstrate why a doctor would actually need to understand these principles, the MCAT now presents the topic in a passage on the proper treatment of frostbite (slow rewarming through a convection current in a rotating water bath at 40°C–42°C).

Some schools are better than others at establishing these connections for students; integrated and clinically based courses are extremely helpful with this goal. By making this application of hard science in a biological context a priority, however, the MCAT can increase this exposure among students even before they arrive for their white-coat ceremony.

A LONG (AND POWERFUL) EXAM

The length of the MCAT actually reflects its use in admissions decisions. Historically, the total score was the most important for admissions committees; section subscores in Physical Sciences, Verbal Reasoning, and Biological Sciences merely showed the breakdown in this total score so schools could pick up on students who were highly lateralized toward one section. Thus, the increased number of questions on the current MCAT is large enough to give reliable, valid data both for section scores and for an overall score—while still being manageable for a test taken in only one day.

Table 1.1 shows the structure of the four sections of the MCAT.

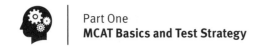
Chemical and Physical Foundations of Biological Systems	
Time	95 minutes
Format	• 59 questions • Score range: 118 to 132 • 44 questions are passage based, and 15 are discrete (stand-alone) questions
What It Tests	• Biochemistry: 25% • Biology: 5% • General Chemistry: 30% • Organic Chemistry: 15% • Physics: 25%
Critical Analysis and Reasoning Skills (CARS)	
Time	90 minutes
Format	• 53 questions • Score range: 118 to 132 • All questions are passage based; there are no discrete (stand-alone) questions
What It Tests	Disciplines: • Humanities: 50% • Social Sciences: 50% Skills: • Foundations of Comprehension: 30% • Reasoning Within the Text: 30% • Reasoning Beyond the Text: 40%
Biological and Biochemical Foundations of Living Systems	
Time	95 minutes
Format	• 59 questions • Score range: 118 to 132 • 44 questions are passage based, and 15 are discrete (stand-alone) questions
What It Tests	• Biochemistry: 25% • Biology: 65% • General Chemistry: 5% • Organic Chemistry: 5%
Psychological, Social, and Biological Foundations of Behavior	
Time	95 minutes
Format	• 59 questions • Score range: 118 to 132 • 44 questions are passage based, and 15 are discrete (stand-alone) questions
What It Tests	• Biology: 5% • Psychology: 65% • Sociology: 30%
Total	
Testing Time	375 minutes (6 hours, 15 minutes)
Questions	230
Score Range	472 to 528

Table 1.1. The Four Sections of the MCAT

EIGHT COMMON MISCONCEPTIONS ABOUT THE MCAT

#1 The MCAT Is a Content Test, Summing Up the Courses I Took in Undergrad

Yes, the MCAT does test a lot of content—two semesters each of physics, general chemistry, organic chemistry, and biology plus a semester each of biochemistry, psychology, and sociology. Although you do need to know about the Doppler effect, the Henderson-Hasselbalch equation for buffers, acyl substitution reactions, and the hormones that govern the menstrual cycle (sometimes called the HPO, or hypothalamic-pituitary-ovarian axis), content alone is not sufficient for excellent MCAT performance.

Rather, critical thinking—the ability to reason, to integrate, to look at a problem in a creative way and find efficient methods to solve it—is the primary driver of a high score.

Why is this? Well, schools can get a sense of your content knowledge by looking at your undergraduate or post-baccalaureate grades. However, the thinking process and ability to use these sciences is not tested evenly across schools. Thus, the MCAT acts as a great equalizer, testing your ability to think—not just memorize. Perhaps most importantly, critical thinking underlies your ability to succeed as a physician.

Consider the patient coming into the emergency department with acute abdominal pain of four hours' duration. Sure, you could memorize all of the possible diagnoses, workups, and treatments for every condition that causes abdominal pain . . . or could you? The differential diagnosis (list of likely causes) is extensive. However, considering the age of the patient, the patient's gender, comorbidities (other illnesses he or she has), and the description of the pain, you can reason what questions would be best to ask to determine the diagnosis.

#2 The MCAT Likes to Test Exceptions, Unusual Examples, and Esoteric Content

This is a common misconception about the MCAT, which leads many pre-medical students to take additional coursework that is not necessary for success on Test Day. Although advanced organic synthesis, anatomy and physiology, and modern physics can show up in an MCAT passage, the outside knowledge required by the AAMC still adheres to the eleven-semester sequence previously mentioned.

It's certainly not a bad idea to take more advanced science courses if your schedule permits. For example, having an understanding of anatomy and physiology before you get to medical school will undoubtedly make cadaver dissection a bit easier. However, recognize that these courses should not be taken specifically for the MCAT. All of the information necessary to answer the questions will be in the passages or in outside knowledge as listed by the AAMC's content outlines.

#3 Passages Are Included on the MCAT to Slow Me Down

Students sometimes assume that passages are included as background information for those unfamiliar with the content covered in a given set of questions. Therefore, they misinterpret the passages as merely introducing a time crunch rather than being a critical part of the test.

The change to passage-based questions in 1992 came from a far more sophisticated drive than timing; these questions require you to integrate new information with the corpus of knowledge you already have and see how they jive together. MCAT passages frequently challenge common assumptions about a given scientific process or introduce an experiment testing the validity of a scientific idea. Only by reading the passage and actually seeing what happens can you be prepared for the accompanying questions.

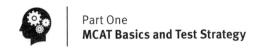
Medicine is a field that requires continuous learning. Our advancements in technology belie our advancements in understanding the human body. Much like how you have to integrate new information with what you already know while reading MCAT passages, as a physician you will have to stay abreast of the newest studies in medicine through academic journals, conferences, and trainings. Admissions committees (and your future patients!) are very interested in your ability to adjust to new data, manipulate it, and absorb it into your schemata of how the world works.

#4 I'll Never Use This Information Again—Especially as a Doctor!

Both the concepts and critical thinking that underlie the MCAT are important to decisions you'll make as a doctor. We've discussed the critical thinking, but why are these concepts important? There's probably no better way to prove it than with a few examples.

When a patient breaks a bone, the translational forces and torques still acting on the bone can be used to predict what structures might be damaged if the fracture is angulated or displaced (moved from its starting position). We also must understand these forces and torques if we are to reset the bone correctly.

Acid-base chemistry dictates the blood disturbances seen in a variety of cases, such as chronic obstructive pulmonary disease, altitude sickness, and acute kidney failure. We further use the principles of acid-base chemistry and the semipermeable membrane to increase the excretion of toxins. For example, a patient who has overdosed on aspirin (acetylsalicylic acid) can excrete more of the toxin when it is deprotonated because it takes on a negative charge and thus cannot cross the cell membrane to reenter the body from the renal tubules. Urinary alkalization (when titrated correctly) can therefore help avoid a toxic overdose.

The continuity equation and Bernoulli's principle explain the pathophysiology of a number of valvular and vascular disorders in the body. In fact, one of the diagnostic findings in valvular stenosis (the narrowing of a heart valve) is an increased velocity of blood flow. Physicians know from the continuity equation that as cross-sectional area decreases, velocity increases (assuming a constant flow rate/cardiac output).

Isomerism is a critical consideration in drug design. Consider the proton pump inhibitor omeprazole (used for gastroesophageal reflux disease, peptic ulcers, and other acid-excess states). When this medication was going to come off patent, a new drug was developed: esomeprazole. Take a look at the names there. Omeprazole is a racemic mixture; esomeprazole is only the *S*-enantiomer of the same drug. Yet the receptor here is achiral! Thus, for a huge difference in cost, the patient sees very little difference when taking one drug versus the other. Yet a patient will be thankful when the therapy you prescribe doesn't break the bank!

There are countless additional examples. To be clear, drawing out these connections between science and medicine—and making them more explicit—is a critical component of the MCAT.

#5 The MCAT Is Not Particularly Predictive of My Success in Medical School

Although it may have been a bit harder to draw a correlation between your SAT score and success in undergraduate school, the MCAT has been demonstrated multiple times to be highly predictive of first- and second-year grades in medical school and success on the United States Medical Licensing Examination, Step 1 (USMLE, or the "Boards"). A landmark study by Ellen Julian in 2005 found that the MCAT was 59 percent correlated with first- and second-year grades, 46 percent correlated with clerkship (third-year) grades, and 70 percent correlated with Step 1 scores. This was significantly higher than the undergraduate grade point average alone, at 54 percent, 36 percent, and 49 percent, respectively. The brief takeaway: dominating the MCAT bodes well for your success in medical school.

#6 There Isn't Enough Time to Use Strategies on the MCAT

The MCAT is a timed test. Under the pressure of the clock, many test takers abandon their strategies. This is the last thing you want to do! The Kaplan strategies are designed to help you finish each section on time while maximizing your number of correct answers. Having a methodical approach to every level of the test (section, passage, question, and answer) ensures that you never have to waste time wondering how to get started or what to do next. In order to get the full benefit of the strategies, they must be internalized. If you have to think about the strategies, that's an indication that they have not been practiced enough to become second nature.

#7 The MCAT Is Curved

A curved test is one in which an individual's performance is gauged by the performance of other test takers. If everyone who takes the MCAT on the same day as you does really well, that does not affect your score. Conversely, if everyone does really poorly, that has no bearing on your score because the MCAT isn't curved—it's scaled and equated. Each test form is slightly different, and the raw to scaled score conversion is adjusted to compensate. That means that on Test Day, you're not competing against other test takers; you're competing against the test.

#8 If I Don't Do Well, I Can Just Retake the MCAT

Although you *can* take the MCAT multiple times, this is not recommended. For one, the MCAT is an investment of your time (nearly a full day), money (over $300), and energy (emotionally and physically!). Additionally, the AAMC follows a full disclosure policy, meaning they send all scores earned after April 2003. How multiple scores are interpreted vary from school to school, but medical schools do see them all. Finally, there are actually limits to the number of times you can take the MCAT: three times in a single year, four times in two consecutive years, and seven times in a lifetime.

SCORING

Each of the four sections of the MCAT is scored between 118 and 132, with the mean and median at 125. This means the total score ranges from 472 to 528, with the mean and median at 500. Why such peculiar numbers? The AAMC stresses that this scale emphasizes the importance of the central portion of the score distribution, where most students score (around 125 per section, or 500 total), rather than putting undue focus on the high end of the scale.

Note that there is no wrong answer penalty on the MCAT. So you should select an answer for every question—even if it is only a guess.

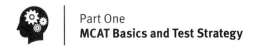

The AAMC has released the 2018–2019 correlation between scaled score and percentile, as shown in Table 1.2. It should be noted that the percentile scale is adjusted and renormalized over time and thus can shift slightly from year to year.

Total Score	Percentile Rank	Total Score	Percentile Rank
472	<1	501	50
473	<1	502	53
474	<1	503	57
475	<1	504	60
476	1	505	64
477	1	506	67
478	2	507	70
479	2	508	74
480	3	509	77
481	4	510	80
482	5	511	82
483	6	512	85
484	7	513	87
485	8	514	89
486	10	515	91
487	11	516	93
488	13	517	94
489	15	518	96
490	17	519	97
491	20	520	98
492	22	521	98
493	25	522	99
494	28	523	99
495	30	524	100
496	33	525	100
497	37	526	100
498	40	527	100
499	43	528	100
500	46		

Table 1.2. 2020–2021 Correlation between Scaled Score and Percentile

Source: AAMC. (2020). Summary of MCAT total and section scores. Accessed June 2020. https://students-residents.aamc.org/advisors/article/percentile-ranks-for-the-mcat-exam/.

The MCAT is a computer-based test and is offered at Pearson VUE centers seven months of the year. There are optional breaks between each section and a lunch break between the second and third sections of the exam.

Register online for the MCAT at **www.aamc.org/mcat**.

For further questions, contact the MCAT team at the Association of American Medical Colleges (AAMC):

MCAT Resource Center
Association of American Medical Colleges

(202) 828-0690
www.aamc.org/mcat
mcat@aamc.org

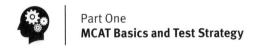

1.2 Medical School Admissions

The path to medical school takes years to complete. However, if you are thinking about taking the MCAT, then congratulations! It's likely that you are near the finish line. The timeline in Figure 1.1 shows a few key events in the final stretch, with an emphasis on timely completion of the primary and secondary applications. That said, the best timeline is the one that gets you into your dream school, and that often means deviating from the ideal.

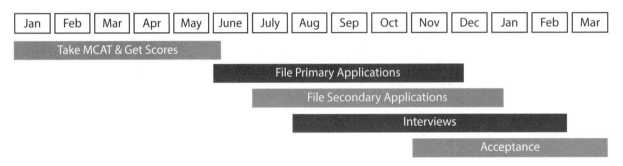

Figure 1.1. Timeline for MCAT and Acceptance to Medical School

THE PRIMARY APPLICATION

Your primary application for the majority of allopathic medical schools is submitted through the American Medical College Application Service, or AMCAS. Those who are additionally, or alternatively, applying to osteopathic medical school should submit a primary application through the American Association of Colleges of Osteopathic Medicine Application Service, or AACOMAS. Those applying to medical school in Texas (allopathic and/or osteopathic) need to submit their application through the Texas Medical and Dental Schools Application Service, or TMDSAS. Although there are some differences among each of these application services, for the most part they require the same information. For the purpose of brevity, this review focuses on the AMCAS, breaking down each of the nine sections and what you can do to be prepared for each section.

Sections 1 to 3: Background Information
The first three sections of the AMCAS application want to know your background. This includes your name, birthday, the college or colleges you've attended, and information about your family, languages you speak, military service, any criminal record, etc.—all kinds of things that will help admissions departments get a better picture of you as a potential medical school candidate.

It also asks for your contact information. Per AMCAS's website, they will contact you primarily via email. So make sure to provide an address you check frequently. If you primarily use an address provided by your undergraduate institution, ensure that you will be able to use this address after graduation.

Section 4: Coursework

Official transcripts are required, but AMCAS also asks that you personally provide them with a list of your undergraduate courses and grades. Each course will also be marked with a particular classification according to content. Based on your grades, standardized AMCAS GPAs will be generated. One GPA is calculated using biology, chemistry, physics, and math classes (BCPM GPA). Another GPA is calculated using the rest of your classes, or all other classes (AO GPA).

Make sure you enter the course name exactly as it is written on your transcript! If the information submitted about coursework does not match up with the official record, you may have your application returned. This means a delay in getting it sent to medical schools. So be sure to double-check that everything is correct before you submit.

Section 5: Work and Activities

The work and activities section is where you get a chance to shine. You can list up to 15 experiences that make you stand out as a medical school candidate. Anything goes here: volunteering, research, shadowing at a hospital, even hobbies. The objective in this section is to show a diversity of pursuits that have prepared you for medical school. In this section, you can choose up to three of your activities that were most meaningful for you and expand on those.

When completing the AMCAS work and activities section, you should have **a full list of 15 significant experiences**. If you're struggling to come up with a full 15 activities, consider how you can break up certain activities into multiple entries. For example, you may have one entry about a research experience. Could you also write a second entry about the publication of a research paper or a poster presentation you gave on that research experience at a conference?

If you're early enough in your undergraduate career, consider keeping a journal of potential activities to include on your list. Write down who you worked with, how many hours you worked, a summary of the experience as a whole, and a description of the impact it had on you. If you're already preparing to fill out your medical school application without a journal, take some time to write out a list of impactful experiences so that you have plenty of things to choose from. Start by listing every activity you can think of, aiming for an initial list of 20 activities, and then trim the list down to 15.

Section 6: Letters of Evaluation

The letters of recommendation section is one where the majority of the content won't be provided by you. Instead, you'll be asked to provide the names of your letter writers and where they can be contacted. Be sure you've spoken to those you're asking for letters of recommendation before putting them on your AMCAS application. You can request up to ten letters, though the number that individual medical schools accept varies.

In choosing the people to ask for letters, consider what they can add to your application. Above all, ask people who know you well and will provide a great—nay, glowing—letter of recommendation. Keep in mind that you can submit your application before the requested letters are received by AMCAS; so don't panic if everything else is ready but your letters are not. Each letter will go out with an ID that will allow it to be matched up to your application.

Section 7: Medical Schools

This section is where, after you've done your initial research to find the schools that best fit your wants, needs, and career goals, you'll make a list of the schools where you want your application sent. This is also where you'll indicate if you want to be an early decision candidate, apply for a combined degree program, etc.

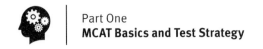

How to Build Your School List

The Medical School Admission Requirements (MSAR) website is one of the most definitive places to go for medical school information. It costs $28 for a year-long subscription, but it's among the best resources you'll have for researching medical schools. It includes important information about acceptance rates, average MCAT scores and GPAs of applicants and accepted students, numbers of out-of-state students, application requirements, and crucial application deadlines.

Another nice feature of MSAR is that you can easily search for schools you want to learn about. All of the information is standardized, accessible, and up-to-date, and the site allows you to compare and contrast medical schools easily. This is an especially useful resource for taking a preliminary look and narrowing down your options.

The equivalent to the MSAR for osteopathic medical schools is the Osteopathic Medical College Information Book, or CIB for short, which is actually available as a free PDF on the AACOM (American Association of Colleges of Osteopathic Medicine) website.

Medical School Websites

Each medical school provides key information through its website. Although most of this will have some overlap with what's available on the MSAR or CIB, it'll give you a feel for how the program describes itself in promotional materials—beyond the numbers. You can typically read about the school's mission statement and will often find testimonials from alumni and students. Each school's website also includes pictures of the campus and details about the curriculum.

The downside when comparing medical schools via their respective websites is the lack of standardization. Because these sites vary among medical schools, it's not always easy to compare. So plan on investing some time to research information that's relevant to you. Individual medical school sites can be an especially great resource after you've already started to narrow your search and have a short list of programs to consider.

MD vs. DO

Both allopathic (MD) and osteopathic (DO) medical programs involve the same level of schooling and training. They both provide similar career opportunities in terms of specialization and salary expectations. Medical school admissions is tough, whether you go the allopathic or osteopathic route. However, osteopathic admissions is slightly less competitive with respect to average GPA and MCAT scores.

Like allopathic schools, osteopathic medical schools emphasize holistic admissions. In other words, they want to know what you've done in your life and the unique talents and experiences you may bring to their programs. When taken together with (slightly) lower average scores, osteopathic programs can be attractive to nontraditional applicants, many of whom have been away from school for years but can boast unique life experiences.

Unlike allopathic medical schools, osteopathic schools require students to study osteopathic manipulative medicine (OMM), which posits the idea that every tissue in the body is connected to every other part through an entity called the myofascia. Therefore, a problem in one area can affect the function of another area, thereby affecting the overall health of the patient. Osteopathy students are taught to palpate and manipulate bones, joints, and muscle to relieve impediments to function or to coax poorly functioning tissues to function properly, which then enhances the proper functioning of other body parts. This unique approach to medicine may be of particular interest to students who plan to pursue orthopedics, sports medicine, physical medicine (physiatry), or physical therapy and pain management. Those who wish to enter primary care may also wish to pursue osteopathic medicine, as back and knee pain, arthritis, and all kinds of chronic pain are common presenting complaints.

Having said this, graduates of DO programs are well-represented in all of the specialties, including cardiology, dermatology, otorhinolaryngology, and surgery. Furthermore, DO students who are interested can take the same standardized exams as MD students and can apply to MD residencies.

Public vs. Private

There are many major differences between public and private medical schools—especially when it comes to cost and availability of scholarships. When choosing medical schools, it's prudent to find out what percentage of students receive scholarships and, on average, how much it decreases their tuition. Another component of public *vs.* private institutions is their acceptance rate of in-state *vs.* out-of-state students. Often the public institutions favor taking more students from their state since those students are more likely to stay in the state after graduation and practice medicine there. Private institutions don't have as much stake in refueling the state's workforce and are oftentimes more likely to accept out-of-state students.

In-State vs. Out-of-State

Schools have varying acceptance rates and levels of preference for in-state *vs.* out-of-state applicants. The number of target schools that are in your state will also affect the number of applications you submit. For instance if you live in California, where there are a lot of medical schools, you'll want to apply to as many programs as possible that give you in-state preference. Unfortunately, some states have one medical school and others have none. If your state doesn't have a medical school, find out if there are schools in neighboring states that will give you in-state preference. Limited in state options mean you should increase the number of applications you submit.

Go with Your Gut

All of these factors are important, but the most important factor is fit. Where do you feel the most comfortable? Which school do you think will help you become the best physician you can be? You can fill columns in your application pros and cons spreadsheet, but your gut is actually the best judge of where you belong.

Section 8: Essays

As with the work and activities section, the essays section really gives you an opportunity to sell yourself. Here you must write a personal statement: why do you want to go to medical school? On the AMCAS application, you have 5,300 characters to showcase why you'll be a great asset to whatever school you choose to attend. The TMDSAS application gives you 5,000 characters, and the AACOMAS application gives you 4,500.

Don't write your personal statement as you're filling out your application. Write drafts, have others review and critique them, and proofread, proofread, proofread! By the time you actually submit your essay, it should be polished and professional.

If you're applying for an MD/PhD program, you are required to submit two additional essays. So keep that in mind if you're considering a combined degree.

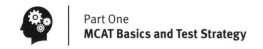

Tips for the Personal Statement

- Be very personal. Always provide support for what you say. Give an example from your work, volunteer activities, or special contact with doctors, through your own experiences or those of family or friends. Never just make a statement about yourself and expect the reader to take it at face value.
- Don't make general, sweeping statements ("I want to help people"). Instead, be very specific.
- Write from the heart, but don't make it mushy. Keep it real, and support what you write.
- Medical schools want diversity in their classes, so write about your particular educational experience, interests, life challenges, etc.
- Use the first person pronoun "I," but don't let your writing get too informal. Avoid slang, jargon, and trite clichés.
- Don't rewrite your resume, honors, or any information that is in other parts of the application.
- You want to show yourself as a thoughtful person, but don't get into controversial issues. This is not the time or place to be confrontational.
- Your personal statement should give the admissions committee a strong sense of you as an individual. However, one of the hardest questions to answer is exactly that—who am I? Try asking three people—perhaps one family member, one good friend, and one acquaintance—to describe you using just two or three adjectives. You'll get a good idea of how other people see you. Now reflect. Is this how you see yourself? If so, use that insight to write about yourself. If not, consider why there's a difference between how you see yourself and how others see you, and use that as a thoughtful starting point.
- After you have written a first draft, ask a trusted friend or relative to read it and, based on what you wrote, tell you what he or she has learned about you. Did you express yourself as you wanted to? Will the schools now know who you really are and why you want to be a doctor?
- Try to have a theme. If you're a marathon runner who is also passionate about patient care, tie these together. Perhaps talk about the long but satisfying training, the exultation at the end of a race, the lessons learned from coming in first or last—essentially, the intersection between sports and medicine specific to your own life.
- Keep writing drafts until you are completely satisfied that you've clearly discussed the significant life experiences that showcase your top qualities and that demonstrate you will make an excellent physician.

Section 9: Standardized Tests

Of course, no medical school application is complete without an MCAT score! Like your BCPM GPA, the MCAT is a standardized way for medical schools to consider applicants from diverse backgrounds and undergraduate institutions. Most schools will only accept an MCAT score received within the last three years, but this does vary by school.

If you're applying for a combined degree program, schools may require additional standardized tests, such as the Graduate Management Admission Test (GMAT) for an MBA/MD program. If this is the case, you can submit those scores on this section of the application as well.

SECONDARY APPLICATIONS

Fees and Deadlines

Nearly every secondary application comes with a fee, ranging from $30 to $250. Before you shell out the money, be sure to check out the AAMC's Fee Assistance Program to see if you qualify.

The sooner you can submit your primary application, the sooner you can work on secondary applications and get those in. Time is critical. Medical schools use rolling admissions, and the slots (anywhere from 25 to about 200) fill up very quickly. Don't forget: You could be a stellar candidate, but if you're at the bottom of the pile because your application was received late, it might not even get looked at. Additionally, there is an expectation that you **return any secondary application that you receive within two weeks**. Otherwise, medical schools will interpret the delayed return as a lack of interest in their school or possibly not accept the application at all.

Essays

Nearly every school asks a version of "Why do you want to go to our school?" This sounds challenging. To make answering the question easier, you should compile a list of your interests and what you want out of medical school. Then tailor that information for each school. This means that you need to research each school's program and curriculum so you can figure out how each school might provide you with the opportunities you want.

Secondary applications range from a few questions to ten or more. Here are some examples:

What are you interested in?
How would you add to the diversity of our school?
What is a challenging situation you've had to overcome?
What is one nonmedical activity that has had a significant impact on you?
If you have already graduated, what have you done since undergrad?
If you didn't become a doctor, what would you do?

These questions might seem challenging (and a bit annoying), and it's especially overwhelming if a school asks a lot of them. However, if you look closer, they're all a version of "What unique talents and experiences would you bring to our school?" Remember, you already answered this when writing a list of your activities and interests and them tailoring them to different schools.

Sometimes the questions do get weird, but the Internet has your back—or more specifically, friendly pre-meds who post the questions on message boards have your back. Be sure you check these out while waiting for those secondary apps.

Finally, the secondary application is a good place to update schools about your current activities, especially if it's been a few months since you sent in the primary application. In fact, some schools have a space for current activities; if not, it's pretty easy to work it into responses for questions.

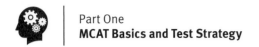
INTERVIEWS

Getting an interview is a major milestone in the medical school admissions process. There are two main types of medical school interviews: traditional and multiple mini interviews (MMI).

Traditional

The traditional interview is generally one or two interviews, often with one faculty member and one current student, each lasting between 30 and 45 minutes. Approaches vary by school. So be sure to do your research so you know what to expect when you arrive for the big day.

How much will interviewers know about you when you walk into the room? This too may vary. They may have seen all of your application, part of it, or none of it. You should therefore be prepared to summarize your background and draw upon your experiences when speaking with your interviewer. It's always a good idea to glance through your AMCAS and secondary applications before interview day to make sure you're able to communicate your strengths effectively during your sessions.

Multiple Mini Interviews

In the MMI, you'll be given anywhere from six to ten scenarios or questions. You will be given a couple of minutes to study each question and then about eight minutes to respond. You will be observed and critiqued on how you choose to handle each situation presented. The scenarios often deal with ethical/moral issues, interpersonal skills, and/or professionalism. Although it may seem like a daunting situation to be placed into, keep in mind that the MMI can help level the playing field on interview day. Rather than presenting yourself to just one or two individuals, you'll likely interact with different interviewers for each new scenario you're given. That means you have more opportunities to make a great first impression and show off your personal talents and skills.

Some schools hybridize interviews to include both formats. Some provide one-on-one interviews with a faculty member or with a student. Others interview with two or more faculty members or a combination of faculty and students. At still others, you appear before a panel of evaluators. Sometimes there may be silent observers who don't interact directly with you at all.

With all that in mind, make sure you're operating at your professional best throughout interview day with everyone you meet, from your first encounter with the admissions office staff onward.

DEVELOPING INTERVIEWING SKILLS

Draw on Real-World Interviewing Experience

You may not realize it, but you're hitting the ground running. As a pre-med student, you already have a wealth of interviewing experience: volunteering jobs, research positions, paid employment, scholarships, shadowing, and so on. Reflect on your interviews for these positions. Make a note of what you did right and how you can improve. Chances are you still have a number of positions in the pipeline (before applying to medical school), so make sure you get comments from your interviewers. Feedback from real-world interviews, even if the position isn't health related, is arguably more valuable than feedback from mock interviews for medical school.

Familiarize Yourself with Common Interview Questions

Our articles on interviewing contain lists of interview questions; be sure to check these out. First, though, make sure you can answers the questions that come up in almost every interview:

> *Why do you want to become a doctor?*
> *Why do you want to go to our medical school?*
> *What specific talents and experiences would you bring to our program?*
> *Tell me about yourself.*

Avoid Scripted Responses

Prepare thoughtful responses, but do not memorize them word for word. Focus on content, not specific lines. Otherwise, you will seem rehearsed and stiff, which will make you seem less believable and therefore less convincing. You must at least appear as if you are answering the question in the moment so that you are actually conversing with the interviewer. This will help you build a rapport with him or her.

Practice, Practice, Practice

The goal is not to memorize responses but to be so prepared that you know an interviewer can throw everything but the kitchen sink at you and you won't be rattled. Then you will project confidence and make the interviewer have confidence in you.

Start by answering questions by yourself. Get a bunch of $3'' \times 5''$ note cards, and write one interview question per card. Shuffle them, and pick a card without looking. Then read the question aloud and answer it. It helps to look at yourself in the mirror so you can monitor your facial expressions.

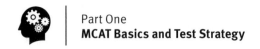
Practice with a Friend or Colleague

Ask a friend to pepper you with weird or unexpected questions and to play the devil's advocate. ("Didn't you get a 'B–' in organic chemistry? Why should I take you over someone with a perfect record?") Ask your friend to give feedback on the content of your answers, delivery, and level of confidence and poise. Most importantly, ask your friend whether you convinced him or her that you would make a great doctor.

Videotape the Interview

Watch with a friend (or, ideally, a mentor who has experience as an interviewer) who can critique your answers and help you pick up on nonverbal cues, tics, and other behaviors that might detract from your overall presentation. The advantage of videotaping is that some nonverbal signs are missed by interviewers during the course of an interview but nonetheless affect them. A careful review of the session can reveal such behaviors.

Be Ready for Unusual, Tricky Questions

Log onto the Internet message boards for unusual interview questions from specific schools. Then create responses to these questions and rehearse them. Again, do not memorize responses word for word but, rather, focus on content.

Boost Your Improvisational Skills

If your crazy pre-med schedule allows for it, consider enrolling in an improvisational comedy or an acting class. This will train you to stay loose, think on your feet, adapt to changing situations, and pick up on nonverbal cues and play off of them (in this case, those coming from your interviewer). At the very least, doing improv will help you blow off steam. (As a pre-med student, you definitely need that.)

Aim for *I Would Make a Great Doctor*

Impart the feeling that you would make a great doctor, not just a great med student. This isn't just another interview. You're making a case for your chosen career—your calling.

CHAPTER 2

Reading the Kaplan Way

MCAT reading is unlike any other reading that you have done in the past. In the same way that one reads a novel differently than a textbook, MCAT reading requires its own unique approach. At its core, the MCAT is a critical-thinking exam. In fact, one section is even titled Critical Analysis and Reasoning Skills (also called the CARS section). Whether in a science section or the CARS section, to be successful on the MCAT, you must read passages actively. Active reading consciously considers how and why passage information is presented, which then provides insight on how the information is tested. This chapter, *Reading the Kaplan Way*, is a strategic framework that facilitates active reading and helps you avoid common pitfalls such as accidentally glazing over text or forgetting what you had read. In this chapter, you will learn the Kaplan Method for Passages (Preview, Choose, Read, and Distill) and how to apply it on all sections of the MCAT.

2.1 How to Read Strategically Using Keywords

MCAT passages are packed with dense academic prose. There are several distinct levels for which the text should be evaluated: content, purpose, and reasoning. Addressing all three modes of reading is essential for Test Day success.

Read for content: Extract the information from the text, discovering precisely *what* is being said. This includes understanding the ideas and concepts presented in the passage.

Read for purpose: Examine the purpose of the text by asking, *why* did the author write this? Reading for purpose can be applied at various levels of the passage: *Why did the author include this term or phrase? Why did the author include a paragraph? Why did the author write the entire passage?*

Read for reasoning: Consider *how* the different ideas presented in the passage relate to one another. In argumentative passages, this involves identifying how the author supports and challenges his/her claims. If the informational content is the *what* of the text and if the purpose of writing is the *why,* then the reasoning is the *how.*

Being comfortable with all three modes of reading will give you the flexibility needed when reading the wide variety of passages you'll encounter on Test Day. For instance, you may find yourself reading a passage that discusses concepts that are incomprehensible, as you lack the academic background of the author. In that case, you will be better suited reading the passage for purpose and reasoning.

KEY CONCEPT

Any passage can be understood in three different ways, which we call the modes of reading. Each mode answers at least one vital question:
- Content: *What does the text say? What does this mean?*
- Purpose: *Why does the author write? Why does the author include a specific piece of information? How does the author feel?*
- Reasoning: *How do sentences connect? How do ideas relate? How are the arguments built?*

RELATION KEYWORDS

Relation keywords are words or phrases used by the author to connect ideas within a text. When tackling a passage, you must understand how the text you're currently reading fits into the bigger picture of the paragraph or passage. Paying attention to these Relation keywords can accomplish this. Although ideas might be related to one another in many ways, the vast majority of **Relation keywords** fall into one of two subcategories: Continuation or Contrast.

- **Continuation keywords** indicate that more of the same idea is coming in the text.
- **Contrast keywords** signify a change in the author's focus or a direct contrast between two things.

More Complex Relationships
- **Opposition keywords** indicate an outright conflict between ideas.
- **Sequence keywords** suggest a series of events advancing in time.
- **Comparison keywords** are used to evaluate ideas and rank them relative to others.

Table 2.1 lists examples of Relation keywords in each category. Note that some words can fit into more than one category; for example, the word *not* reveals a contrast and can also create a direct opposition.

Continuation	Contrast	Opposition
and	but	not/never/none
also	yet	either . . . or
moreover	however	as opposed to
furthermore	although	on the contrary
like	(even) though	versus
same/similar	rather (than)	on one hand . . . on the other hand
that is	in contrast	otherwise
in other words	on the other hand	**Sequence**
for example	otherwise	before/after
take the case of	nevertheless	earlier/later
for instance	whereas	previous/next
including	while	initially/subsequently/finally
such as	different	first/second/third/last
in addition	unlike	historically/traditionally/used to
plus	notwithstanding	now/currently/modern
at the same time	another	**Comparison**
as well as	instead	better/best
equally	still	worse/worst
this/that/these/those	despite	less/least
: [colon]	alternatively	more/most
; [semicolon]	unless	-er/-est
— [em dash]	not	primarily
( ) [parentheses]	conversely	especially
" " [quotes]	contrarily	above all

Table 2.1. Common Relation Keywords

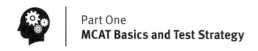
MCAT EXPERTISE

The relationships seen in the sciences differ from those in the CARS section. Concepts in science passages are often related through quantitative means and are highly testable on the MCAT. As such, noting words that denote trends are vital for MCAT success. These words include *increasing*, *decreasing*, *required*, *inhibited*, and many others.

MCAT EXPERTISE

Most CARS passages on the MCAT contain strong but not extreme opinions. Rarely will an author be completely neutral because there is little reasoning to test if the author does not express at least a moderately positive or negative opinion.

KEY CONCEPT

Although they are both overall neutral, these two attitudes are very different:
• Ambivalent = having both a positive and a negative opinion.
• Impartial = having neither a positive nor a negative opinion.

AUTHOR KEYWORDS

Author keywords are verbs, nouns, adjectives, and adverbs that hint at the author's opinions. Author keywords have a connotation of either approval or disapproval. Authors may use characteristic words and short phrases to make their claims more extreme as well as others that moderate their claims. Noting the presence and function of Author keywords facilitates *reading for purpose*.

Positive *vs.* Negative

- **Positive keywords** include nouns such as *masterpiece*, *genius*, and *triumph*; verbs such as *excel*, *succeed*, and *know*; adjectives such as *compelling*, *impressive*, and *elegant*; and adverbs such as *correctly*, *reasonably*, and *fortunately*.
- **Negative keywords** include nouns such as *disaster*, *farce*, and *limitation*; verbs such as *miss*, *fail*, and *confuse*; adjectives such as *problematic*, *so-called*, and *deceptive*; and adverbs such as *questionably*, *merely*, and *purportedly*.

Note that in addition to positive, negative, or neutral, an author can also be **ambivalent**. Ambivalence literally means "feeling both ways," and it is different from **impartiality**.

EXTREME

Extreme keywords are words that enhance the charge of what the author is saying, forcing the author into one extreme or the other.

MODERATING

Moderating keywords are words that set limits to claims to make those claims easier to support. These keywords are moderating because a stronger statement is usually more difficult to prove than a weaker one.

Table 2.2 lists examples of Author keywords in each category.

Positive	Negative	Extreme	Moderating
masterpiece	disaster	must	can/could
genius	farce	need/necessary	may/might
triumph	limitation	always	possibly
excel	miss	every	probably
succeed	fail	any	sometimes
know	confuse	only	on occasion
compelling	problematic	should/ought	often
impressive	so-called	indeed	tends to
elegant	deceptive	very	here
correctly	questionably	especially	now
reasonably	merely	obviously	in this case
fortunately	purportedly	above all	in some sense

Table 2.2. Common Author Keywords

LOGIC KEYWORDS

Reading for reasoning focuses on identifying the connections between different claims and ideas stated in the passage. *Logic keywords* aim to reveal specific connections between evidence and conclusions. In this way, Logic keywords can clarify the reasoning of a passage. Logic keywords tend to be relatively rare, occurring less frequently than either Relation or Author keywords in most passages.

Evidence and Conclusion

A **conclusion** is a claim that the author is trying to convince the audience to believe, whereas pieces of **evidence** are the reasons that are given for believing the conclusion. When applied to CARS passage reading, conclusions, not evidence, capture the main takeaway of a paragraph. Thus, let Logic keywords, when present, help you identify the author's conclusions.

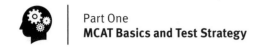

Refutation

Refutation keywords are the opposite of evidence; they are countervailing reasons for rejecting a conclusion.

Table 2.3 lists examples of Logic keywords in each category.

Evidence	Conclusion	Refutation
because (of)	therefore	despite
since	thus	notwithstanding
if	then	challenge
for	so	undermined by
why	consequently	object
the reason is	leading to	counter(argument)
as a result of	resulting in	critique/criticize
due to	argue	conflict
as evident in	conclude	doubt
justified by	imply	problem
assuming	infer	weakness
after all	suggest	called into question by

Table 2.3. Common Logic Keywords

2.2 How to Analyze Passages Critically

THE KAPLAN METHOD FOR CARS PASSAGES

The Kaplan Method for critically reading CARS passages consists of four steps: **Preview, Choose, Read,** and **Distill**.

- **Preview:** Spend approximately 10 seconds noting the presence or absence of key passage patterns. Use these patterns to determine passage difficulty and whether you should do the passage now or later.
- **Choose:** Using the patterns noted in the Preview step, Choose an appropriate Distill approach for the passage (Interrogate, Outline, or Highlight).
- **Read:** Use keywords and the three reading modes to read strategically.
  - Identify **Relation keywords** (to connect different ideas in the text), **Logic keywords** (to reveal the passage's arguments), and **Author keywords** (to offer glimpses of the writer's intentions).
  - Don't reread text excessively.
- **Distill:** While reading the passage, your aim is to distill the major takeaway of each paragraph using one of the following approaches.
  - **Interrogate**: Thoroughly examine each major idea presented in the paragraph by asking interrogative questions, such as, *why* did the author include this piece of information and *how* does it connect to the surrounding text.
  - **Outline**: Create a brief label for each paragraph that summarizes the major takeaway of the paragraph.
  - **Highlight**: Highlight one to three terms per paragraph that capture the major takeaway.

  Before moving onto the questions, consider what was the author's goal when writing the passage.

PREVIEW

A lot can happen in 10 seconds, especially when Previewing a passage! Although 10 seconds may seem incredibly short, with practice you will be able to spot key passage patterns that will set you up for a successful passage read through. Look out for the following fixed patterns in your Preview step to help you establish the difficulty of a passage.

- **Passage type**: Is the passage type humanities or social sciences?
- **Passage language**: Is the terminology familiar? Is the passage written in a clear voice? Is the author's voice academic or social?
- **Passage structure**: Does the passage follow a clear argument structure or does it wander? Can the purpose of individual paragraphs be determined at a glance from their first sentence?
- **Sentence structure**: Is the author's sentence structure clear? Does the author include many complicated/long sentences or unusual punctuation?

These patterns can be seen by glancing at the first one to two sentences of the passage and the first several words of the later paragraphs. Using the patterns found, determine the difficulty of the passage and decide whether you will attack the passage *now* or *later*.

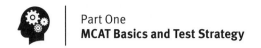
CHOOSE

Perhaps it goes without saying that choosing which Distill approach you use for a passage is ultimately up to you. However, avoid simply defaulting to the approach you find most comfortable as this can limit your growth as a critical reader. Instead, let the passage patterns revealed in your Preview step influence your choice.

- **Interrogation** is the most thorough of the Distill approaches and therefore requires a major time investment, taking up to six minutes to complete. When choosing to Interrogate a passage, you should be confident that your time investment will be rewarded with a deeper understanding of the passage.
  - ○ *Consider interrogation* for passages with clearer sentence structure, as it is likely that spending the extra time interrogating will provide a deeper passage understanding.
  - ○ *Consider interrogation* for passages that cover more abstract topics, as these ideas must often be explored through interrogation to be fully understood.
  - ○ *Avoid interrogation* for passages that are exceptionally difficult to read, as the extra time spent interrogating may not result in a deeper understanding.
- **Outlining** aims to Distill the major takeaway of a paragraph into a briefly written label. Implicit in this action is that each paragraph has a clear defined takeaway, but this is not always the case.
  - ○ *Consider outlining* for passages that have a clear passage structure as seen in the Preview step.
  - ○ *Consider outlining* for passages that are heavy in details or evidence, as they can often be distilled to a key takeaway or conclusion.
  - ○ *Avoid outlining* for passages that have unusual passage structure. These include passages with paragraphs that differ greatly in length, passages with oddly few but very long paragraphs, or passages with an absurd amount of very short paragraphs.

- **Highlighting** spends a minimal amount of time distilling the passage and thus only provides the most shallow level of passage understanding. However, this is offset by allowing most of your passage time to be spent on the passage questions.
  - *Consider highlighting* for difficult passages where you are unsure whether a more thorough read through will provide deeper understanding. Often these are passages with unclear sentence and passage structure.
  - *Avoid highlighting* passages that may be better suited for outlining or interrogation, such as passages with clear passage structure or abstract concepts, respectively.

READ AND DISTILL

Earlier in this chapter, we explored the three modes of reading (content, purpose, and reasoning). Each of the three Distill approaches (Interrogate, Outline, and Highlight) uses all three modes of reading. Therefore, no matter which Distill approach is chosen, readers should be looking to leverage keywords while they read.

The difference between the Distill approaches is depth of understanding. Each approach distills the major takeaway of the paragraphs and passage, but they do so to varying degrees. As such, the time investment of the approaches greatly differs. Interrogation may take up to six minutes. Outlining may take up to four minutes. Highlighting should take no more than two to three minutes.

Interrogation

This approach borrows its name from the learning science term *elaborative interrogation*, which describes the process of asking *why* and *how* questions to deepen one's understanding and strengthen one's memory of a concept (or a passage). In the CARS section, this takes the form of asking in-depth questions aiming to understand the author's intent and purpose in his or her writing as well as how the author chose to structure the passage. If done properly, interrogating a passage should provide not only a deeper understanding of the author's perspective and passage, but also stronger recall of the major ideas in the passage. In many cases, a strong interrogation means questions can be answered without returning back to the passage.

At its core, interrogation is all about asking yourself the right questions about each passage to deepen your understanding. For many, the hardest part of this process is not answering these questions but, rather, generating the interrogative questions in the first place. Below presents a series of steps you can use to generate interrogative questions and develop your interrogation skills.

Interrogative Questions through Chunking

In learning science, *chunking* is the process of breaking down a complex set of information into smaller pieces or *chunks* for easier digestion, such as remembering the number 3710 as two chunks, "thirty-seven and ten." When applied to the Interrogation approach, chunking means to parse a paragraph into chunks based on purpose. For example, if the next sentence serves a different purpose from the previous sentence, the next sentence can be seen as a new chunk. If a paragraph defines a moral theory and then provides an example, the paragraph could be parsed into two chunks. Most paragraphs can be parsed into two to three chunks.

MCAT EXPERTISE

Part of your passage and question review should include the self-reflective question, "Did I choose an appropriate Distill approach for this passage?" This will allow you to refine your methodology as you gain more experience. With practice, you may find that the decisions make in your Choose step diverge from the general advice of this book. This is OK and may even be expected, as your individual CARS development and experience will differ from that of others.

MCAT EXPERTISE

If you're like most readers, the majority (if not all) of your reading has been for content. Whether it was reading the newspaper to stay up to date with the latest events or reading the *Kaplan MCAT Biology Review Notes* for high-yield concepts, your aim was to learn *what* the recent news items were and *what* the textbook was explaining. As a result, you may be more familiar and comfortable in reading for content. If this is the case, you're not alone! For most students getting ready for the MCAT, reading for purpose and reasoning is a new skill. Be sure to practice these modes of reading deliberately so they come to naturally to you on Test Day!

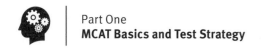
The very task of parsing a text into its chunks demands the interrogator to ask the first type of interrogative question, *why did the author include this?* This can be taken further by asking, *how does the current chunk connect to the chunk before it and how does it predict what will come after?* Finally, the interrogator can take advantage of the self-referencing effect and ask, *how can the ideas in this chunk be applied to my life or the real world?*

Outlining

Outlining aims to capture the major takeaway of a paragraph and write it down in a succinct manner. This act of paraphrasing is the secret behind outlining, as it demands the reader to think actively about what he or she just read in the paragraph in order to generate a label for each paragraph.

Although the goal is always to capture the major takeaway in the outline, this can be achieved in several different ways. The three modes of reading can serve as guidelines for the kind of material to include in each label.

- **Content:** Write down the key ideas of each paragraph.
- **Purpose:** Write down how the paragraph functions within the larger whole of the passage.
- **Reasoning:** Write down how the paragraph relates to those around it. Identify whether each paragraph bolsters or objects to an argument.

In a single passage, you may find that specific paragraphs lend themselves to be outlined based on content while others must be outlined based on reasoning. This is fine, as each label still captures the major takeaway of the paragraph. However, be sure to keep labels concise. Generally, five to seven words are ideal, but labels of up to ten to twelve words are acceptable for more complex passages.

When answering passage questions using the Outline approach, you will most likely need to refer back to the passage more frequently than if you had interrogated the passage. Fortunately, your written outline in your noteboard should allow you to identify quickly which paragraph contains the information needed to answer the question.

Noteboard Strategy

Once you've chosen to Outline a passage, begin to construct your outline. Each paragraph should be numbered using a brief notation, such as *P4*. For instance, you could set up your noteboard for a five-paragraph passage as follows:

P1.

P2.

P3.

P4.

P5.

Highlighting

In comparison to the other Distill approaches, the Highlight approach can be the most passive due to the ease of using the highlighting tool available on the MCAT testing interface. However, you never want to read a CARS passage passively! Because of this, the Highlight approach may seem the easiest at a first glance. However, it is deceptively hard to master and thus should be practiced regularly.

The Highlight approach aims to capture the major takeaway of a paragraph by thoughtfully highlighting specific terms or phrases. This method of highlighting is different from how it is typically used in academia: to highlight important facts or items you wish to remember. This practice can result in paragraphs being oversaturated with yellow ink. To avoid this, let's consider the purpose of highlighting in CARS, which is *to pull your attention back to relevant information when needed for a question*. To achieve this effect, you must be thoughtful in selecting what to highlight. When put another way, to highlight terms that capture the major takeaway of the passage, you must first find the major takeaway. This leads us an important realization: when reading CARS passages, highlight terms after you read and understand the paragraph, not while you are reading.

Aggressively Leveraging Keywords

One aspect of the Highlight approach that we haven't discussed yet is its short time allotment of two to three minutes to Read and Distill the passage. This is very aggressive timing. In order to fit your Distill step within this time limit, aggressive use of keywords must be a crucial part of your reading.

Most paragraphs in a passage have only one or two key ideas that make up a relatively small portion of the paragraph. The remaining text supports, elaborates, or provides context for the key ideas. When reading aggressively, your goal is to spend time identifying these key concepts while skimming over the supporting text. Reading for purpose and reasoning play a role in this task, but more directly, your application of keywords actually achieves this goal.

Keywords indicating a major takeaway:

- Contrast
- Conclusion
- Author
- Comparison

Keywords indicating supporting details:

- Continuation
- Evidence

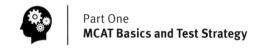

How to Highlight

On Test Day, the testing interface will have an array of computer-based testing tools, including a highlight function. To highlight text:

1. Ensure the **Highlight** option is selected in the top left corner, indicated by a yellow box (this is the default setting).
2. Use the cursor to left-click and hold while dragging over the desired text.
3. Press Alt + H or, alternatively, left-click on the **Highlight** button at the top left of the screen.

THE KAPLAN METHOD FOR SCIENCE PASSAGES

The Kaplan Method for critically reading science passages consists of the same four steps: **Preview, Choose, Read,** and **Distill**.

- **Preview:** Spend approximately 10 seconds to determine the passage topic and whether the passage is *information* or *experiment*. Use these patterns to determine passage difficulty and whether you should do the passage *now* or *later*.
- **Choose:** Using the patterns noted in the Preview step, Choose an appropriate Distill approach for the passage (Interrogate, Outline, or Highlight).
    - Interrogation should be chosen for experiment passages.
    - Outlining should be chosen for information passages that are dense or detail heavy.
    - Highlighting should be chosen for information passages that are light on details.
- **Read:** Use keywords and science terms to identify the most important and testable content.
    - Identify passage information that can be applied or connected to your MCAT science content.
    - Note causal relationships between terms or processes, indicated by words such as *increases, inhibited,* and *required*.
- **Distill:** While reading the passage, your aim is to distill the major takeaway of each paragraph using one of the following approaches.
    - **Interrogate**: Thoroughly examine the experiment passage by identifying the key components of experimental design. Interrogate *why* specific procedures were done and *how* they connect to the overall purpose of the experiment.
    - **Outline**: Create a brief label for each paragraph that summarizes the contents of the paragraph and allows you to return quickly to the passage when demanded by a question.
    - **Highlight**: Highlight one to three terms per paragraph that can pull your attention back to testable information when demanded by a question.

PREVIEW

Similar to CARS, your first 10 seconds or so of a passage should be spent noting key passage patterns to determine your ideal choice using the Distill approach and whether to attack the passage *now* or *later*.

- **Passage type**: Is the passage information or experiment?
- **Passage topic**: What science topic is the passage discussing? What is your comfort in the topic?
- **Passage structure**: Is the passage primarily text? Does it have a figure or graphic?

CHOOSE

Choosing an appropriate Distill approach in the sciences is considerably more clear-cut than in the CARS section.

- **Interrogation**, which is the most thorough Distill approach, is best utilized for experiment passages where one must consider the experimenter's purpose in writing and the reasoning behind experimental conclusions.
- **Outlining** aims to Distill the major takeaway of a paragraph into a briefly written label. Information passages that are dense in detail can be summarized into clear and succinct labels. Therefore, outlining should be done for these passage.
- **Highlighting** spends a minimal amount of time distilling the passage and thus provides only a shallow level of passage understanding. Information passages that are brief in detail or passages where you are confident in your content knowledge can be highlighted.

MCAT EXPERTISE

Part of your passage and question review should include the self-reflective question, "Did I choose an appropriate Distill approach for this passage?" This will allow you to refine your methodology as you gain more experience.

READ AND DISTILL

In the sciences, the overarching goal in the Read and Distill step is to identify test-worthy information. Although this sounds like a lofty goal, there are a couple MCAT patterns to notice that can make this goal more attainable.

- Passage concepts that relate or can be applied to your MCAT science knowledge often appear in passage questions.
- Passage information that can be directly used to answer MCAT questions or information that you've previously used to answer MCAT questions will likely be needed in a passage question.
- Passage information that describes experimental setups, or experimental design as a whole, are highly testable.

Each of these patterns will be expanded upon below in our discussion of the Distill approaches.

Interrogation

Recall that the Interrogation approach includes stopping to ask *why* and *how* the author included passage information. For many science passages, these questions lead to the unremarkable conclusion of *the author included this information to explain a concept*. On Test Day, this is not very helpful. However, for experiment passages specifically, exploring the *why* and *how* of passage information is vital as this will lead to a deeper understanding of the experiment, which is needed for passages on Test Day.

Key Components of Experimental Design

Like the MCAT, scientific studies and experiments follow specific patterns. If you've read any scientific papers or articles, whether for course credit or just general interest, you've probably noticed that it gets easier the more often you do it! With a little experience, you begin to anticipate what will come up next in the article and begin to look out for results and subsequent discussion. The patterns in these articles have their analogs in the experiment passages on the MCAT as both follow the steps of the scientific method. Although the scientific method is not explicitly tested on the MCAT, having a thorough understanding of the scientific method and experimental design will better equip you to Read and Distill experiment passages on Test Day.

Experiments are done with a *purpose* in mind, often one clinical in nature. For instance, experiments can be done to gain a deeper understanding of disease pathology, to evaluate the efficacy of treatments, or to understand a novel regulatory pathway. No matter the case, on Test Day once the purpose of the experiment has been distilled, identifying the remaining experimental components will be easier as they can be related back to the experimental purpose. Experiment purposes are often found in or near the beginning of a passage.

The next components of the experimental design to consider are the independent variable, dependent variable, and hypothesis. The *independent variable (IV)* is manipulated during the experiment in hopes of seeing an effect in the *dependent variable (DV)*, which is measured in the experiment for this reason. A simple definition of a *hypothesis* is an idea that is to be tested in an experiment. For the MCAT experiment passages, though, we can get more specific. Here the hypothesis is a proposed connection between the independent and dependent variable. In other words, the hypothesis proposes that the dependent variable is dependent on the independent variable.

Some passages, typically biochemistry and psychology passages, include *experimental procedures* that explain how the IVs are manipulated and DVs are measured. The most difficult experiment passages have procedures that are incredibly information dense or require highly specific knowledge of biochemical assays. However, keeping the IV, DV, hypothesis, and purpose in mind while distilling the passage will allow you to understand the most important steps.

The last components of experimental design are the results and conclusion. The *results* are often given as data related to the dependent variables. If given experimental results on Test Day, be sure to analyze them for any clear trends. A *conclusion* takes the results a step further and connects them and their trends back to the experimental hypothesis and purpose. These final two components often go hand in hand in the passage; however, some passages may omit one of these components. In that case, expect questions to appear that demand you to reason about the omitted information.

KEY TAKEAWAY

Key components of experimental design:

- *Purpose:* The purpose of the study/experiment, often clinical.
- *Independent variables (IV):* These are variables manipulated by the experimenters between the different study arms.
- *Dependent variables (DV):* These are the variables measured by the experimenters.
- *Hypothesis:* This is a proposed connection between the IV and DV that is tested by the experiment.
- *Experimental procedures:* The steps of the experiment that describe how the IVs are manipulated and how the DVs are measured.
- *Results:* The data from the dependent variables.
- *Conclusions:* The implicit findings that connect the independent and dependent variables, often relating back to the purpose of the experiment.

Outlining

Similar to the CARS Outline approach, in the sciences Outlining involves writing a succinct label of each paragraph while working through the passage. With the goal of the Read and Distill step being to identify test-worthy material, your labels should adequately capture what is found in the paragraph. However, be sure to not include every detail. For instance, if a paragraph describes a multi-step biochemical pathway producing prostaglandins, instead of labeling each step, simply label *prostaglandin pathway*. In this way, capturing what can be found in a paragraph is a mixture of reading for content and reading for purpose.

An effective Outline should allow you to return quickly to the relevant parts of a passage when demanded by a question. Therefore, it's unlikely in the sciences that your Outline will contain the needed information itself. As long as your Outline points you to the relevant paragraph, though, it's serving its function.

Highlighting

Similar to Outlining, Highlighting should allow you to return quickly to test-worthy information when demanded by a question. In order to achieve this, aim to Highlight the test-worthy material itself. Consider the previously mentioned example. If a paragraph describes a multi-step biochemical pathway producing prostaglandins, focus your highlighting on terms around the products or the steps that you deem important.

Of course, there are diminishing returns when it comes to Highlighting. The more you highlight in a passage, the less useful it becomes! If you find yourself needing to highlight more than one to three terms per paragraph in a science passage, perhaps Outlining would have been a better choice for the passage.

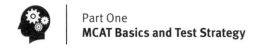

2.3 How to Attack Different Passage Types

CARS PASSAGES

The AAMC lists ten different fields in the humanities and a dozen different social sciences, as shown in Table 2.4. Quickly identifying the type of passage during the Preview step of the Kaplan Method can help shape your expectations about what the passage will include and what the accompanying questions will test.

Humanities	Social Sciences
Architecture	Anthropology
Art	Archaeology
Dance	Cultural Studies
Ethics	Economics
Literature	Education
Music	Geography
Philosophy	History
Popular Culture	Linguistics
Religion	Political Science
Theater	Population Health
	Psychology
	Sociology

Table 2.4. Humanities and Social Sciences Disciplines in the CARS Section

HUMANITIES

Passages in the humanities tend to fall into two broad categories. The first category, which includes most of the passages from architecture, art, dance, literature, music, popular culture, and theater, could be considered **arts passages**. The second category, **philosophical passages,** includes ethics, philosophy, and many religion passages.

- **Arts passages** often use quotations from both artists and critics, include strong opinions, and use descriptive language to illustrate artistic examples.
- **Philosophical passages** tend to be abstract and heavy on logic as well as focus on concepts and the relations between them.

Keep in mind that plenty of humanities passages mix characteristics of arts and philosophical passages.

SOCIAL SCIENCES

When it comes to the social sciences, some passages take what might be called a **scientific** form, such as passages in anthropology, education, linguistics, population health, psychology, and sociology. The counterpart to scientific form would be **historical passages**, which may include topics like archaeology, cultural studies, economics, geography, history, and political science.

- **Scientific passages** include heavy references to empirical studies. Usually the author's opinion is subtle.
- **Historical passages** tend to draw on historical events and quotations from sources alive at the time of the events they discuss. Sometimes empirical studies are referenced.

SUPPORT IN PASSAGES

Because a majority of questions in the CARS section have some connection to logical support, it's essential to understand the different kinds of support that can be found in CARS passages.

Categories of Support

- **Unsupported claims:** Not every assertion in a passage is backed up with evidence. Unsupported claims lack logical connections to other parts of the passage.
- **Empirical evidence:** Whenever the author appeals to experience, particularly in the context of scientific studies, he or she is using empirical evidence.
  - Historical accounts and case studies draw on experience but are limited in value because they represent only single cases.
  - Surveys, statistical analyses, and controlled experiments are more solid evidence because variables can be isolated and evidence can be gathered by examining a wide swath of experience.
- **Logical appeals** refer to the use of logic, claims, or evidence to argue for a point.
  - **Analogical reasoning:** Two things known to be alike are declared to be alike in a different respect for which there may not be direct evidence.
  - **Reduction to absurdity** is supporting a position by the elimination of alternative possibilities.
- **Appealing to authority** draws on another person or test to support a claim.
  - The level of support depends on the credibility of the authority.
    - **Primary sources provide the most support.**
    - **Secondary sources** are dubious in value and vary based on the expertise of the authority being cited.
- **Appeals to the reader:** In this case, the author uses the reader to help ground an argument. Sometimes the author begins an argument with points that the reader is likely to agree with. Another possibility is that the author uses charged language and colorful descriptions to evoke particular responses from the reader.
- **Faulty support** involves backing up a controversial claim with another claim that is similarly controversial. This kind of assertion is extremely weak at best.

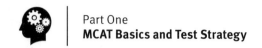

ANTICIPATING QUESTIONS

While reading CARS passages, it is essential to anticipate the questions. Certain passage characteristics lend themselves to specific question types. The following are a few examples of passage types and what types of questions typically accompany each.

- **Heavily opinionated** passages lend themselves to questions that require understanding what the author would agree or disagree with.
- Passages that are **abundant in detail** are likely to have questions that necessitate combing through the passage while searching for particular bits from the text.
- Passages **lacking in support** probably have questions that incorporate new information.
- Passages that **use numerous Logic keywords** tend to have questions that ask about the author's argumentative structure.
- When the author introduces **new terminology or concepts**, the questions likely test for understanding of the novel information.
- When passages **offer two opposing viewpoints**, expect questions that ask you to compare and contrast the viewpoints.

SCIENCE PASSAGES

The science sections on the MCAT generally present content in two types of passages. The first type is best described as information passages, where you need to pay attention to definitions and relationships. The second—and most common—type are experiment passages. For these passages, your job is to pay attention to why the experiment was done and what the overall findings are. It is important to note that any figures or tables are also worth labeling for the science passages because they also contain testable information. More details on science passages are provided in Part Three of this book.

2.4 Concept and Strategy Summary

HOW TO READ STRATEGICALLY USING KEYWORDS

- Passages on Test Day must be read actively, questioning the passage as it is read. Active reading can be facilitated by consciously reading via three modes.
  - Read for **content**: Understand the ideas and concepts presented by the author by asking, *what is the author saying?*
  - Read for **purpose**: Understand the perspective and motivations of the author by asking, *why did the author write this text? Why did he or she include a specific piece of information?*
  - Read for **reasoning**: Understand the relationships within the passage by asking, *how do the sentences connect? How do the ideas relate?*
- **Keywords** should be leveraged to read the passage actively for content, purpose, and reasoning.
- **Relation** keywords indicate how passage ideas are related to each other.
  - **Continuation** keywords indicate that more of the same idea is coming in the text.
  - **Contrast** keywords signify a change in the author's focus or a direct contrast between two things.
- **Author** keywords indicate the author's opinions and motivations.
  - **Positive** and **negative** keywords indicate the author's approval or disapproval of an idea, respectively.
  - **Extreme** keywords indicate a strong opinion held by the author.
  - **Moderating** keywords indicate a weaker opinion held by the author.
- **Logic** keywords indicate connections of support between passage claims.
  - **Conclusion** keywords indicate a conclusion is being presented. Conclusions are statements or claims that are supported with evidence.
  - **Evidence** keywords indicate evidence is being presented. Evidence involves statements, facts, or data that support a conclusion.
  - **Refutation** keywords are the opposite of evidence and actually attack or weaken a conclusion.

HOW TO ANALYZE PASSAGES CRITICALLY

The Kaplan Method for CARS Passages
- **Preview** for difficulty.
  - Look for passage patterns: topic, language, sentence structure, and passage structure.
  - Determine the relative difficulty of the passage.
  - Decide to attack the passage now or later.
- **Choose** your approach.
  - **Interrogation** is ideal for passages where you are confident a larger time investment in the Distill step will deepen your understanding of the passage.
  - **Outlining** is ideal for passages that have clear passage structure or are heavy in details.
  - **Highlighting** is ideal for passages with difficult topics or structure where a larger time investment may not produce a deeper understanding of the passage.

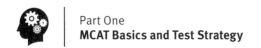
- **Read** the passage strategically using the keywords.
- **Distill** the major takeaway of the paragraphs and passage.
  - **Interrogate**: Read actively by questioning *why* the author included the information and *how* it relates to the information around it.
  - **Outline**: Read actively by writing a brief label on your noteboard that captures the major takeaway of each paragraph.
  - **Highlight**: Read actively by highlighting one to three key terms that capture the major takeaway of each paragraph.

The Kaplan Method for Science Passages
- **Preview** for difficulty.
  - Determine the passage topic and whether the passage is *information* or an *experiment.*
  - Determine passage difficulty and whether you should do the passage *now* or *later.*
- **Choose** your approach.
  - Interrogation should be chosen for experiment passages.
  - Outlining should be chosen for information passages that are dense or detail heavy.
  - Highlighting should be chosen for information passages that are light on details.
- **Read and Distill** the passage to identify testable information.
  - **Interrogate**: Thoroughly examine the experiment passage by identifying the key components of experimental design and by interrogating *why* specific procedures were done and *how* they connect to the overall purpose of the experiment.
  - **Outline**: Create a brief label for each paragraph that summarizes the contents of the paragraph, thereby allowing you to return quickly to the passage when demanded by a question.
  - **Highlight**: Highlight one to three terms per paragraph that can pull your attention back to testable information when demanded by a question.

HOW TO ATTACK DIFFERENT PASSAGE TYPES

CARS Passages
- CARS passages fall into two general categories **humanities** and **social sciences**.
- **Humanities** can be further divided into two categories: arts and philosophical.
  - **Arts passages** often use quotations from both artists and critics, include strong opinions, and use descriptive language to illustrate artistic examples.
  - **Philosophical passages** tend to be abstract, heavy on logic, and focus on concepts and the relations between them.
- **Social sciences** can be further divided into two categories: scientific and historical passages.
  - **Scientific passages** include heavy references to empirical studies. Usually the author's opinion is more subtle.
  - **Historical passages** tend to draw on historical events and quotations from sources alive at the time of the events they discuss. Sometimes empirical studies are referenced.
- Quickly identifying the passage type can shape your expectations of the passage and allow you to anticipate accompanying questions.

Science Passages

- **Information passages** require noting definitions, concepts, and relationships. Accompanying questions often require connecting passage information to your studied MCAT content.
- **Experiment passages** require understanding of the experimental procedure and its results. Accompanying questions often require understanding of the internal logic of the experimental procedure and drawing conclusions from presented data.

CHAPTER 3

Kaplan's Question and Answer Strategies

In this chapter, we shift our strategic focus away from the passages to consider the treatment of question stems and answer choices. We begin by outlining the Kaplan Method for MCAT questions. Subsequently, we will look at the recurring traps that the test makers set for the unwary student, which we call Wrong Answer Pathologies. In the final portion of the chapter, we'll consider the counterpart to Wrong Answer Pathologies: patterns common in correct answers.

3.1 Kaplan Method for Questions

In the previous chapter, we saw how the general Kaplan Method for tackling MCAT passages could be refined to the needs of the CARS section. In this section, we'll do the same with our question method, which takes the basic form shown in Figure 3.1.

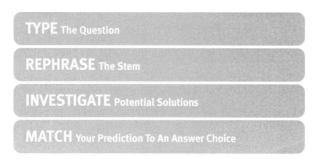

Figure 3.1. The Kaplan Method for Questions

This same four-step approach should be used on all questions on the MCAT—in both the CARS section and the science sections. The CARS-specific version is shown in Figure 3.2.

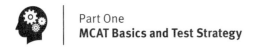

MCAT EXPERTISE

The Kaplan Method for questions will slow you down at first, but with practice, it will become second nature. When the method is internalized, you will be armed with a plan of attack that will allow you to maximize your potential no matter what the AAMC presents on Test Day.

TYPE The Question

- Read the question, **NOT** the answers
- Identify the question type and difficulty
- Decide to attack *now* or *later* in the same passage

REPHRASE The Stem

- Determine the task to be accomplished based on the question type
- Simplify the phrasing of the original question stem
- Translate the question into a specific piece of information you can either locate or infer

INVESTIGATE Potential Solutions

- Search for the answer in your interrogation, your outline, or the passage
- Predict what you can about the answer
- Be flexible if your initial approach fails: when in doubt, refer back to the passage itself

MATCH Your Prediction To An Answer Choice

- Search the answer choices for a response that is synonymous with your prediction
- Eliminate answer choices that diverge from the passage
- Select an answer and move on

Figure 3.2. Detailed Steps of the Kaplan Question Method

It is important to note that the worked-out practice passages in Parts Three and Four of this book all focus on how to implement the four steps of this question strategy effectively.

MCAT EXPERTISE

For most questions in the CARS section, reading the answer choices will only mislead you. However, peeking at the answer choices in the science sections can provide valuable information about the correct answer. *Are the answers numbers? If so, how do they relate to each other? Are the answers logic based? If so, what concepts are mentioned?* Gathering this information in the Type step will help streamline the rest.

STEP ONE: TYPE

You might notice that the first step of the question method is in many ways similar to the Preview step of the Kaplan Method for passages. This is not a coincidence; it is a consequence of the timing constraints posed by the section. Because every question is worth the same number of points, there's no reason to get derailed by any one question. Be honest with yourself: at least a few questions in each section are so difficult that you're likely to get them wrong, no matter how many minutes you spend on them. Wouldn't it be better to recognize which questions those are right away, so you can instead use that precious time where it will actually pay off?

To that end, your first task with any question is to read the stem, and only the stem, for the sake of making the decision either to work on the question *now* or to triage (to use an apt medical metaphor) and save it for *later in the passage*. Gauging the difficulty is made easier if you can identify the **question type**. Through extensive research of all released MCAT material, we've discovered that almost all of the CARS section's Foundations of Comprehension questions fall into one of four categories. In addition, the CARS section's Reasoning Within the Text questions and Reasoning Beyond the Text questions can each be split into two predominant types with assorted others making rare appearances. Starting each question with the Typing step not only allows for proper assessment of difficulty but also makes Rephrasing and Investigating a question much easier. We will discuss how question type indicates difficulty and how to apply the Type step most effectively to each question type in Chapter 15.

Why avoid looking at the answer choices in the CARS section? The primary reason is that most of them are wrong. If you glance at just one of them, for instance, it's three times more likely to be incorrect than correct and could seriously mislead you about the question. Inexperienced test takers immediately jump to the answers, and the AAMC punishes them for it by wording wrong options seductively. Selecting the first answer that looks good without really formulating an approach is a recipe for failure. Thus, until you get into the habit of ignoring the answers entirely until the Match step, use your hand or a sticky note to cover up the answer choices whenever you start to work on a question.

While avoiding looking at the answer choices is a sound strategy for CARS, the Type step is different for science questions. Taking advantage of the patterns in the answer choices for science will really help narrow the scope when you get to the Investigate step. However, glancing at the answers is not the same as analyzing them. Look to see what form the answer choices are in so that you will know what form the prediction should take. If you see numbers in the answer choices and the topic of the question stem looks like it's going in the direction of math, that's enough information to consider triaging that question for the end, as math questions very often take longer than the usual allotted time for a question. Another instance where you may consider triage is a question with lengthy answer choices and no clear pattern.

STEP TWO: REPHRASE

Once you've decided to attack a question, it's time to rephrase it. The **Rephrase** step goes beyond simply restating the question stem. The purpose of the Rephrase step is to provide you with a clear **task** and direction that you can use to attack the question. To this end, rephrase the question stem, focusing on the task itself and any relevant context given in the stem, to identify clearly what the question is demanding of you. Simpler question types, such as Main Idea and Definition-in-Context, always involve one specific task (recognizing the big picture and explaining the meaning of part of the text as used in the passage, respectively). Even the most complex question types will have one major task to accomplish, though it may involve multiple steps. For example, Apply questions involve one of three tasks: gauging the author's response, predicting a likely outcome, or finding a good example. One of the most common causes of missed questions in the CARS section is misreading the question stems; taking the additional time to Rephrase will earn you valuable points on Test Day.

Sometimes rephrasing is more difficult to accomplish, such as when the task is obscured by unclear language or by extraneous information in the stem. In either of these cases, try working your way backward, starting with the part of the question directly before the question mark or colon (in a question that requires completing a sentence). Try to simplify the phrasing of that part first and then connect it to any other relevant information in the stem. If you still

MCAT EXPERTISE

If you ever find yourself playing the word search game, save the question for later! Tackling the other questions in a passage set can often give you an opportunity to see the relevant detail or often hint at the correct answer. Question triaging doesn't mean you're giving up on the question but, instead, being savvy with your time management.

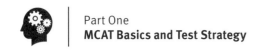
struggle to identify the task of the question, consider the question type you found in the Type step, because different instances of the same question type often have similar tasks. Finally, don't waste time on Test Day writing out the rephrased question; simplifying the question in your head is usually sufficient.

For more straightforward questions, rephrasing may not be necessary. For others, it is very useful. For instance, "LEAST likely to disagree" can be converted to *agree*. Other troublesome phrases, such as double negatives, should also be simplified to avoid careless misreading errors.

It is worth pointing out that Rephrasing the stem into a task can be done without any passage knowledge, due to the standardization of CARS questions. Taking notice of common patterns will allow you to devise a plan of attack even if you have difficulty mastering the passage itself. This skill of Rephrasing will require practice to master, but it's worth the time and effort. After the Rephrase step, you should have a clear understanding of the task(s) to be completed in order to reach the correct answer. *How* you go about accomplishing those objectives is the focus of the Investigate step.

On a similar note, the Rephrase step for the science questions is focused on simplifying the question in order to make clear the task. Of note, many question stems have extraneous science background information that is not related to the underlying question being asked. So in addition to the tips above about paraphrasing tricky question stems, the Rephrase step works to narrow the scope of focus and can turn a seemingly complex question into something much more straightforward.

STEP THREE: INVESTIGATE

The next step in the question and answer strategy is to **Investigate** potential solutions using your Rephrasing of the question. Specifically, you will follow the directives in your rephrase to **predict** what the correct answer should look like. How you use the passage to make this prediction depends on your passage approach (**Highlight**, **Outline**, or **Interrogate**).

A **Highlight** approach to the passage should provide the location of important pieces of information and central ideas but typically lacks details. Thus, the corresponding Investigate step should include rereading specific portions of the passage, as directed by the Rephrase step and the ideas highlighted. Ensure that you are not scanning the entirety of the passage during this step; instead, consider the task of the question and you're highlighting to determine where you should look. Keep in mind that due to the nature of this Distill method, Investigating questions may take longer on average than for other Distill methods.

An **Outline** approach to the passage should not only note the location of important pieces of information but should also summarize the central ideas of each paragraph. Thus, you should expect your written outline to be sufficient to form predictions for questions that require understanding of the main ideas. However, questions that ask about a specific detail or require inferences from passage information often require you to return to the passage. Again, ensure you are not scanning the entirety of the passage to make your prediction—use your outline to determine where to look.

An **Interrogate** approach to the passage is usually in-depth enough to leave you with a solid understanding of the central ideas of the passage and how those ideas are related. As a result, you'll find you can answer many questions without even referring back to the passage. Of course, a quick double check of the passage is always allowed. Keep in mind that with an Interrogate approach, though, not much time will be left for passage research during the questions.

When investigating your predictions, it's important to be mindful of how specific or in-depth your prediction should be. Predictions lie along a spectrum from focused to general. Focused predictions should be specific enough to allow you to match your prediction directly to an answer choice. In contrast, general predictions just set broad expectations about what the correct answer should include or exclude. Where your predictions falls on this spectrum primarily depends on the question type and question task. Your mantra for predicting should be *predict what you can.*

When armed with predictions, you are better prepared to evaluate the gauntlet of misleading answer choices. Perhaps you're wondering: why bother with the Investigate step and with making predictions? After all, you've taken multiple-choice tests before that included reading comprehension sections, and perhaps you've never needed much strategy to do well on them. There are several reasons why Investigating is key to success in CARS. For one, the CARS section is quite different from postsecondary reading comprehension exams. CARS passages are less likely to be on topics that you have familiarity with, so you're less likely to have an intuitive sense of the answers to the questions. In addition, the answer choices in the CARS section are designed to lure testers who do not use the passage to answer the question. They often sound like something you read in the passage, or they appeal to outside information that seems right but is irrelevant. Without first making a thoughtful prediction, you are more likely to fall for these alluring yet incorrect answer choices.

What should you do if you can't locate relevant information in the passage or don't know where to look? Typically, such questions are best to try later on, at the very end of the passage set, after you've researched the other questions and have already reviewed some of the text. You may find that by the time you return to the questions you've skipped, the effort you put into other questions ended up revealing a difficult question stem's correct answer. When you ultimately attempt these questions, a general prediction and process of elimination usually end up being the best plan. As a final note, you should answer all of the questions associated with a CARS passage before moving on—even if it means guessing. It is more effective to answer questions while the passage is still fresh rather than returning to them at the end of the section.

Just as in CARS, the Investigate step in science questions is where you decide where you have to go to predict the answer. You need to use the question stem, passage information, and an additional component—your content background. Because of this added variable, generating predictions can be more complex in science questions compared to CARS. It's common for students to be unbalanced with their sources initially. For instance, students often rely too much on passage information and do not know enough content background or, alternatively, depend too heavily on content knowledge when the passage contains the required information.

STEP FOUR: MATCH

The final step of **Matching** to the correct answer is the same in CARS as it is in the sciences. First evaluate the choices. If you see an item that closely resembles what you expected, reread every word of that answer carefully to make sure it says precisely what you think it does. Rarely will you find a word-for-word match for your prediction. Instead, your best bet is to look for a correspondence between ideas by searching for a choice that shares a similar meaning with your prediction but uses different words. Once you have found such an answer, select it and move on to the next question. At that point, *reading the other choices will not be worth your time*—be confident that you've answered the question when you find that conceptual match.

MCAT EXPERTISE

On the MCAT, you can strike out an answer by selecting text in the answer and then selecting the strikethrough button on the top left side of the screen.

MCAT EXPERTISE

If you read a question stem and it doesn't give you very much to work with, don't just say *I don't know* and jump straight to the answer choices. Use your outline to remember the main themes of the passage, and then use those themes to help with the process of elimination. This will help you avoid being distracted by answer choices that are seductive but do not fit the passage.

MCAT EXPERTISE

Should I compare answer choices?

Your default assumption should be that only one answer choice is correct and that the others contain at least one flaw each, sufficient for ruling them out. However, you may occasionally find questions containing superlatives (*strongest challenge*, *most supported*, *best example*, and so on) in which you need to compare two or more answers that have the same effect but to different degrees. When making such comparisons, don't assume that an extreme answer is necessarily wrong, especially if the question stem includes the words *if true* or similar language. A stronger answer that nevertheless produces the desired outcome would actually be the correct choice.

If you aren't able to find a choice that is synonymous with your prediction, don't feel that you immediately need to resort to the process of elimination (although that is a valid strategy). Part of being flexible is being able to revise your initial prediction and to set a new expectation if the answer choices point you in that direction. The answer choices could technically be considered an additional source of information for arriving at the correct answer, but keep in mind that they include a lot of misinformation and so should be treated with caution.

Sometimes the question stem just doesn't give you very much to work with. On other occasions, you'll search through the answers but find no likely match. In these cases, you have to use the process of elimination, which may require multiple returns to the text as you research each choice individually. If you were able to set expectations during the Investigate step for wrong choices, however, less additional research will be required. Keep in mind that an answer requires only one major flaw for elimination, so the Wrong Answer Pathologies described later can greatly expedite the process.

When all else fails, you can fall back on educated guessing. Eliminate whatever you can, and then go with your gut among the remaining options. Never make a blind guess unless you're completely out of time and need to fill in an answer choice. Even crossing off just one wrong answer increases your chances of randomly choosing the correct one by 33 percent. Crossing off two wrong answers doubles your chances. If possible, work on any unanswered questions for the passage and see if that allows you to return to rule out additional wrong options.

3.2 Wrong Answer Pathologies

The AAMC, the maker of the MCAT, has designed the sections of the exam to be fair tests of critical-thinking skills. The need for fairness is great news because it means that the questions don't play tricks on you! There is never a question with two correct answer choices or one in which all of the options are wrong. Each question you encounter on Test Day has one and only one right answer and three that are incorrect for at least one reason. Even better, there can be only so many of these reasons: in fact, a few of them are found so frequently that you can treat them similar to recurring signs and symptoms of answer choice "illness." Naturally, we call them **Wrong Answer Pathologies**.

A choice needs only one fatal flaw to be worth eliminating, but wrong answer options often have many issues. So don't necessarily be alarmed if you ruled out a wrong answer for a different reason than the one mentioned in a practice question's explanation. In addition to having some occasional overlap, the following list of pathologies is not meant to be exhaustive; it includes the four patterns we've identified as the most common through researching all of the released MCAT material. As the previous section details, pathologies function as recurring expectations for wrong answers, which you can assume fit for most of the questions you encounter (with a few significant departures).

FAULTY USE OF DETAIL

The test makers often include accurate reflections of passage details in wrong answers, primarily to appeal to those students who jump at the familiar language. This is a Faulty Use of Detail (FUD). What makes the use of a detail faulty is that it simply doesn't answer the question posed. It may be too specific for a question that requires a general answer, the detail may come from the wrong part of the passage, or it might be a factually correct statement in the science section. Even if a choice comes from the right paragraph, the detail cited might not be relevant to the question posed, as is often the case in Strengthen–Weaken (Reasoning Within the Text) questions. A thorough prediction makes catching these FUDs much easier.

OUT OF SCOPE

With the noteworthy exception of Reasoning Beyond the Text questions (for which this pathology does not apply), an answer choice that is Out the Scope (OS) of the passage is inevitably wrong. Typically, such answers are on topic but bring in some element that the text does not discuss. For instance, if an author never makes comparisons when discussing different ideas, an OS answer choice might involve the author ranking two or more of the ideas. Another common OS pattern is the suggestion that a view was the first of its kind or the most influential, when the author entirely avoids discussing its historical origins or relative popularity. Keep in mind that information can be unstated by the passage but not count as Out of Scope, as is the case with the correct answers to many Reasoning Within the Text questions. So don't be too quick to reject a choice as OS just because the author does not explicitly say it.

KEY CONCEPT

Wrong Answer Pathologies are the most frequent patterns found in incorrect answer choices. They are so common that you'll find at least one in just about every CARS question and even in many of the questions in the three science sections!

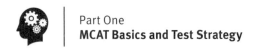
OPPOSITE

Whenever an answer choice contains information that directly conflicts with the passage, we call it an Opposite (OPP). Often the difference results simply from the presence (or absence) of a single word such as *not* or *except*, a prefix such as *un-* or *a-*, or even a suffix like *-less* or *-free*. Be especially careful when stems or choices involve double (or triple) negatives; they're much easier to assess if you reword them with fewer negations. Moreover, don't assume that just because two answer choices contradict, one of them has to be correct. For example, suppose an author argues that it is impossible to prove whether a divine being exists, a variant of the religious view known as *agnosticism*. If a question accompanying the passage asks for a claim the author agreed with, *God exists* and *There is no God* would both be OPP of the correct answer.

DISTORTION

Extreme answers and others that twist the ideas in the passage further than the author would prefer are what we call Distortions (DIST). Although they do not automatically make a choice incorrect, the following are common signals of distorted claims:

- Strong words such as *all*, *always*, *none*, *never*, *impossible*, or *only*
- A prefix such as *any-* or *every-*
- A suffix such as *-est* or *-less*

MCAT authors typically do not take radical positions on issues, so it's worth noting whenever they do. In those rare cases, extreme choices would not actually be DISTs of the author's view and would actually be more likely to be correct. The other major case in which extreme answer choices should not be immediately ruled out is when the question stem tells you that you can treat the answer choices as true, and your task is to gauge only which would have the greatest impact on a particular argument. This often is the case with Strengthen–Weaken (Beyond the Text) questions.

In science questions, Distortions can often be signaled by incorrect science facts, which can allow for an additional level of analysis that cannot be done in CARS. Challenging the scientific truth of an answer choice allows for the possibility of eliminating answer choices even without fully understanding the question or passage.

MISCALCULATION

Miscellaneous (MISC) is a wrong answer pathology that is unique to the science section and occurs only in questions that involve math. The test makers do not randomly create wrong answer choices to calculation questions. Rather, wrong answer choices result from specific errors that the test makers expect students to make, such as using the wrong units or forgetting to multiply by a constant. One small math error made early on in calculation can carry through the entire problem, which can match to a wrong answer choice. Therefore, triaging math questions and working through them slowly and carefully is a great strategy.

3.3 Signs of a Healthy Answer

If you're like most students prepping for the MCAT, you've had a dispute with at least one question explanation. *Hey, what about what the author says in the first paragraph?* you may have wondered or perhaps said to yourself (or aloud!), *But couldn't you think of it like **this** instead?* Even though you may be in the habit of arguing for points with college professors, it does you no good to try to argue with the MCAT. The test makers are extremely deliberate about how they word correct answers, always taking care to include exactly one per question.

Correct answer choices can vary widely in appearance, but there also are patterns in how they are written. If the traps that can lead you astray on Test Day are appropriately called Wrong Answer Pathologies, then the corresponding traits of correct answers can be thought of as indications of good health. Even though the following signs are not enough by themselves to make an answer right, you can treat them as general expectations for the correct choices in most types of questions.

APPROPRIATE SCOPE

You might say correct answers follow the "Goldilocks principle" when it comes to scope: not too broad, not too specific, but just right. The **scope** defines the limits of the discussion, or the particular aspects of the larger topic that the author really cares about. Considering the purpose of the passage as you Read and Distill should give you an idea of the scope of the passage overall. As a general rule (with one important exception), correct answers to MCAT questions remain within the scope of the passage. However, you can formulate a more precise expectation of what scope the correct answer needs to have by identifying the question's type and task.

Main Idea questions always have correct answers that match the scope of the entire passage. They typically include at least one wrong answer choice that is too focused (FUD) and at least one that goes outside the passage entirely (OS). In contrast, Detail and Definition-in-Context questions usually require more refined scopes for their correct answer choices. If a clue directs to a particular portion of the passage, the correct answer more often than not has the same scope as the referenced text (or what immediately surrounds it).

The important exception to the rule that answers must remain within the scope of the author's discussion applies to Reasoning Beyond the Text questions, addressed in Chapter 15. Like their name suggests, these broaden the scope to new contexts, sometimes appearing to have no connection to the passage whatsoever. Note, however, that some Reasoning Beyond the Text questions present new information in the stem but have answers that stick to the scope of the passage anyway. So be savvy with the answer choices in Reasoning Beyond the Text questions. Although the correct answer choice tends to move slightly outside the scope of the passage, don't automatically rule out an answer choice just because it happens to be in scope.

MCAT EXPERTISE

The scope of a text refers to the particular aspects of a topic that the author addresses. Every paragraph in a CARS passage has its own scope, and together you can think of them as constituting the scope of the whole passage. Similarly, each answer choice has its own scope, which could mimic any part of the author's discussion or depart from the passage entirely. It is essential to note that having the same scope doesn't necessarily mean having identical content. For instance, unstated assumptions in an argument are definitely within the scope of the passage, even though the information they contain is left unsaid by the author.

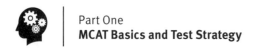

AUTHOR AGREEMENT

Unless a question stem explicitly asks about an alternative viewpoint or a challenge to the information presented in the passage, a correct answer choice is consistent with what the author says. This is one reason why considerations of **tone** (most clearly reflected by Author keywords) are usually important enough to be worth including as you Read and Distill the passage. Generally, a correct answer should not contradict anything that the author says elsewhere in the passage, with the possible exception of sentences that speak in a different voice than the author's (such as quotes or references to others' opinions). In short, if an answer choice doesn't sound like something the author would say, you'll most likely want to rule it out.

SYNONYMOUS PHRASING

The correct answer should match the prediction made in your Investigate step, be it a focused or general prediction. When evaluating answer choices using your prediction, keep in mind that the AAMC often phrases correct answers with different terms than those presented in the passage. This can mistakenly lead students to rule out correct answers as OS simply because they contain unfamiliar language. Thus, when evaluating answer choices, it is key to remember that consistency of meaning is more important than consistency of phrasing.

WEAKER IS USUALLY BETTER

One final consideration is a consequence of the fact that the AAMC tends to select passages in which the authors do not take extreme views. You may find one or two passages on Test Day with more radical writers; for them, a stronger claim in the answer choices may actually be a good sign. However, for most of the passages you'll encounter, authors tend to use numerous Moderating keywords to limit the strength of their claims. Because a stronger claim has a higher burden of proof (that is, stronger evidence must be provided to support the claim), most authors avoid them to make what they write more plausible. Thus, you should generally give preference to answer choices that use weaker language, such as *can*, *could*, *may*, *might*, *is possible*, *sometimes*, *often*, *likely*, *probably*, and *in some sense*. Exceptions to this tendency are questions that instruct you to consider the answer choices as true and gauge their effect on an argument. These were addressed previously in the discussion of the DIST Wrong Answer Pathology.

3.4   Getting the Edge Using the Question Strategy

This chapter is only an introduction to the question method; the worked examples that follow in Part Three are a necessary supplement for seeing how the method functions in practice. Specific strategy suggestions and worked examples are included for each of the most common question tasks, which together constitute a large proportion of what you'll encounter on Test Day. The explanations accompanying these sample questions also identify their Wrong Answer Pathologies, giving you some concrete examples to go with the explanations provided here.

3.5   Concept and Strategy Summary

KAPLAN METHOD FOR QUESTIONS

- **Type** the question.
  - Read the question, not the answers for CARS.
  - Read the question and scan for patterns in the answer choices for science.
  - Identify the question type and difficulty.
  - Decide to attack *now* or *later in the same passage.*

- **Rephrase** the stem.
  - Establish the task set forth by the question type.
  - Simplify the phrasing of the original question stem.
  - Translate the question into a specific piece of information you can either locate or infer.

- **Investigate** potential solutions.
  - Search for the answer in your interrogation, your outline, or highlight of the passage.
  - For science questions, recall the relevant content background.
  - Predict what you can about the answer.
  - Be flexible if your initial approach fails; when in doubt, refer back to the passage itself.

- **Match** your prediction to an answer choice.
  - Search the answer choices for the response that is synonymous with your prediction.
  - Eliminate the answer choices that diverge from the passage.
  - Select an answer and move on.

WRONG ANSWER PATHOLOGIES

- **Faulty Use of Detail** answer choices may be accurate statements but fail to answer the question posed.
  - The answer choice may be too specific for a question that requires a general answer.
  - The answer choice may use a detail from the wrong part of the passage.
  - The answer choice may be from the right paragraph but still not be relevant to the question posed.

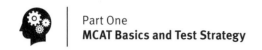

- **Out of Scope** answer choices usually bring in some element that the passage does not discuss (and that cannot be inferred from the passage).
  - The answer choice may make connections or comparisons that the author does not discuss.
  - The answer choice may make a statement about the significance of the history of an idea that the author does not.
  - The answer choice may otherwise bring in information that does not fall within the constraints of the passage.

- **Opposite** answer choices contain information that directly conflicts with the passage.
  - The answer choice may contain (or omit) a single word, such as *not* or *except*.
  - The answer choice may contain a prefix, such as *un-* or *a-*, or a suffix, such as *-less* or *-free*.
  - The answer choice may say that a given claim is true when the author is actually ambivalent.

- **Distortion** answer choices are extreme or twist the ideas in the passage further than the author would prefer.
  - The answer choice may use a strong word, such as *all*, *always*, *none*, *never*, *impossible*, or *only*.
  - The answer choice may contain a prefix, such as *any-* or *every-*, or a suffix, such as *-est* or *-less*.
  - The answer choice is usually more radical than the author because radical positions are rare in MCAT passages.

- **Miscalculation** answer choices are the result of common errors in math questions.
  - The answer choice may result from using the wrong units.
  - The answer choice may result from forgetting about conversion factors like *milli-* or *micro-*.

SIGNS OF A HEALTHY ANSWER

- Correct answers tend to have the right **scope**—not too broad, not too specific, but just right.
- Correct answers tend to be consistent with what the author said.
- Correct answers use language that differs from the passage but is still consistent with the ideas discussed.
- Correct answers tend to use Moderating keywords, such as *can*, *could*, *may*, *might*, *is possible*, *sometimes*, *often*, *likely*, *probably*, and *in some sense*.

PART TWO

Scientific Inquiry and Reasoning Skills

CHAPTER 4

Skills 1 and 2

There is no question that a high score on the MCAT requires extensive content knowledge in biology, biochemistry, general chemistry, organic chemistry, physics, psychology, and sociology. However, the MCAT is not a content test. One of the most common mistakes that test takers make when studying for the MCAT is treating it as if it is a content test and studying for it as if it is an undergraduate course. The MCAT is actually a critical-thinking test, designed to test your ability to apply your knowledge to new situations. In addition, questions on the MCAT have been expanded to include additional skills, such as the evaluation of experimental design and execution as well as the interpretation of data and statistical reasoning. The AAMC has separated these categories into four skills, appropriately called Skills 1, 2, 3, and 4. In this chapter, we will discuss how the MCAT tests Skills 1 and 2.

4.1 What Are Skills 1 and 2?

Unlike many tests administered to undergraduates, MCAT questions are carefully crafted and tested to ensure that they test the specific skills and content areas that the AAMC believes are most essential for success in medical school. To do this, the AAMC creates questions reflecting four different skills. Skills 1 and 2 are designed to evaluate your scientific knowledge and reasoning ability.

SKILL 1

Skill 1 is the simplest of the skills, testing knowledge of scientific concepts and principles. These questions are fairly straightforward, asking you to identify relationships between related concepts. Essentially, Skill 1 questions test your content knowledge in a very specific manner. Skill 1 questions are designed to test the following:

- Knowledge and recognition of scientific principles
- Ability to identify relationships between related concepts
- Ability to identify relationships among graphical, symbolic, and verbal representations of information
- Ability to identify observations that illustrate specific scientific principles
- Application of mathematical principles to solve problems

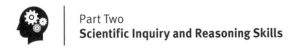
SKILL 2

Skill 2 is more complex than Skill 1 in that Skill 2 tests your scientific reasoning and problem-solving skills. Essentially, Skill 1 tests your content knowledge, whereas Skill 2 tests your ability to apply that knowledge. Skill 2 questions ask you to reason about scientific principles, models, and theories as well as evaluate and analyze predictions and explanations related to scientific concepts.

Overall, Skill 2 questions test your critical-thinking skills. What, though, are "critical-thinking skills"? Critical thinking is a method of processing and using information. It is defined as "the process of actively and skillfully conceptualizing, applying, analyzing, synthesizing, and evaluating information to reach an answer or conclusion." Critical thinking is not just memorizing information; it is using this information through higher-order processing. However, critical thinking requires some level of knowledge about a topic beyond basic memorization.

One of the ways that students can tackle critical thinking is by changing how they learn information. Many students use memorization as a primary method of learning and are successful in passing undergraduate-level science courses. However, medical school is very different from undergraduate science courses. The volume of information is astounding, often covering the same volume of information in an entire semester of an undergraduate science course in two weeks or less. Medical students are expected to learn this information and be able to apply this information systematically to patient care. Without the gift of superhuman photographic memory, getting through medical school by brute force memorization is just not realistic. Instead, as with the MCAT, better performance results from the ability to think, analyze, and apply information you already know to situations and concepts you may not know. This particular skill is essential for medicine; you will have to apply the information you know about the human body to a patient about whom you may know little.

So, how can you improve your ability to learn and apply information? You need to focus on your learning behavior.

One of the tools used in educational psychology for assessing learning is known as Bloom's taxonomy (see Figure 4.1). In this taxonomy, there are six levels of intellectual behavior that are important for learning, which are as follows:

- **Remembering**: Can you recall the information?
- **Understanding**: Can you explain the information to a classmate?
- **Applying**: Can you apply the information to a new situation?
- **Analyzing**: Can you compare and contrast different parts of the concept? Can you differentiate among the details within the concept?
- **Evaluating**: Can you use the information to support a judgment based on the information?
- **Creating**: Can you incorporate the information to create another structure/document/theory?

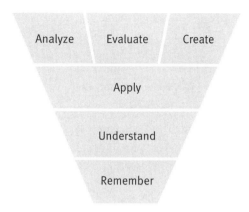

Figure 4.1. Bloom's Taxonomy

In each content area on the MCAT, one or more elements of Bloom's taxonomy are being tested, regardless of the skill. When evaluating your knowledge of a particular subject, you can use Bloom's taxonomy to determine your level of learning and increase your level of learning. Try this step-by-step method for deepening your learning of a concept:

- Do you think you remember and understand a particular concept? Then explain it to a friend or classmate.
- If you can do that, then try to find situations that are different but to which the same concept applies.
- Then compare and contrast the concept to a similar theory or concept.
- Once you can see the differences and the similarities, work through a passage and questions, explaining why each answer choice is correct or incorrect.
- Finally, can you write something about a concept? Try to write a passage similar to one seen on the MCAT.

Although it is unrealistic to do this for every topic on the MCAT because it would be highly inefficient, the levels of Bloom's taxonomy represent the different levels of learning that the MCAT requires. It also explains why so many students spend thousands of hours studying for the MCAT but are not successful on Test Day. Many focus almost exclusively on the "remembering" part of learning and only a little bit on the "understanding" part.

The secret to success on Test Day is not just in remembering the content; it is having a higher level of understanding of the content. If you can complete all levels of Bloom's taxonomy with a concept, you not only really know that topic but also are far more likely to recall that topic on Test Day. Memorized information does not have nearly the same level of recall as information that is deeply understood, is able to be synthesized, and is actively used to solve problems. In other words, you are not going to remember everything you study for Test Day. In fact, it is unlikely that you will be comfortable with every single topic on Test Day. However, if you build your knowledge to such a degree that you focus on a deeper level of learning, you will be able to use logic to go from what you do know to determine answers to questions you may not specifically "know" the answer to.

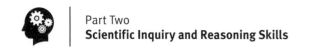

Scientific Inquiry and Reasoning Skills

Skill 2 questions specifically test the skills mentioned in Bloom's taxonomy. Skill 2 questions are designed to test the following abilities:

- To reason about scientific models, principles, and theories
- To evaluate and analyze scientific predictions and explanations
- To interpret and evaluate arguments regarding causes and consequences
- To unify observations, theories, and evidence to come to conclusions
- To recognize scientific findings that pose a challenge or invalidate a scientific theory or model
- To identify and use scientific formulas to solve problems

Table 4.1 compares and contrasts Skill 1 and Skill 2.

	Skill 1	**Skill 2**
What the Skill Tests	Basic scientific knowledge	Scientific reasoning skills
Tasks in Questions	Identifying the task Selecting the correct answer	Identifying the task Planning an attack that involves a multi-step process to determine an answer Selecting the correct answer

Table 4.1. Skill 1 *vs.* Skill 2

K

4.2   How Will Skills 1 and 2 Be Tested?

The differences between Skills 1 and 2 require a different approach to assess whether you have acquired the reasoning skills that will help you be successful in medical school and as a physician. This section explores how the skills are tested for each of the four question types as well as how these questions will appear on Test Day.

SKILL 1

Skill 1 questions are fairly simple. These are often easy points on Test Day as long as you have conducted a thorough and effective content review prior to Test Day. However, getting Skill 1 questions correct on Test Day is only a small piece of earning a high score; you will have to be proficient in all four skills. Skill 1 questions can be separated into the following categories:

- **Discrete questions**
  - Straightforward, direct questions, either addressing relationships between concepts or identifying a single detail or characteristics regarding a concept.

- **Questions that could stand alone from the passage**
  - Very similar to discrete questions, often thematically related to the passage.
  - Require identification of a single concept or relationship without a multi-step reasoning process.

- **Questions that require data from the passage**
  - Require minimal analysis of data from the passage, often connecting information from the passage to scientific concepts
  - Identification of a scientific concept with a graph or table may be required.
  - A mathematical equation may be presented, and you may be requested to use this equation to solve a problem.

- **Questions that require the goal of the passage**
  - Skill 1 questions are unlikely to require this level of analysis. When they do, the questions are simple and require identification of a relationship between a scientific concept and a fundamental piece of information in the passage.

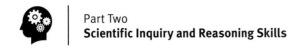

SKILL 2

Skill 2 questions are extremely common on Test Day. In fact, this was an extremely common question type on previous versions of the MCAT. Skill 2 questions can be separated into the following categories:

- **Discrete questions**
  - Require you to understand a particular concept and then link that concept with the task of the question.
  - No passage is associated; thus, the scope of the answer is limited to the scope of the question.

- **Questions that stand alone from the passage**
  - Much like discrete questions but often thematically related to the passage.
  - May require application of knowledge related to the passage but not specifically mentioned in it.

- **Questions that require data from the passage**
  - Likely to require calculations, evaluation of data, connection of the data with scientific principles, and use of scientific data and knowledge to draw conclusions related to information presented in the passage.
  - May require interpretation or analysis of graphs, tables, or diagrams.
  - May require you to apply information obtained from the passage to a new situation not presented in the passage.
  - May ask you to analyze the relationship between two variables in terms of causation and correlation.

- **Questions that require the goal of the passage**
  - Will require you to interpret the passage as a whole and connect the passage with your knowledge about scientific principles or your knowledge about a natural or social phenomenon.
  - May require you to identify arguments about cause and effect as supported by the passage or new evidence provided in the question stem.
  - Information may be presented in the question stem that either strengthens or weakens the argument made in the passage. You will be asked to identify how this new information is related to the passage as a whole.
  - May expect you to draw conclusions from the information presented in the passage or evaluate the validity of a conclusion based on evidence from the passage.

4.3 Getting the Edge in Skill 1 and Skill 2 Questions

Content knowledge is required for the MCAT, especially for Skill 1 questions. However, content knowledge is not enough for success on Test Day. The MCAT uses science as a vehicle to test critical-thinking skills, especially on Skill 2 questions. To get the edge on Skills 1 and 2, a thorough and efficient content review must be coupled with a significant number of practice questions. A common mistake made by students when studying for the MCAT is focusing too heavily on content review and not enough on practice questions and passages. The only way to be successful on Test Day is to integrate content review with practice questions and passages. Success on Skill 2 questions requires that you acquire a deeper level of learning than what is required in undergraduate science courses. To do this, ensure that you review content and then immediately apply content to practice passage and questions.

Every question that you answer incorrectly on a practice passage or question is an opportunity to review how you approached the question. Systematically reviewing questions to determine weaknesses in your critical-thinking skills will help you identify and address those weaknesses. If you find that you are stuck at a score plateau on practice tests, it is essential that you take an honest look at your critical-thinking skills to break through that plateau.

When the AAMC released the specifications for the current version of the MCAT, it established the expected distribution as **35 percent Skill 1** and **45 percent Skill 2** questions for each science section.

CHAPTER 5

Skill 3

Modern medicine requires the practical application of research. As a physician, you will constantly be seeking answers in research to determine prognoses, assess the appropriateness of a treatment modality for a given patient, and answer patients' questions. Evaluation of research is critical to the progress of all fields of medicine and will be a key component of your life as a physician.

To practice medicine in this way, certain basic skills are required, such as the ability to reason about the design and execution of research, otherwise known as Skill 3. In this chapter, we will discuss the specific characteristics of Skill 3 as well as how Skill 3 will be tested on the MCAT.

5.1 What Is Skill 3?

Skill 3 is divided into two main components: concepts behind scientific research and reasoning about ethical issues in research. You must understand how studies are designed using the scientific method as a guiding principle, and also the ethical issues present in research, especially in the use of human subjects.

SKILL 3

Skill 3 questions are designed to test the following:

- Identification of the roles of past findings, theories, and observations in scientific inquiry
- Identification of testable hypotheses and research questions
- Ability to distinguish between samples and populations and to identify results that support generalizations about populations
- Identification of independent and dependent variables
- Ability to reason about the features of research studies that suggest relationships among variables, including causality
- Ability to draw conclusions from results produced by research studies
- Identification of how results from research may apply to real-world situations
- Reasoning skills with respect to ethical issues in scientific research

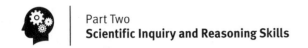

5.2 Fundamental Concepts of Skill 3

Skill 3 questions ask you to apply scientific concepts to your understanding of research in both the life sciences and the behavioral sciences. However, this information is rarely, if ever, covered in your undergraduate science classes. The scientific method is usually mentioned, but it is unlikely that it is covered in the level of detail that you will need on Test Day. This section discusses the basic concepts that you need to be successful on Skill 3 questions.

THE SCIENTIFIC METHOD

The scientific method is the basic paradigm of all scientific inquiry. It is the established protocol for transitioning from a question to a new body of knowledge. The steps in the scientific method are as follows.

Generate a Testable Question
- Occurs after observing something anomalous in another scientific inquiry or daily life.

Gather Data and Resources
- Phase of journal and database searches and information compilation.
- Look at all information, not just those consistent with the opinion of the investigator.

Form a Hypothesis
- Often in the form of an if-then statement, which will be tested in subsequent steps.

Collect New Data
- Collect data by experimentation (manipulation and control of variables of interest) or by observation (usually involves no changes in the subject's environment).

Analyze the Data
- Look for trends.
- Perform mathematical manipulations to solidify the relationship(s) among the variables.

Interpret the Data and Existing Hypothesis
- Consider whether the data analysis is consistent with the original hypothesis.
- If data are inconsistent, consider alternate hypotheses.

Publish
- Provide an opportunity for peer review.
- Summarize what was done during the previous steps in the publication.

Verify Results
- Repeat the experiment to verify results under new conditions.

BASIC CONCEPTS IN SCIENTIFIC RESEARCH

Basic science research—the kind conducted in a laboratory, not on people—is generally the easiest to design because the experimenter has the most control. Often, a causal relationship is being examined because the hypothesis generally states a condition and an outcome. To make generalizations about our experiments, the outcome of interest must not be obscured. In addition, there must also be a method by which causality may be demonstrated, which is relatively simple in basic science research but less so in other research areas. This requires the use of a control, or standard, and an identified set of variables.

Controls

In basic science research, conditions are applied to multiple trials of the same experiment that are as near to identical as possible.

- A control or standard is included as a method of verifying results.
- Controls can also be used to separate experimental conditions.
- Positive and negative controls are used as points of comparison, or a group of controls can be used to create a curve of known values.
  - Positive controls are those that ensure a change in the dependent variable when it is expected. For example, if a new assay is developed for the detection of a human immunodeficiency virus (HIV) infection, a number of blood samples known to contain HIV virus can act as a positive control.
  - Negative controls ensure that the dependent variable does not change when no change is expected. For example, the same new HIV assay would be used to test samples known to be without the virus. In pharmaceutical trials, a negative control could be used to assess the placebo effect. An observed or a reported change when an individual is given an inactive substance, such as a sugar pill, is an example of the placebo effect.

Causality

By manipulating all of the relevant experimental conditions, basic science researchers can often establish causality. Causality is an if-then relationship and is often the hypothesis being tested.

- **Independent variable:** the variable that is manipulated or changed.
- **Dependent variable:** the variable that is measured or observed.
- If a change in the independent variable always causes a change in the dependent variable and if the change in the dependent variable does not occur without a change in the independent variable, a relationship is said to be causal.

Error Sources

In basic science research, experimental bias is usually minimal. The most likely way for an experimenter's personal opinions to be incorporated is through the generation of a faulty hypothesis from incomplete early data and resource collection. Other sources of error include the manipulation of results by eliminating trials without appropriate background or by failing to publish works that contradict the experimenter's own hypothesis.

The low levels of bias introduced by the experimenter do not eliminate all error from basic science research. Measurements are especially important in the laboratory sciences, and the instruments may give faulty readings. Instrument error may affect accuracy, precision, or both. Accuracy, also called validity, is the ability of an instrument to measure a true value. Precision, also called reliability, is the ability of an instrument to read consistently or within a narrow range. Because bias is a systematic error in data, only an inaccurate tool will introduce bias. However, an imprecise tool will still introduce error.

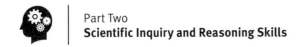

HUMAN SUBJECTS RESEARCH

Research using human subjects is considerably more complex, and the level of experimental control is invariably lower than in basic science research. In human subjects research, there are both experimental and observational studies.

EXPERIMENTAL APPROACH

Experimental research, similar to basic science research, attempts to establish causality. An independent variable is manipulated, and changes in a dependent variable are identified and quantified (if possible). Because subjects are in less-controlled conditions, the data analysis phase is more complicated than in laboratory studies. Two of the most fundamental concepts of the experimental approach are randomization and blinding.

Randomization

- Method used to control for differences between subject groups in biomedical research.
- Uses an algorithm to place each subject into either a control group that receives no treatment (or a sham treatment) or one or more treatment groups.
- Results are measured in all groups.
- Ideally, each group is perfectly matched on conditions such as age and gender.

Blinding

- Many measures in biomedical research are subjective. The perception of the subject and the investigator may be biased by knowing the group to which the subject has been assigned.
- When a study is blinded, the subject and/or the investigator are not aware of the group in which the subject has been placed.
- In single-blind experiments, only the patient or the assessor is blinded.
- In double-blind experiments, neither the subject nor the assessor (or even the investigator) is aware of the group into which a subject has been placed.
- The lack of blinding results in a diminished placebo effect in the control group, but the presence of the placebo affects the treatment group.

In biomedical research, data analysis must account for variables outside the independent and dependent variables. Most often, these include gender and age, lifestyle variables such as smoking, body mass index, and other factors that may affect the measured outcomes. Confounding variables, or variables that are not controlled or measured, also may affect the outcome.

OBSERVATIONAL APPROACH

The observational approach is often adopted to study certain causal relationships for which an experiment is either impractical or unethical. Observational studies in medicine fall into three categories: cohort studies, cross-sectional studies, and case-control studies.

Cohort Studies

- Subjects are sorted into two groups based on differences in risk factors (exposures) and then assessed at various intervals to determine how many subjects in each group have a certain outcome.

Cross-Sectional Studies

- Patients are categorized into different groups at a single point in time based on the presence or absence of a characteristic, such as a disease.

Case-Control Studies

- Subjects are separated into two groups based on the presence or absence of some outcome.
- The study looks backward to assess how many subjects in each group had exposure to a particular risk factor.

Identifying causality isn't necessarily simple. Hill's criteria describe the components of an observed relationship that increases the likelihood of causality in that relationship, as shown in Table 5.1. Although only the first criterion, temporality, is necessary for the relationship to be causal, it is not sufficient. An increased likelihood of causality is signified by an increased number of met criteria. Hill's criteria do not provide an absolute guideline on causality of a relationship. Thus, for any observational study, the relationship should be described as a correlation.

Criterion	Description
Temporality	Exposure (independent variable) must occur before the outcome (dependent variable).
Strength	Greater changes in the independent variable will cause a similar change in the dependent variable if the relationship is causal.
Dose-response Relationship	As the independent variable increases, there is a proportional increase in the response (dependent variable).
Consistency	The relationship is found in multiple settings.
Plausibility	The presence of a reasonable mechanism for the relationship between the variables is supported by existing literature.
Consideration of Alternate Explanations	If all other plausible explanations have been eliminated, the remaining explanation is more likely.
Experiment	An experiment can confirm causality.
Specificity	Change in the outcome (dependent) variable is produced only by an associated change in the independent variable.
Coherence	New data and hypotheses are consistent with the current state of scientific knowledge.

Table 5.1. Hill's Criteria

ERROR SOURCES

In addition to the measurement error found in basic science research, we must be aware of bias and error introduced by using human subjects as part of an experimental or observational model. As mentioned earlier, bias is a systematic error. As such, it generally does not impact the precision of the data but, rather, skews the data in one direction or the other. Bias is a result of flaws in the data collection phase of an experimental or observational study. Confounding is an error during analysis (see Figure 5.1).

Selection Bias

- Most prevalent type of bias.
- Occurs when subjects used for the study are not representative of the target population.
- May apply in cases where one gender is more prevalent than another or when there are differences in the age profile of the experiment group and the population.
- Measurement and the assessment of selection bias occur before any intervention.

Detection Bias

- Results from educated professionals applying knowledge in an inconsistent manner.
- Often occurs when prior studies have indicated that there is a correlation between two variables; when the researcher finds one of the variables, then he or she is more likely to search for the second, possibly related variable. That makes the second variable more likely to be found because the investigator is looking for it.

Observation Bias

- Also known as the Hawthorne effect.
- Occurs when the behavior of study participants is altered when the participants are aware that they are being studied.
- Systematic and occurs prior to data analysis.

Confounding

- Data analysis error.
- Data may or may not be flawed, but an incorrect relationship is characterized.
- Variables that are not controlled or measured but are present.

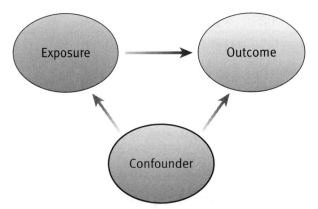

**Figure 5.1. Relationship Between Confounder,
Exposure, and Outcome**

ETHICAL ISSUES IN RESEARCH

In medicine, there are four core ethical tenets: beneficence, nonmaleficence, patient autonomy, and justice.

- Beneficence: an obligation to act in the patient's best interest
- Nonmaleficence: an obligation to avoid treatments or interventions in which the potential for harm outweighs the potential for benefit
- Patient autonomy: the responsibility to respect patients' decisions and choices about their own health care
- Justice: the responsibility to treat similar patients with similar care and to distribute health care resources fairly

In research, these principles are replaced by a slightly modified set as defined by the Belmont Report, a landmark document published by the National Commission for the Protection of Human Subjects in Biomedical and Behavioral Research. According to the Belmont Report, the three necessary pillars of research include respect for persons, justice, and a slightly more inclusive version of beneficence.

Respect for Persons

- Includes the need for honesty between the subjects and the researcher and generally—but not always—prohibits deception.
- Also includes the process of informed consent, in which a patient must be adequately counseled about the procedures, risks, benefits, and goals of a study to make a knowledgeable decision about whether or not to participate. Consent may be withdrawn at any time.
- Prohibits a coercive influence over the subjects.
- Institutional review boards are in place to provide systematic protections against unethical studies.
- Vulnerable persons, including children, pregnant women, and prisoners, require special protections above and beyond those taken with the general population.
- Confidentiality is generally considered to be part of respect for persons during research.

Justice

- Applies to both the selection of a research topic and the execution of the research.
- Morally relevant differences are defined as those differences among individuals that are considered an appropriate reason to treat the individuals differently. These differences include age and population size. Race, ethnicity, sexual orientation, and financial status are not considered morally relevant differences. However, religion is a special case in that certain interventions are prohibited by a given religion. Thus, avoidance of that treatment in individuals of that religion is consistent with patient autonomy.
- Risks inherent in the study must be distributed fairly so as to not impose undue harm on a particular group. However, when there is a population that is likely to receive a greater benefit from a study, this group may necessarily bear a greater proportion of the risk. Thus, the likelihood of benefit may be a morally relevant difference among individuals in certain situations.

Beneficence

- The intent of a study must be to cause a net positive change for both the study population and the general population. The study must be conducted in such a way as to minimize any potential harm.
- Research should be conducted in the least invasive, least painful, or least traumatic way possible. When choosing between two methods of measurement, the less painful and less invasive method should be employed.

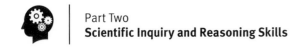
5.3   How Will Skill 3 Be Tested?

Skill 3 questions require a considerable amount of background information because study design and execution are generally not coverable in a single question stem. Thus, the more complex and nuanced Skill 3 questions are likely to require either data from the passage or the goal of the passage. These Skill 3 questions are also likely to require the scientific reasoning skills tested in Skill 2. It is important to note that even though the four skills have been separated neatly into categories by the AAMC, the separations may not be quite so distinct on Test Day; most questions still require some level of scientific reasoning. Skill 3 questions can be separated into the following categories:

- **Discrete questions**
  - Questions that are not associated with a descriptive passage.
  - Likely to focus on basic research concepts, including the identification of variables and the concepts of measurement, including accuracy and precision.

- **Questions that stand alone from the passage**
  - Similar to discrete questions.
  - Likely to focus on more basic concepts of study design and execution.

- **Questions that require data from the passage**
  - Be prepared for questions that require you to use data from the passage to identify variables and relationships among variables and that test your ability to distinguish between causation and correlation.

- **Questions that require the goal of the passage**
  - These questions require you to have an understanding of the passage as a whole and be able to identify the goal of the passage.
  - May ask for alternative explanations for the phenomena described in the passage as well as examination of evidence presented in the passage.
  - Questions may require you to draw conclusions from evidence presented in the passage as well as identify conclusions that are not supported by the passage.
  - Expect you to evaluate study design in light of results and conclusions drawn from the information.
  - Identification of independent and dependent variables as well as confounding variables and types of bias.

5.4   Getting the Edge in Skill 3 Questions

Much of what is tested in Skill 3 is not necessarily presented in introductory-level courses. Some test takers will have taken courses with more emphasis in research, whereas others may have little to no experience in this area. You can maximize your score by developing a thorough understanding of the topics discussed in this chapter. The MCAT assumes you have a certain level of knowledge in the area of research. It is essential that you develop that knowledge by reading research articles and becoming comfortable with the general format and discussion present in all research studies, including background, the literature review, procedure, results, and discussion. As you read more research studies, you will gain increasing comfort with research as a part of scientific inquiry. Be sure to read research in all subject areas tested on the MCAT, including biology, biochemistry, general chemistry, organic chemistry, physics, psychology, and sociology. Most students are comfortable with lab research but are less comfortable with research involving human subjects. Focus your review of study design in the areas that are more likely to involve human subjects, including biology, psychology, and sociology.

When the AAMC released the specifications for the current version of the MCAT, it established the expected distribution as **10 percent Skill 3** for each science section.

CHAPTER 6

Skill 4

By now, you have no doubt realized that the MCAT places a high level of importance on your ability to understand the process by which new scientific and medical knowledge is acquired by research. As discussed previously, Skill 3 questions test your ability to reason about the design and execution of research in the life sciences and the behavioral sciences. However, Skill 4 questions test your ability to understand and draw conclusions using the data collected by research.

6.1   What Is Skill 4?

Academic papers are extremely predictable. A research paper generally starts with an abstract—a few short paragraphs reflecting the major points of the rest of the paper. The authors then provide an expanded introduction, materials and methods, data, and discussion. The key to a high-quality research paper is making this discussion unnecessary; any scientists, when given the prior sections, should be led to the same conclusions as those given by the author. The test makers are keenly aware of this fact. On Test Day, you may be presented with research in the form of an experiment-based passage. Part of your task will be inferring the important conclusions that can be supported by the findings of the study.

Skill 4 questions test your ability to draw conclusions using both raw data and graphical representations of data. Skill 4 can be divided into two main components: (1) interpretation of patterns in tables, figures, and graphs and (2) drawing conclusions from the data presented. However, you are expected to use statistical reasoning skills to draw conclusions. Although the identification of patterns is important, you must also be able to determine if these patterns are statistically significant.

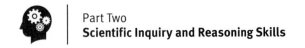
SKILL 4

Skill 4 questions are designed to test the following:

- Use, analyze, and interpret data in tables, graphs, and figures.
- Determine the most effective way to represent data for specific scientific observations and data sets.
- Use central tendency (mean, median, and mode) and dispersion (range, interquartile range, and standard deviation) measures to describe data.
- Identify and reason regarding random and systematic error.
- Determine the statistical significance and uncertainty of a data set using statistical significance levels and confidence intervals.
- Identify relationships and explanations of those relationships using data.
- Predict outcomes using data.
- Draw conclusions and answer research questions using data.

6.2   Fundamental Concepts of Skill 4

Many students take biostatistics or some other statistics class in preparation for a major in biology or the life sciences. However, many students who take the MCAT have not taken a statistics course. Thus, the basic information required to answer these questions is briefly covered in this section. Keep in mind that the AAMC does not permit the use of calculators on any section of the MCAT.

MATH WITHOUT A CALCULATOR

Math on the MCAT is about more than remembering the correct formula and facts. Without an available calculator, you need to be able to efficiently calculate the correct answer by hand. This skill requires familiarity with such topics as arithmetic, significant figures, exponents, logarithms, trigonometry, unit conversions, and dimensional analysis.

The following question illustrates the first way you can make your life easier: **look for ratios.**

One mole of helium gas is taken from standard temperature and pressure to a temperature of 546 K and a volume of 67.2 L. Assuming ideal behavior, what is the new pressure of the gas?

The numbers 546 K and 67.2 L are very specific, and there's a reason for that. They are related to other numbers implied within the question stem. The gas begins at standard temperature and pressure (STP), which you're required to know is 273 K and 1 atm. The temperature change to 546 K is a common one you'll see because it's exactly twice the standard temperature. Similarly, you are required to know that an ideal gas at STP occupies 22.4 L per mol, so you'll often see volume changes that are a multiple of this number. Sure enough, 67.2 L is three times the initial volume. In other words, the question is *really* asking you, "What effect will doubling the temperature and tripling the volume have on the pressure of an ideal gas?"

This analysis leads to the second important math tip for the MCAT: **know your variable relationships.**

The formula for two sets of conditions with the ideal gas law, $\frac{P_1V_1}{n_1T_1} = \frac{P_2V_2}{n_2T_2}$, can certainly get the job done here, but performing a computation using that formula is not the most efficient way. Rather, consider the relationships represented by that formula. Pressure and temperature are on opposite sides of the fraction line on the same side of the equation and thus are directly related. Therefore, doubling the temperature will double the pressure (assuming everything else is kept constant). Pressure and volume are both in the numerator on the same side of the equation, indicating that they are inversely related. Therefore, tripling the volume will cut the new pressure to $\frac{1}{3}$ its value. Combining these two effects with the initial volume of 1 atm yields the new volume:

$$1 \text{ atm} \times 2 \times \frac{1}{3} = \frac{2}{3} \text{ atm}$$

Let's take a look at another example:

Calculate the pressure exerted by the fluid on a scuba diver at a depth of 58.4 m in ocean water of density 1,025 kg/m^3.

Again, understanding the appropriate formula is prerequisite knowledge. The formula for pressure exerted by a fluid is $P = \rho g z$, where ρ is density of the fluid, g is gravity (9.8 m/s^2), and z is depth. The exact calculation for the pressure would be $P = (1,025 \text{ kg/m}^3)(9.8 \text{ m/s}^2)(58.4 \text{ m})$. With a calculator in hand, this would be a cinch. However, you could easily get bogged down doing this calculation by hand.

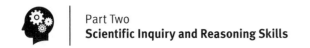

Here's where the next tip comes into play: **estimate wherever possible.**

This calculation becomes much more manageable with a few simple changes to the numbers. If instead you consider $P = (1{,}000 \text{ kg/m}^3)(10 \text{ m/s}^2)(60 \text{ m})$, you can quickly get an estimate of 600,000 pascals, which isn't far off from the exact answer of 586,628 pascals.

Keep in mind a few other considerations when doing math on the MCAT:

- Use the answer choices as an indication for how much you can estimate. If the answer choices are all incredibly far apart, you can be comfortable being liberal with your rounding. If they're close together, keep your rounding to a minimum.
- Track the effect your estimations will have on the final answer. In the above problem, one number was rounded down while two numbers were rounded up, which offset the error. However, if you only rounded numbers up, expect to end up with a larger number than the actual answer. If you only rounded down, expect to have a smaller number.
- Don't forget the effects of rounding are reversed when rounding a number in the denominator. Rounding up a number in the denominator makes your estimate smaller than the actual answer, while rounding down in the denominator leads to a number that is larger.
- When dealing with large or small numbers (including numbers less than 100), use scientific notation! Depending on the calculation, it's often easier to work with two or more numbers in scientific notation.
- Know common decimal to fraction conversions and convert to fractions whenever convenient. One common example deals with the Hardy–Weinberg equilibrium. If p^2 is 0.04, then what is p? It's a common mistake to calculate the square root of 0.04 as 0.02. It's much easier to see that the correct answer is $\frac{2}{10}$ when the square root of $\frac{4}{100}$ is taken.

MEASURES OF CENTRAL TENDENCY

Measures of central tendency describe a central value around which the other values in the data set are clustered. However, this central value can be described in multiple ways, including the mean, median, and mode.

Mean

The mean, or average, of a set of data is calculated by adding the individual values within the data set and dividing the result by the number of values. Mean values are a good indicator of central tendency when all of the values tend to be fairly close to one another. Having an outlier, or an extremely large or extremely small value compared with the other data values, can shift the mean toward one end or the other.

Median

The median value for a set of data is its midpoint, where half of the data points are greater than the median value and half are smaller. In data sets with an odd number of values, the median is actually one of the data points. In data sets with an even number of values, the median is the mean of the two central data points. To calculate the median, a data set must first be listed in increasing order. The median position can be calculated with the following equation, where n is the number of data values:

$$\text{median position} = \frac{(n + 1)}{2}$$

In a data set with an even number of data points, this equation results in a number such as 9.5. This result indicates that the median lies between the ninth and tenth value of the data set and is the average of the ninth and tenth values.

The median tends to be the measure of central tendency that is the least susceptible to outliers. However, the median may not be useful for data sets with very large ranges (the distance between the largest and smallest data points) or with multiple modes.

If the mean and median are far from each other, this difference implies the presence of outliers or a skewed distribution, as discussed later in this chapter. If the mean and the median are very close, this proximity implies a symmetrical distribution.

Mode

The mode, quite simply, is the number that appears most often in a data set. There may be multiple modes in a data set, or—if all numbers appear equally—there can even be no mode for a data set. When we examine distributions, the peaks represent modes. The mode is not typically used as a measure of central tendency for a data set. However, the number of modes, and the distance between the modes, is often informative. If a data set has two modes with a number of values between the modes, it may be useful to analyze these portions separately or look for confounding variables that may be responsible for dividing the distribution into two parts.

DISTRIBUTIONS

Often, a single statistic for a data set is insufficient for a detailed or relevant analysis. In this case, it is useful to look at the overall shape of the distribution as well as specifics about how that shape impacts our interpretation of data. The shape of a distribution impacts all of the measures of central tendency as well as some measures of distribution.

Normal Distributions

In statistics, normal distributions are the most common. Even when we know that a distribution is not quite normal, we can use special techniques so that our data will approximate a normal distribution. This normalization is very important because the normal distribution has been "solved" in the sense that we can transform any normal distribution to a standard distribution with a mean of zero and a standard deviation of one and then use the newly generated curve to get information about probability or percentages of populations. The normal distribution is also the basis for the bell curve seen in many scenarios and in Figure 6.1, including exam scores on the MCAT.

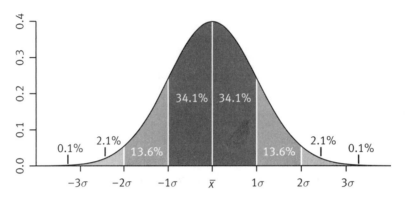

Figure 6.1. The Normal Distribution
The mean, median, and mode are at the center of the distribution.
Approximately 68 percent of the distribution is within one standard deviation
of the mean, 95 percent within two standard deviations, and 99 percent within three standard deviations.

Skewed Distributions

Distributions are not always symmetrical. A skewed distribution is one that contains a tail on one side or the other of the data set (see Figure 6.2). On the MCAT, skewed distributions are most often tested by identifying the type of skewed distribution. Skewed distributions are often an area of confusion for students because the visual shift in the data appears opposite the direction of the skew. A negatively skewed distribution has a tail on the left (or negative) side, whereas a positively skewed distribution has a tail on the right (or positive side). In summary, use the tail (not the peak) to determine the direction of the skew.

Because the mean is more susceptible to outliers than the median, the mean of a negatively skewed distribution is generally lower than the median. In contrast, the mean of a positively skewed distribution is generally higher than the median.

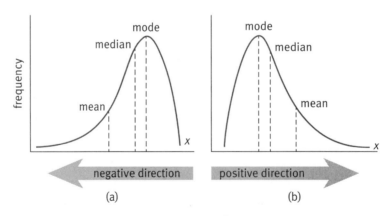

Figure 6.2. Skewed Distributions
(a) Negatively skewed distribution, with mean lower than median
(b) Positively skewed distribution, with mean higher than median

Bimodal Distributions

Some distributions have two or more peaks. A distribution containing two peaks with a valley in between is called bimodal (see Figure 6.3). It is important to note that a bimodal distribution might have only one true mode if one peak is slightly higher than the other. The presence of two peaks of different sizes does not discount a distribution from being considered bimodal. If there is sufficient separation between the two peaks or a sufficiently small amount of data within the valley region, bimodal distributions can often be analyzed as two separate distributions.

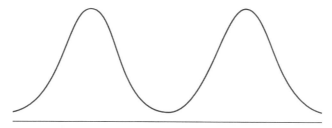

Figure 6.3. Bimodal Distribution

MEASURES OF DISTRIBUTION

Distributions can also be characterized by the distance between the highest and lowest values as well as by the distance from the mean value.

Range

Range is an absolute measure of the spread of a data set. The range of a data set is the difference between the highest and lowest values. Range does not consider the number of items in the data set, nor does it consider the placement of any measures of central tendency. Therefore, range is heavily affected by the presence of data outliers. In cases where it is not possible to calculate the standard deviation for a normal distribution because the entire data set is not provided, it is possible to approximate the standard deviation as one-fourth of the range.

Standard Deviation

Standard deviation is the most informative measure of distribution, but it is also the most mathematically laborious. It is calculated relative to the mean of the data. On Test Day, you may be asked to calculate a standard deviation. However, it is more likely that you will have to apply the concept of the standard deviation to identify an outlier. In addition, standard deviation can also be used to describe the distance from the mean of a particular value.

- Sixty-eight percent of the data points fall within one standard deviation of the mean.
- Ninety-five percent of the data points fall within two standard deviations of the mean.
- Ninety-nine percent of the data points fall within three standard deviations of the mean.

Interquartile Range

Before defining interquartile range, we must define quartiles. If we were to divide an ordered set of numbers (arranged from smallest to largest) into four equal quarters, we would need three boundaries. These boundaries are known as **quartiles**, specifically Q_1, Q_2, and Q_3.

(Note that Q_0 and Q_4 are also defined as the first and last data point, respectively. However, they are rarely tested on the MCAT.)

- Q_1 separates the first and second quarters of data. Q_1 can be found by multiplying the total number of data points (n) by $\frac{1}{4}$.
- Q_2 is the median and separates the data in half. Q_2 should be calculated the same way as when calculating the median.
- Q_3 separates the third and fourth quarters of data. Similar to Q_1, the position of Q_3 can be found by multiplying the total number of data points (n) by $\frac{3}{4}$.

If the calculation for the position of Q_1 or Q_3 produces a whole number, the quartile is the mean of the value at this position and the next highest position. Alternatively, if the calculation produces a decimal, round up and take that position as the quartile. It is worth noting that there are several different methods to calculate quartiles, any of which will work on Test Day.

Interquartile range (IQR) is a measure of distribution defined as the difference between the value of third quartile and the first quartile.

$$IQR = Q_3 - Q_1$$

Outliers

Outliers are data points that fall outside of the general trend of the data. More precisely, outliers are defined as data points that are $1.5 \times$ IQR below the first quartile or $1.5 \times$ IQR above the 3rd quartile. To summarize, outliers are the following:

- Data points $< Q_1 - (1.5 \times IQR)$
- Data points $> Q_3 + (1.5 \times IQR)$

Standard deviation (SD) can also be used to approximate these outlier boundary points. Data points above or below three standard deviations are often considered outliers.

Outliers typically result from one of three causes:

- A true statistical anomaly
- A measurement error
- A distribution that is not approximated by the normal distribution

When an outlier is found, this discovery should trigger an automatic investigation to determine which of the three causes applies. You will likely be asked to determine the most likely cause of an outlier on Test Day. If there is a measurement error, the data point should be excluded from analysis. However, two other situations, described below, are less clear.

If an outlier is the result of a true measurement but it is not representative of the population, the outlier may be weighted to reflect its rarity or may be excluded from the analysis depending on the purpose of the study and the preselected protocols. The decision should be made before a study begins—not after an outlier has been found. When outliers are an indication that a data set may not approximate the normal distribution, repeated samples or larger samples will generally demonstrate if this is true.

STATISTICAL TESTING

Hypothesis testing and confidence intervals allow us to draw conclusions about populations based on our sample data. Both are interpreted in the context of probabilities and what we deem an acceptable risk of error.

Hypothesis Testing

Hypothesis testing begins with an idea about what may be different between two populations. We have a null hypothesis (H_0), which is always a hypothesis of equivalence. In other words, the null hypothesis says that two populations are equal or that a single population can be described by a parameter equal to a given value. The alternative hypothesis (H_a) may be nondirectional (saying that the populations are not equal) or directional.

The most common hypothesis tests are z-tests or t-tests, which rely on the standard distribution or on the closely related t-distribution. From the data collected, a test statistic is calculated and compared with a table to determine the likelihood that the statistic was obtained by random chance (under the assumption that our null hypothesis is true). This is our p-value. We then compare our p-value to a significance level (α); 0.05 is commonly used. For a directional test, if the p-value is greater than α, we fail to reject the null hypothesis. This result means that the two populations are not statistically significantly different. If the p-value is less than α, we reject the null hypothesis and state that there is a difference between the two groups. When the null hypothesis is rejected, we state that our results are statistically significant.

The value of α is a level of risk that we are willing to accept for incorrectly rejecting the null hypothesis (also called a type I error). In other words, a type I error is the likelihood that we report a difference between two populations when one does not actually exist. A type II error occurs when we incorrectly fail to reject the null hypothesis. In other words, a type II error is the likelihood that we report no difference between two populations when one actually exists. The probability of a type II error is sometimes symbolized by β. The probability of correctly rejecting a false null hypothesis (reporting a difference between two populations when one actually exists) is referred to as power and is equal to $1 - \beta$. Finally, the probability of correctly failing to reject a true null hypothesis (reporting no difference between two populations when one does not exist) is referred to as confidence. Table 6.1 summarizes all of these scenarios for your review.

		Truth About the Population	
		H_0 True (No Difference)	H_a True (Difference Exists)
Conclusion based on sample	Reject H_0	Type I error (α)	Power ($1 - \beta$)
	Fail to reject H_0	Confidence	Type II error (β)

Table 6.1. Results of Hypothesis Testing

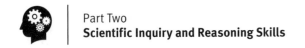
Confidence Intervals

Confidence intervals are essentially the reverse of hypothesis testing. With a confidence interval, we determine a range of values from the sample mean and the standard deviation. Rather than finding a p-value, we begin with a desired confidence level (95 percent is standard) and use a table to find its corresponding z-score or t-score. When we multiply the z-score or t-score by the standard deviation and then add or subtract this number from the mean, we create a range of values. For example, consider a population for which we wish to know the mean age. We draw a sample from that population and find that the mean age of the sample is 30, with a standard deviation of 3. If we wish to have 95 percent confidence, the corresponding z-score (which would be provided on Test Day) is 1.96. Thus, the range is $30 \pm (3)(1.96) = 24.12$ to 35.88. We can then report that we are 95 percent confident that the true mean age of the population from which this sample is drawn is between 24.12 and 35.88.

APPLYING DATA

In an academic paper, the discussion portion is where the gathered and interpreted data are applied to the original problem. We can then begin drawing conclusions and creating new questions based on our results.

Correlation and Causation

Correlation refers to a connection—direct relationship, inverse relationship, or otherwise—between data. Correlation does not necessarily imply causation; we must avoid this assumption when there is insufficient evidence to draw such a conclusion. If an experiment cannot be performed, we must rely on Hill's criteria. Remember, the only one of Hill's criteria that is universally required for causation is temporality.

In the Context of Scientific Knowledge

When interpreting data, it is important that we not only state the apparent relationship between data but also begin to draw connections to other concepts in science and our background knowledge. At a minimum, the impact of the new data would be integrated into all future investigations on the topic. Additionally, we must develop a plausible rationale for the results. Finally, we must make decisions about our data's impact on the real world and determine whether our evidence is substantial and impactful enough to necessitate changes in understanding or policy.

6.3 How Will Skill 4 Be Tested?

Skill 4 questions are likely to appear in a variety of scenarios on Test Day. This skill easily lends itself to a variety of scenarios and levels of information. Skill 4 questions can be separated into the following categories:

- **Discrete questions**
  - Questions are not associated with a descriptive passage.
  - Likely to ask fairly simple questions related to Skill 4.
  - Calculations of a mean, median, mode, or range are likely to appear.
  - May be related to fundamental concepts, including types of error or bias.

- **Questions that stand alone from the passage**
  - Very similar to discrete questions.
  - Likely to be fairly simple and not require a large amount of analysis.

- **Questions that require data from the passage**
  - May require analysis or interpretation of a chart, graph, or table.
  - Calculations may be required.
  - Comparisons between variables may be required.

- **Questions that require the goal of the passage**
  - These questions are the most in-depth of all the Skill 4 question types.
  - Likely to require you to evaluate data to determine if the data support the conclusion presented in the passage.
  - May ask you to draw conclusions from the data and information presented in the passage, requiring integration of the passage, data, and statistical analysis.
  - Expect that some Skill 4 questions in this category will require you to identify relationships between variables or evaluate the study for error or bias based on your statistical analysis.

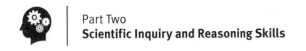

6.4 Getting the Edge in Skill 4 Questions

Skill 4 requires an understanding of how research data are evaluated. The best way to identify your strengths and weaknesses in this area is actually to read academic papers. However, just reading academic papers is not enough. You have to go through each calculation that has been performed and interpret each paper in light of your own statistical analysis. Think of yourself like a teacher grading a research paper. Read critically, and identify any flaws in the authors' analysis of data, including miscalculations. Finally, after reading each paper, summarize the value of the information. If you had a patient whose disease or treatment course could be affected by the information in the paper, do you believe that the information in the paper is reliable? Is it statistically significant? Did the discussion in the paper actually address the questions set forth at the beginning of the paper? As you read more papers, these questions will become easier to answer.

In addition to reading papers, it is essential that you answer a considerable number of practice questions in this area. Often, passages that are steeped in research also present a number of Skill 3 questions. Although we present these skills separately here, both are essential to understanding academic research papers. By seeking out practice passages and question sets that use both of these skills, these question types will become easier. You will then be able to maximize your score on Test Day.

When the AAMC released the specifications for the current version of the MCAT, it established the expected distribution as **10 percent Skill 4** questions for each science section.

Science Subject Review

CHAPTER 7

Science Unit Overview

Now that you are more comfortable with the MCAT and the Kaplan Method for the exam, it is time for us to dive into practice mode. The following chapters summarize the most salient takeaways of the test maker's content outlines, with special emphasis on how you can use the information to succeed on Test Day.

For your convenience, each science discipline covered on the exam is presented for your review before the practice. The content review for each subject includes the following:

- What is unique about that topic on the exam
- How you should expect to see the content on the exam
- How you can get the edge by using the Kaplan Method
- A detailed, annotated outline of the topics and subtopics covered

After the overview, you will have an opportunity to see worked examples demonstrating exactly how the Kaplan Method can help tackle a challenge passage. You not only have the opportunity to try the passage on your own, but you can also see the Kaplan Method for questions demonstrated for each worked passage.

Following the science overview and worked examples, you will then have an opportunity to practice the Kaplan Method on your own with practice problems (in the book and online).

To get the most out of your practice, be sure to note question types, Wrong Answer Pathologies, and clues to the correct answer.

CHAPTER 8

Behavioral Sciences

A significant factor influencing a patient's ability to heal from an injury or manage a chronic disease is that person's psychiatric and socioeconomic status. When considering treatment options for a patient, a physician must take into account the patient's ability to understand and adhere to a treatment plan. Patients with a psychiatric disorder or who are unable to afford their prescriptions are not likely to take medications as prescribed, unless the treatment regimen is simple and affordable. In an effort to emphasize the psychological and social aspects of medicine, the AAMC has added a section to the MCAT known as the Psychological, Social, and Biological Foundations of Behavior section. This section is approximately 65 percent psychology, 30 percent sociology, and 5 percent biology. In addition, another 5 percent of the psychology questions cover biologically relevant topics.

8.1   Reading the Passage

Like the other sections, there will be two main passage types: information passages and experiment passages. However, the distinction is not as clear as in the other sections. Behavioral science passages will almost always discuss an experiment or study, even if the passage seems to be more informational. Many of these passages will be designed to test your ability to analyze experimental data and evaluate experimental design. The informational aspects of the passage will provide background or discuss a fundamental concept, and the attached experiment or study will be related to the passage topic. As such, you will be expected to use the same critical reading skills you have been using all along, but in a much more integrated way.

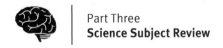

PASSAGE TYPES

Almost all of the passages will contain an experiment. The data from the experiment or study described may be presented in the form of a chart or graph indicating the probability of some outcome or the likelihood of some characteristic among the study population.

MCAT EXPERTISE

For passages with both experimental and informational content, use a combination of distill approaches appropriate to the information presented.

However, the early parts of the passage will often read like an information passage, much like the background portion of a peer-reviewed paper within the scientific disciplines. The passage then will change course to present the hypothesis, variables, and procedure of the study. Finally, the results will be presented. Thus, the early parts of the passage containing information should be treated like an information passage, with reading aimed at getting the gist of the paragraph(s), without spending time analyzing the details. When discussion of the study begins, switch to a more experiment-based reading strategy, seeking out the hypothesis, procedure, and results. Finally, the chart, graph, or table will require more intensive analysis.

What to Expect: Behavioral Sciences

- Almost all passages will contain an experiment, especially psychology passages.
- Any passages that do not contain an experiment are more likely to be sociology passages. These passages will focus primarily on sociological theory.
- Many passages will blend subject matter, and you will be expected to understand the connections between biology, psychology, and sociology.

	The Core Sciences	**Behavioral Sciences**
Topics	Biology, biochemistry, general chemistry, organic chemistry, and physics	Biology, psychology, and sociology
Passage types	Information and experiment	Passages will mainly consist of information and experiment portions, but many passages will not fall neatly into either category
Questions	Will require a variety of skills from basic recall of information, application of information to a new situation, analysis of data, and evaluation of experiment design	Will require a variety of skills, but data analysis and evaluation of experiment design will be emphasized

Table 8.1. The Core Sciences *vs.* Behavioral Sciences

READING AND DISTILLING THE PASSAGE

Regardless of how the passages in this section differ from those found in the other sections, the same Kaplan Method should be applied across all sciences. Read the passage quickly and efficiently, applying the Distill method best suited to the kind of information being conveyed.

- **Preview** for difficulty
    - Note the structure of the passage, the location of the paragraphs, and any figures such as charts, graphs, tables, or diagrams.
    - Determine whether the passage is *experiment* or *information* or a blend of both.
    - Determine the topic and the degree of difficulty.
    - Identify whether this passage will require a large time investment.
    - Decide whether this passage is one to do now or later.

- **Choose** your approach
    - Using information from the Preview step, Choose an appropriate Distill approach for the passage (Interrogate, Outline, or Highlight).
    - **Interrogation** should be chosen for experiment passages.
    - **Outlining** should be chosen for information passages that are dense or detail heavy.
    - **Highlighting** should be chosen for information passages that are light on details.

- **Read and Distill** key themes
    - While reading the passage, your aim is to distill the major takeaway of each paragraph and identify testable information using one of the following approaches.
    - **Interrogate**: Thoroughly examine the experiment passage by identifying the key components of experimental design and interrogating *why* specific procedures were done and *how* they connect to the overall purpose of the experiment.
    - **Outline**: Create a brief label for each paragraph that summarizes the contents of the paragraph, allowing you to quickly return to the passage when demanded by a question.
    - **Highlight**: Highlight one to three terms per paragraph that can pull your attention back to testable information when demanded by a question.

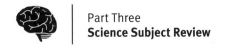

8.2 Answering the Questions

Behavioral sciences questions seek to integrate concepts, especially with regard to data analysis and experimental design. However, the same basic four question types are present:

- **Discrete questions**
  - Questions are not connected to a passage.
  - Are preceded by a warning such as "Questions 12–15 do not refer to a passage and are independent of each other."
  - Often require you to recall or apply a basic concept, such as a theory or a process.
  - Not likely to evaluate experimental design or data analysis.

- **Questions that stand alone from the passage**
  - Questions that accompany a passage but do not require information or data from the passage to identify the correct answer.
  - More likely to require application of a basic concept, theory, or process to a situation presented in the question stem.

- **Questions that require data from the passage**
  - Questions that require a piece of data or information from the passage but do not require the goal of the passage.
  - These questions are likely to focus on data analysis or an evaluation of an experimental procedure.
  - May focus on the information section of the passage and require you to identify a detail presented.

- **Questions that require the goal of the passage**
  - Questions that require the goal of the passage or a fundamental grasp of the passage as a whole.
  - These questions are likely to focus on the results and a discussion of the results of an experiment.
  - May assess your ability to analyze data or evaluate an experimental design but from a broader perspective, such as a change that could be made in the procedure that would affect the results in a particular way.
  - May require you to evaluate the results of an experiment and apply those results to the information presented earlier in the passage.
  - Likely to require the application of basic concepts and theories to understanding the passage as a whole.

ATTACKING THE QUESTIONS

Even though the behavioral sciences passages and questions are somewhat different from those seen in the other two science sections, the questions are still designed to test the same basic analytical skills. Thus, the same Kaplan Methods apply. In addition, having a basic strategy that you go to for each and every question combats any nervousness you may experience, especially as you encounter topics with which you are not as comfortable. The Kaplan Method provides a framework that aids in the identification of the correct answer, prevents hasty selection of incorrect answers, and combats test anxiety.

- **Type** the question
  - Read the question; peek at the answer choices for patterns, but don't analyze them closely.
  - Assess the topic and the degree of difficulty.
  - Identify the level of time involvement: is this question likely to take a tremendous amount of time to identify the answer? If so, skip it and come back after you do the other questions in the passage set.
  - Good questions to do now in the behavioral sciences are those that stand alone from the passage because these are generally quick and easy points.

- **Rephrase** the question stem
  - Rephrase the question, focusing on the task(s) to be accomplished.
  - Simplify the phrasing of the original question stem.
  - Translate the question into a specific set of tasks to be accomplished using the passage and your background knowledge.

- **Investigate** potential solutions
  - Complete the task(s) identified in your Rephrase step.
  - Analyze the data, and evaluate the experimental design; locate the information required; and connect the information, data, and experimental design with the information you already know.
  - Predict what you can about the answer.
  - Be flexible if your initial approach fails.

- **Match** your prediction to an answer choice
  - Search the answer choices for a response that is synonymous with your prediction, or eliminate answers that are not correct.
  - Select an answer and move on.
  - If you cannot find a match to your prediction, eliminate wrong answers, select a response from the remaining choices, and move on.

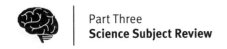
8.3 Getting the Edge in Behavioral Sciences

Earning a high score on Test Day in the behavioral sciences requires the ability to reason and apply what you already know to new situations. This skill requires a level of learning that is often different from that required by undergraduate courses. Not only do you need to understand the definitions and theories, but you also need to know the real-world applications of those theories. Getting the edge in the behavioral sciences requires practice by working through a significant number of questions in the topic to grasp the level of thinking required for this topic.

In addition, some level of flexibility in approaching the passages is required. In the sciences, the passages fall neatly into two categories: experiment and information. In the behavioral sciences, this distinction is no longer possible on many passages. The first half of many passages read like an information passage, and the second half present an experiment related to the information presented earlier in the passage. This forces you, as the test taker, to handle both aspects within one passage. As you distill the passage, read to understand the context or background of the first half, which serves as the framework for understanding the experimental portion.

Identifying the task of the question ensures that you look for information in the correct place in the passage. Some questions require data analysis and evaluation of an experimental procedure, meaning that the experiment portion of the passage is required. More theoretical questions are likely to require the information portion. However, the location of necessary information may vary depending on the task of the question. The task of the question will guide you to the correct location in the passage.

8.4 Preparing for the MCAT: Behavioral Sciences

The following presents the behavioral sciences content you are likely to see on Test Day. The behavioral sciences are among the most important subjects on the MCAT, so be sure to familiarize yourself with all of the content. The High-Yield badges point out the topics that are tested most frequently. You will notice that, given the importance of behavioral sciences on the MCAT, most of the content within this section is considered high yield.

BIOLOGY AND BEHAVIOR

The Nervous System

 High-Yield

Neuropsychology is the study of the connection between the nervous system and behavior. This discipline most often focuses on the functions of various brain regions.

There are three types of neurons in the nervous system: **sensory** (**afferent**) neurons, **motor** (**efferent**) neurons, and **interneurons. Reflex arcs** use the ability of interneurons in the spinal cord to relay information to the source of stimuli while simultaneously routing that information to the brain; these are the most basic complete neural networks.

The nervous system is made up of the **central nervous system** (**CNS**; brain and spinal cord) and **peripheral nervous system** (**PNS**; most cranial and spinal nerves). The PNS is divided into the **somatic** (voluntary) and **autonomic** (automatic) divisions. The autonomic system is further divided into the **parasympathetic** (rest-and-digest) and **sympathetic** (fight-or-flight) branches. (See Figure 8.1.)

KEY CONCEPT

Afferent neurons ascend in the cord toward the brain; efferent neurons exit the cord on their way to an effector.

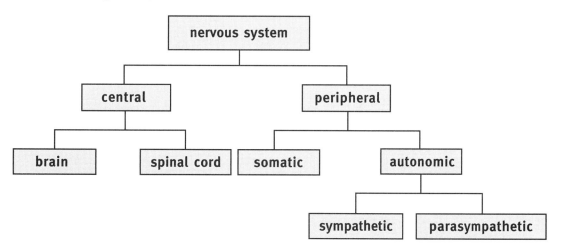

Figure 8.1. Major Divisions of the Nervous System

The brain is divided into two **cerebral hemispheres**, left and right, and also has three subdivisions: hindbrain, midbrain, and forebrain. The **hindbrain** contains the cerebellum, medulla oblongata, and reticular formation. The **midbrain** contains the inferior and superior colliculi. The **forebrain** contains the thalamus, hypothalamus, basal ganglia, limbic system, and cerebral cortex.

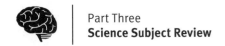
KEY CONCEPT

The functions of the hypothalamus—the four Fs:
• **F**eeding
• **F**ighting
• **F**lighting
• (Sexual) **F**unctioning

The **thalamus** is a relay station for sensory information. The **hypothalamus** maintains homeostasis and integrates with the endocrine system through the **hypophyseal portal system** that connects it to the **anterior pituitary**. The **basal ganglia** smooth movements and maintain postural stability. The **limbic system**, which contains the septal nuclei, amygdala, and hippocampus, controls emotion and memory.

The **cerebral cortex** is divided into four lobes:

- The **frontal** lobe controls executive function, impulse control, long-term planning, motor function, and speech production.
- The **parietal** lobe controls sensations of touch, pressure, temperature, and pain; spatial processing; orientation; and manipulation.
- The **occipital** lobe controls visual processing.
- The **temporal** lobe controls sound processing, speech perception, memory, and emotion.

Neurotransmitters are released by neurons to carry a signal to another neuron or effector. (See Table 8.2.)

Neurotransmitter	Behavior
Acetylcholine	Voluntary muscle control, parasympathetic nervous system, attention, alertness
Epinephrine and norepinephrine	Fight-or-flight responses, wakefulness, alertness
Dopamine	Smooth movements, postural stability
Serotonin	Mood, sleep, eating, dreaming
GABA and glycine	Brain "stabilization"
Glutamate	Brain excitation
Endorphins	Natural painkillers

Table 8.2. Neurotransmitters and Their Functions

The endocrine system is tied to the nervous system through the hypothalamus and the anterior pituitary as well as a few hormones created elsewhere in the body. **Cortisol** is a stress hormone released by the adrenal cortex. **Testosterone** and **estrogen** mediate libido; testosterone also increases aggressive behavior. Both are released by the adrenal cortex. In males, the testes produce testosterone. In females, the ovaries produce estrogen. **Epinephrine** and **norepinephrine** are released by the adrenal medulla and cause physiological changes associated with the sympathetic nervous system.

Nature *vs.* nurture is a classic debate regarding the relative contributions of genetics (nature) and environment (nurture) to an individual's traits. For most traits, both nature and nurture play a role. **Family studies** look at the relative frequency of a trait within a family compared to the general population. **Twin studies** compare concordance rates between monozygotic (identical) and dizygotic (fraternal) twins. **Adoption studies** compare similarities between adopted children and their adoptive parents, relative to similarities with their biological parents.

Development

The nervous system develops through neurulation, in which the notochord stimulates overlying ectoderm to fold over, creating a **neural tube** topped with **neural crest** cells. The **neural tube** becomes the central nervous system (CNS). The **neural crest** cells spread out throughout the body, differentiating into many different tissues.

Primitive reflexes (see Table 8.3) exist in infants and should disappear with age. Most primitive reflexes serve (or served, in earlier times) a protective role. They can reappear in certain nervous system disorders.

Reflex	Behavior
Rooting reflex	Infant turns his or her head toward anything that brushes the cheek
Moro reflex	The infant extends the arms and then slowly retracts them and cries in response to a sensation of falling
Babinski reflex	The big toe is extended and the other toes fan in response to the brushing of the sole of the foot
Grasping reflex	The infant grabs anything put into his or her hand

Table 8.3. Primitive Reflexes

Developmental milestones give an indication of what skills and abilities a child should have at a given age. Most children adhere closely to these milestones, deviating by only one or two months. For example, gross and fine motor abilities progress head to toe and core to periphery, social skills shift from parent-oriented to self-oriented to other-oriented, and language skills become increasingly complex.

SENSATION AND PERCEPTION

Sensation is the conversion, or transduction, of physical, electromagnetic, auditory, and other information from the internal and external environment into electrical signals in the nervous system. **Perception** is the processing of sensory information to make sense of its significance.

Sensory receptors are nerves that respond to stimuli and trigger electrical signals. Sensory neurons are associated with **sensory ganglia**: collections of cell bodies outside the central nervous system. Sensory stimuli are transmitted to **projection areas** in the brain, which further analyze the sensory input. Common sensory receptors include photoreceptors, hair cells, nociceptors, thermoreceptors, osmoreceptors, olfactory receptors, and taste receptors.

A **threshold** is the minimum stimulus that causes a change in signal transduction. The **absolute threshold** is the minimum of stimulus energy that is needed to activate a sensory system. The **threshold of conscious perception** is the minimum of stimulus energy that creates a signal large enough in size and long enough in duration to be brought into awareness. The **difference threshold** or **just-noticeable difference** (**jnd**) is the minimum difference in magnitude between two stimuli before one can perceive this difference. **Weber's law** states that the jnd for a stimulus is proportional to the magnitude of the stimulus and that this proportion is constant over most of the range of possible stimuli.

Signal detection theory refers to the effects of nonsensory factors, such as experiences, motives, and expectations, on perception of stimuli. Signal detection experiments allow us to look at **response bias**. In a signal detection experiment, a stimulus may or may not be given, and the subject is asked to state whether or not the stimulus was given. There are four possible outcomes: hits, misses, false alarms, or correct negatives. **Adaptation** refers to a decrease in response to a stimulus over time.

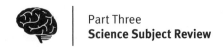
Vision

The eye is an organ specialized to detect light in the form of photons. The **cornea** gathers and filters incoming light. The **iris** contains two muscles that open and close the pupil, in addition to dividing the front of the eye into the **anterior** and **posterior chambers**. The **lens** refracts incoming light to focus it onto the retina and is held in place by **suspensory ligaments** connected to the **ciliary muscle**. The ciliary body produces **aqueous humor**, which drains through the **canal of Schlemm**. The retina contains rods and cones. **Rods** detect light and dark; **cones** come in three forms (short-, medium-, and long-wavelength) to detect colors. The retina contains mostly cones in the **macula**, which corresponds to the central visual field. The center of the macula is the **fovea**, which contains only cones. Rods and cones synapse on **bipolar cells**, which synapse on **ganglion cells**. Integration of the signals from ganglion cells and edge sharpening is performed by **horizontal** and **amacrine cells**. The bulk of the eye is supported by the **vitreous** on the inside and the **sclera** and **choroid** on the outside.

The visual pathway starts from the eye and travels through the **optic nerves, optic chiasm, optic tracts, lateral geniculate nucleus (LGN)** of the thalamus, and **visual radiations** to the **visual cortex**. The optic chiasm contains fibers crossing from the nasal side of the retina (temporal visual fields) of both eyes. The visual radiations run through the temporal and parietal lobes. The visual cortex is in the occipital lobe.

Vision, like all senses, is processed through **parallel processing**: the ability to analyze and combine information simultaneously regarding color, shape, and motion. Shape is detected by **parvocellular cells**, with high spatial resolution and low temporal resolution. Motion is detected by **magnocellular cells**, with low spatial resolution and high temporal resolution.

Other Senses

The ear is divided into the outer, middle, and inner ear. The **outer ear** consists of the **pinna (auricle), external auditory canal**, and **tympanic membrane**. The **middle ear** consists of the **ossicles: malleus** (hammer), **incus** (anvil), and **stapes** (stirrup). The footplate of the stapes rests on the **oval window** of the cochlea. The middle ear is connected to the nasal cavity by the **Eustachian tube**. The **inner ear** contains the **bony labyrinth**, within which is the **membranous labyrinth**. The bony labyrinth is filled with **perilymph**; the membranous labyrinth is filled with **endolymph**. The membranous labyrinth consists of the **cochlea**, which detects sound; **utricle** and **saccule**, which detect linear acceleration; and **semicircular canals**, which detect rotational acceleration.

The auditory pathway goes from the cochlea and through the **vestibulocochlear nerve** and **medial geniculate nucleus (MGN)** of the thalamus to get to the **auditory cortex** in the temporal lobe. Sound information also projects to the **superior olive**, which localizes the sound, and the **inferior colliculus**.

Smell is the detection of volatile or aerosolized chemicals by the **olfactory chemoreceptors (olfactory nerves)** in the olfactory epithelium. The olfactory pathway starts from the olfactory nerves and travels through the **olfactory bulb** and **olfactory tract** to get to higher-order brain areas, such as the limbic system. Taste is the detection of dissolved compounds by **taste buds** in **papillae**. It comes in five modalities: sweet, sour, salty, bitter, and umami (savory).

Somatosensation refers to the four touch modalities: pressure, vibration, pain, and temperature. A **two-point threshold** is the minimum distance necessary between two points of stimulation on the skin such that the points are felt as two distinct stimuli. **Nociceptors** are responsible for pain perception. The **gate theory of pain** states that pain sensation is reduced when other somatosensory signals are present. **Kinesthetic sense (proprioception)** refers to the ability to tell where one's body is in three-dimensional space.

Object Recognition

`High-Yield`

Bottom-up (**data-driven**) **processing** refers to the recognition of objects by parallel processing and feature detection. It is slower but less prone to mistakes. **Top-down** (**conceptually driven**) **processing** refers to recognition of an object by memories and expectations, with little attention to detail. It is faster but more prone to mistakes.

Perceptual organization refers to our synthesis of stimuli to make sense of the world, including integration of depth, form, motion, and constancy. **Gestalt principles** are ways that the brain can infer missing parts of a picture when a picture is incomplete.

- **Law of proximity:** elements close to one another tend to be perceived as a unit
- **Law of similarity:** objects that are similar appear to be grouped together
- **Law of good continuation:** elements following the same path tend to be grouped together
- **Subjective contours:** perception of nonexistent edges in figures based on surrounding visual cues
- **Law of closure:** a space is enclosed by a group of lines is perceived as a complete or closed line
- **Law of prägnanz:** perceptual organization is as regular, simple, and symmetric as possible

LEARNING AND MEMORY

Learning

`High-Yield`

Habituation is the process of becoming used to a stimulus. **Dishabituation** can occur when a second stimulus intervenes, causing a resensitization to the original stimulus. **Associative learning** is a way of pairing together stimuli and responses, or behaviors and consequences. **Observational learning**, or **modeling**, is the acquisition of behavior by watching others.

In **classical conditioning**, an unconditioned stimulus that produces an instinctive, unconditioned response is paired with a neutral stimulus. With repetition, the neutral stimulus becomes a conditioned stimulus that produces a conditioned response.

In **operant conditioning**, behavior is changed through the use of consequences. **Reinforcement** increases the likelihood of a behavior, while **punishment** decreases the likelihood of a behavior. The schedule of reinforcement affects the rate at which the behavior is performed. Schedules can be based either on a ratio of behavior to reward or on an amount of time. Schedules can also be either fixed or variable. Behaviors learned through variable-ratio schedules are the hardest to extinguish.

Memory

Encoding is the process of putting new information into memory. It can be **automatic** or **effortful**. Semantic encoding is stronger than both acoustic and visual encoding. (See Figure 8.2.)

- **Sensory** and **short-term memory** are transient and are based on neurotransmitter activity.
- **Working memory** requires short-term memory, attention, and executive function to manipulate information.
- **Long-term memory** requires elaborative rehearsal and is the result of increased neuronal connectivity and comes in two forms. **Explicit** (**declarative**) **memory** stores facts and stories, while **implicit** (**nondeclarative**) **memory** stores skills and conditioning effects.

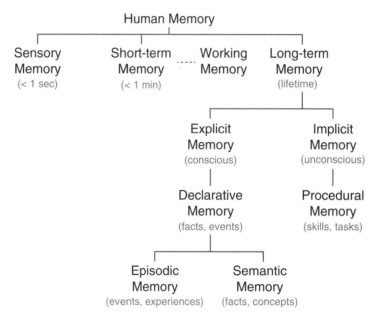

Figure 8.2. Types of Memory

Of note, **recognition** of information is stronger than **recall**, and **retrieval** of information is often based on **priming** interconnected nodes of the semantic network. Memories are also highly subject to influence by outside information and mood at the time of both encoding and recall.

COGNITION, CONSCIOUSNESS, AND LANGUAGE

Cognition

Both learning and memory rely on changes in brain chemistry and physiology, the extent of which depends on **neuroplasticity**, which decreases as we age. **Long-term potentiation**, responsible for the conversion of short-term to long-term memory, is the strengthening of neuronal connections resulting from increased neurotransmitter release and the adding of receptor sites.

The ability to think abstractly develops over the life span. Early cognitive development is limited by brain maturation. Culture, genes, and environment also influence cognitive development. Piaget describes four stages of cognitive development.

- The **sensorimotor stage** focuses on manipulating the environment to meet physical needs through **circular reactions**. **Object permanence** ends this stage.
- The **preoperational stage** focuses on **symbolic thinking**, **egocentrism**, and **centration**.
- The **concrete operational stage** focuses on understanding the feelings of others and manipulating physical (concrete) objects.
- The **formal operational stage** focuses on abstract thought and problem solving.

A mild level of cognitive decline while aging is normal; significant changes in cognition may signify an underlying disorder. Biological factors that affect cognition include organic brain disorders, genetic and chromosomal conditions, metabolic derangements, and drug use.

Problem solving requires identification and understanding of the problem, generation and testing of potential solutions, and evaluation of results. A **mental set** is a pattern of approach for a given problem. An inappropriate mental set may negatively impact problem solving. **Functional fixedness** is the tendency to use objects only in the way they are normally utilized, which may create barriers to problem solving. Types of problem solving include **trial and error**, **algorithms**, **deductive reasoning** (deriving conclusions from general rules), and **inductive reasoning** (deriving generalizations from evidence).

Heuristics, biases, intuition, and emotions may assist decision making, but may also lead to erroneous or problematic decisions. **Heuristics** are shortcuts or rules of thumb used to make decisions. **Biases** exist when an experimenter or a decision maker is unable to evaluate information objectively. **Intuition** is a "gut feeling" regarding a particular decision. However, intuition can often be attributed to experience with similar situations. Emotional state often plays a role in decision making.

Gardner's theory of **multiple intelligences** proposes seven areas of intelligence: linguistic, musical, logical-mathematical, visual-spatial, bodily-kinesthetic, interpersonal, and intrapersonal. Variations in intellectual ability can be attributed to combinations of environment, education, and genetics.

Consciousness

`High-Yield`

States of consciousness include alertness, sleep, dreaming, and altered states of consciousness. **Alertness** is the state of being awake and able to think, perceive, process, and express information. **Beta** and **alpha waves** predominate on **electroencephalography** (**EEG**). **Sleep** is important for brain and body health.

Stage 1 is light sleep and is dominated by **theta waves** on EEG. **Stage 2** is slightly deeper and includes theta waves, **sleep spindles**, and **K complexes**. **Stages 3** and **4** are deep (**slow-wave**) sleep (**SWS**). **Delta waves** predominate on EEG. Most sleep-wake disorders occur during Stage 3 and 4 **non-rapid eye movement** (**NREM**) **sleep**. **Rapid eye movement** (**REM**) **sleep** is sometimes called **paradoxical sleep**: the mind appears close to awake on EEG, but the person is asleep. Eye movements and body paralysis occur in this stage as well as most dreaming.

The **sleep cycle** is approximately 90 minutes for adults; the normal cycle is Stage 1–2–3–4–3–2–REM or just 1–2–3–4–REM, although REM becomes more frequent toward the morning. Changes in light in the evening trigger the release of **melatonin** by the **pineal gland**, resulting in sleepiness. **Cortisol** levels increase in the early morning and help promote wakefulness. **Circadian rhythms** trend around a 24-hour day.

Sleep-wake disorders include **dyssomnias**, such as insomnia, narcolepsy, sleep apnea, and sleep deprivation; and **parasomnias**, such as night terrors and sleepwalking (somnambulism).

Consciousness-altering drugs are grouped by effect into depressants, stimulants, opiates, and hallucinogens (see Table 8.4). Drug addiction is mediated by the **mesolimbic pathway**, which includes the **nucleus accumbens**, **medial forebrain bundle**, and **ventral tegmental area**. Dopamine is the main neurotransmitter in this pathway.

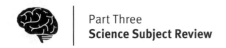
Drug	Effect	Example
Depressants	Promote or mimic GABA activity	Alcohol, barbiturates, benzodiazepines
Stimulants	Increase dopamine norepinephrine and serotonin concentration at synaptic cleft	Amphetamines, cocaine, ecstasy
Opiates	Death by respiratory depression	Heroin, morphine, opium
Hallucinogens	Distortion of reality, sympathetic response	LSD, mushrooms, mescaline

Table 8.4. Effects and Examples of Consciousness-Altering Drugs

Selective attention allows one to pay attention to a particular stimulus while determining if additional stimuli in the background require attention. **Divided attention** uses **automatic processing** to pay attention to multiple activities at one time.

Language
High-Yield

Language consists of phonology, morphology, semantics, syntax, and pragmatics. **Phonology** refers to the actual sound of speech. **Morphology** refers to the building blocks of words, such as rules for pluralization (–s in English), past tense (–ed), and so forth. **Semantics** refers to the meaning of words. **Syntax** refers to the rules dictating word order. **Pragmatics** refers to the changes in language delivery depending on context.

Theories of language development focus on different reasons or motivations for language acquisition.

- The **nativist (biological) theory** explains language acquisition as being innate and controlled by the **language acquisition device (LAD)**.
- The **learning (behaviorist) theory** explains language acquisition as being controlled by operant conditioning and reinforced by parents and caregivers.
- The **social interactionist theory** explains language acquisition as a motivation to communicate and interact with others.

Speech areas in the brain are found in the dominant hemisphere, which is usually the left. The motor function of speech is controlled by **Broca's area**. Damage results in **Broca's aphasia**: nonfluent aphasia where generating each word requires great effort. Language comprehension is controlled by **Wernicke's area**. Damage results in **Wernicke's aphasia**: fluent, nonsensical aphasia with lack of comprehension. The **arcuate fasciculus** connects Wernicke's and Broca's areas. Damage results in **conduction aphasia**, marked by the inability to repeat words heard despite intact speech generation and comprehension.

MOTIVATION, EMOTION, AND STRESS

Motivation
High-Yield

Motivation is the purpose, or driving force, behind our actions. It can be **extrinsic**, based on external circumstances; or **intrinsic**, based on internal drive or perception. The primary factors that influence emotion are instincts, arousal, drives, and needs. **Instincts** are innate, fixed patterns of behavior in response to stimuli. In the **instinct theory** of motivation, people perform certain behaviors because of evolutionarily programmed instincts. In the **arousal theory**, people perform actions to maintain **arousal**, the state of being awake and reactive to stimuli, at an optimal level. The **Yerkes–Dodson law** shows that performance is optimal at a medium level of arousal.

Drives are internal states of tension that produce particular behaviors focused on goals. Primary drives are related to bodily processes. Secondary drives stem from learning and include accomplishments and emotions. Several additional theories of motivation are tested on the MCAT:

- **Drive reduction theory** states that motivation arises from the desire to eliminate drives, which create uncomfortable internal states.
- **Maslow's hierarchy of needs** prioritizes needs into five categories: physiological needs (highest priority), safety and security, love and belonging, self-esteem, and self-actualization (lowest priority).
- **Self-determination theory** emphasizes the role of three universal needs: autonomy, competence, and relatedness.
- **Incentive theory** explains motivation as the desire to pursue rewards and avoid punishments.
- **Expectancy–value theory** states that the amount of motivation for a task is based on the individual's expectation of success and the amount that success is valued.
- **Opponent-process theory** explains motivation for drug use: as drug use increases, the body counteracts the drug's effects, leading to tolerance and uncomfortable withdrawal symptoms.

Emotion

`High-Yield`

Emotion is a state of mind, or feeling, that is subjectively experienced based on circumstances, mood, and relationships. The three components of emotion are **cognitive** (subjective), **behavioral** (facial expressions and body language), and **physiological** (changes in the autonomic nervous system).

The **seven universal emotions** are happiness, sadness, contempt, surprise, fear, disgust, and anger. There are multiple theories of emotion, based on the interactions of the three components of emotion.

- In the **James–Lange theory**, nervous system arousal leads to a cognitive response in which the emotion is labeled.
- In the **Cannon–Bard theory**, the simultaneous arousal of the nervous system and cognitive response lead to action.
- In the **Schachter–Singer theory**, nervous system arousal and interpretation of context lead to a cognitive response.

The **limbic system** is the primary nervous system component involved in experiencing emotion. The **amygdala** is involved with attention, fear, and aggression; helps interpret facial expressions; and is part of the intrinsic memory system for emotional memory. The **septal nuclei** are involved with feelings of pleasure, pleasure-seeking behavior, and addiction. The **thalamus** is a sensory-processing station. The **hypothalamus** releases neurotransmitters that affect mood and arousal. The **hippocampus** creates long-term explicit (episodic) memories and communicates with other parts of the limbic system through an extension called the **fornix**. The **prefrontal cortex** is involved with planning, expressing personality, and making decisions.

Stress

`High-Yield`

The physiological and cognitive response to challenges or life changes is defined as **stress**. Stress appraisal has two stages. **Primary appraisal** is classifying a potential stressor as irrelevant, benign-positive, or stressful. **Secondary appraisal** is directed at evaluating if the organism can cope with the stress, based on harm, threat, and challenge.

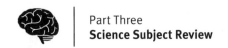

A **stressor** is anything that leads to a stress response and can include environment, daily events, workplace or academic settings, social expectations, chemicals, and biological stressors. Psychological stressors include pressure, control, predictability, frustration, and conflict. Stressors can lead to **distress** or **eustress**. The three stages of the **general adaptation syndrome** are alarm, resistance, and exhaustion. Stress management can include psychological, behavioral, and spiritual aspects.

IDENTITY AND PERSONALITY

Self-Concept and Identity
High-Yield

Self-concept is the sum of the ways in which we describe ourselves: in the present, who we used to be, and who we might be in the future. Our **identities** are individual components of our self-concept related to the groups to which we belong. Religious affiliation, sexual orientation, and ethnic and national affiliations are examples of identities. Our self-concept depends in part on our **reference group**, or the group to which we compare ourselves. Two individuals with the same qualities might see themselves differently depending on how those qualities compare to their reference groups.

Self-esteem describes evaluation of ourselves. Generally, the closer our **actual self** is to our **ideal self** (who we want to be) and our **ought self** (who others want us to be), the higher our self-esteem will be. **Self-efficacy** is the degree to which we see ourselves as being capable of a skill or in a given situation.

When placed into a consistently hopeless scenario, self-efficacy can be diminished to the point where **learned helplessness** results. **Locus of control** is a self-evaluation that refers to the way we characterize the influences in our lives. People with an internal locus of control see their successes and failures as a result of their own characteristics and actions. In contrast, those with an external locus of control perceive outside factors as having more of an influence in their lives.

Formation of Identity
High-Yield

Freud's psychosexual stages of personality development are based on the tensions caused by the **libido**. Failure at any given stage leads to **fixation** that causes personality disorders. Freud's phases (oral, anal, phallic, latent, and genital) are based on erogenous zones that are the focus of each phase of development.

Erikson's stages of psychosocial development stem from conflicts that occur throughout life (trust *vs.* mistrust, autonomy *vs.* shame and doubt, initiative *vs.* guilt, industry *vs.* inferiority, identity *vs.* role confusion, intimacy *vs.* isolation, generativity *vs.* stagnation, integrity *vs.* despair). These conflicts result from decisions we make about ourselves and the environment around us at each phase of our lives.

Kohlberg's stages of moral development describe the approaches of individuals to resolving moral dilemmas. Kohlberg believed that we progress through six stages divided into three main phases: **preconventional**, **conventional**, and **postconventional**.

Imitation and **role taking** are common ways children learn from others. Children first reproduce the behaviors of role models. Then they learn to see the perspectives of others and practice taking on new roles.

Personality
High-Yield

The **psychoanalytic** perspective views personality as resulting from unconscious urges and desires. Freud's theories are based on the **id** (base urges of survival and reproduction), the **superego** (the idealist and perfectionist), and the **ego** (the mediator between the two and the conscious mind). Other psychoanalysts disagree with Freud's theories, claiming that the unconscious is motivated by social rather than sexual urges.

The **humanistic** perspective emphasizes the internal feelings of healthy individuals as they strive toward happiness and self-realization. Maslow's **hierarchy of needs** and Rogers's therapeutic approach of **unconditional positive regard** flow from the humanistic view of personality.

Type and **trait** theorists believe that personality can be described as a number of identifiable traits that carry characteristic behaviors. Type theories of personality include the ancient Greek notion of humors, Sheldon's **somatotypes**, division into **Types A** and **B**, and the **Myers-Briggs Type Inventory**.

The Eysencks identified three major traits that could be used to describe all individuals. The acronym for these traits is PEN: **psychoticism** (nonconformity), **extraversion** (tolerance for social interaction and stimulation), and **neuroticism** (arousal in stressful situations). Later trait theorists expanded these traits to the **Big Five**: openness, conscientiousness, extraversion, agreeableness, and neuroticism.

Allport identified three basic types of traits: cardinal, central, and secondary. **Cardinal traits** are the traits around which a person organizes his or her life; not everyone develops a cardinal trait. **Central traits** represent major characteristics of the personality, while **secondary traits** are more personal characteristics and are limited in occurrence.

The **social cognitive** perspective holds that individuals interact with their environment in a cycle called **reciprocal determinism**: people mold their environments according to their personalities, and those environments in turn shape our thoughts, feelings, and behaviors. The **behaviorist** perspective, based on the concept of operant conditioning, holds that personality can be described as the behaviors one has learned from prior rewards and punishments. **Biological** theorists claim that behavior can be explained as a result of genetic expression.

PSYCHOLOGICAL DISORDERS

High-Yield

The **biomedical approach** to psychological disorders takes into account only the physical and medical causes of a psychological disorder. Thus, treatments in this approach are of a biomedical nature. The **biopsychosocial approach** considers the relative contributions of biological, psychological, and social components to an individual's disorder. Treatments also fall into these three areas. The *Diagnostic and Statistical Manual of Mental Disorders* is used to diagnose psychological disorders. Its current version is the DSM-5 (published May 2013). It categorizes mental disorders based on symptom patterns. Psychological disorders, especially anxiety, depressive, and substance use disorders, are very common.

Schizophrenia is the prototypical psychotic disorder, characterized by both positive and negative symptoms. **Positive symptoms** add something to behavior, cognition, or affect and include delusions, hallucinations, disorganized speech, and disorganized behavior. **Negative symptoms** are the loss of something from behavior, cognition, or affect and include disturbance of affect and avolition. Schizophrenia may be associated with genetic factors, birth trauma, and family history. There are high levels of dopaminergic transmission.

Depressive disorders include major depressive disorder and seasonal affective disorder.

- **Major depressive disorder** contains at least one major depressive episode.
- **Persistent depressive disorder** is **dysthymia** for at least two years that does not meet the criteria for major depressive disorder.
- **Seasonal affective disorder** is the colloquial name for major depressive disorder with seasonal onset, with depression occurring during winter months.

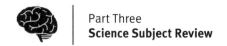

Depression is accompanied by high levels of glucocorticoids and low levels of norepinephrine, serotonin, and dopamine.

Bipolar and related disorders have manic or hypomanic episodes. **Bipolar I disorder** contains at least one manic episode. **Bipolar II disorder** contains at least one hypomanic episode and at least one major depressive episode. **Cyclothymic disorder** contains hypomanic episodes with dysthymia. Bipolar disorders are accompanied by high levels of norepinephrine and serotonin. They are also highly heritable.

Anxiety disorders include generalized anxiety disorder, specific phobias, social anxiety disorder, agoraphobia, and panic disorder.

- **Generalized anxiety disorder** is a disproportionate and persistent worry about many different things for at least six months.
- **Specific phobias** are irrational fears of specific objects or situations.
- **Social anxiety disorder** is anxiety due to social or performance situations.
- **Panic disorder** is marked by recurrent panic attacks: intense, overwhelming fear and sympathetic nervous system activity with no clear stimulus. It may lead to agoraphobia.

Obsessive-compulsive disorder is characterized by **obsessions** (persistent, intrusive thoughts and impulses) and **compulsions** (repetitive tasks that relieve tension but cause significant impairment in a person's life).

Body dysmorphic disorder is characterized by an unrealistic negative evaluation of one's appearance or a specific body part. The individual often takes extreme measures to correct the perceived imperfection.

Post-traumatic stress disorder (**PTSD**) is characterized by intrusion symptoms (reliving the event, flashbacks, nightmares), avoidance symptoms (avoidance of people, places, objects associated with trauma), negative cognitive symptoms (amnesia, negative mood and emotions), and arousal symptoms (increased startle response, irritability, anxiety).

Dissociative disorders include dissociative amnesia, dissociative identity disorder, and depersonalization/derealization disorder.

- **Dissociative amnesia** is an inability to recall past experience without an underlying neurological disorder. In severe forms, it may involve **dissociative fugue**, a sudden change in location that may involve the assumption of a new identity.
- **Dissociative identity disorder** is the occurrence of two or more personalities that take control of a person's behavior.
- **Depersonalization/derealization disorder** involves feelings of detachment from the mind and body or from the environment.

Somatic symptom and related disorders involve significant bodily symptoms.

- **Somatic symptom disorder** involves at least one somatic symptom, which may or may not be linked to an underlying medical condition, that causes disproportionate concern.
- **Illness anxiety disorder** is a preoccupation with thoughts about having, or coming down with, a serious medical condition.
- **Conversion disorder** involves unexplained symptoms affecting motor or sensory function and is associated with prior trauma.

Personality disorders (**PD**) are patterns of inflexible, maladaptive behaviors that cause distress or impaired functioning in at least two of the following: cognition, emotions, interpersonal functioning, or impulse control. They occur in three **clusters**: **A** (odd, eccentric), **B** (dramatic, emotional, erratic), and **C** (anxious, fearful), as shown in Table 8.5.

Cluster A	**Paranoid PD**	Pervasive distrust and suspicion of others
	Schizotypal PD	Ideas of reference, magical thinking, and eccentricity
	Schizoid PD	Detachment from social relationships and limited emotion
Cluster B	**Antisocial PD**	Disregard for the rights of others
	Borderline PD	Instability in relationships, mood, and self-image; **splitting** is characteristic, as are recurrent suicide attempts
	Histrionic PD	Constant attention-seeking behavior
	Narcissistic PD	Grandiose sense of self-importance, need for admiration
Cluster C	**Avoidant PD**	Extreme shyness and fear of rejection
	Dependent PD	Continuous need for reassurance
	Obsessive–compulsive PD	Perfectionism, inflexibility, preoccupation with rules

Table 8.5. Personality Disorders (PD) Based on Cluster

Alzheimer's disease is associated with genetic factors, brain atrophy, decreases in acetylcholine, senile plaques of β-amyloid, and **neurofibrillary tangles** of hyperphosphorylated tau protein. **Parkinson's disease** is associated with **bradykinesia**, **resting tremor**, **pill-rolling tremor**, **masklike facies**, **cogwheel rigidity**, and a **shuffling gait**. There is decreased dopamine production by cells in the **substantia nigra**.

SOCIAL PROCESSES, ATTITUDES, AND BEHAVIOR

Group Psychology

High-Yield

Social facilitation describes the tendency of people to perform at a different level based on the fact that others are around. **Deindividuation** is a loss of self-awareness in large groups, which can lead to drastic changes in behavior. The **bystander effect** describes the observation that when in a group, individuals are less likely to respond to a person in need. **Peer pressure** refers to the social influence placed onto individuals by others they consider equals.

Group decision making may differ from individual decision making. Group **polarization** is the tendency toward making decisions in a group that are more extreme than the thoughts of the individual group members. **Groupthink** is the tendency for groups to make decisions based on ideas and solutions that arise within the group without considering outside ideas. Ethics may be disturbed as pressure is created to conform and remain loyal to the group.

Culture describes the beliefs, ideas, behaviors, actions, and characteristics of a group or society of people. **Assimilation** is the process by which a group or an individual's culture begins to melt into another culture. **Multiculturalism** refers to the encouragement of multiple cultures within a community to enhance diversity. **Subcultures** refer to a group of people within a culture who distinguish themselves from the primary culture to which they belong.

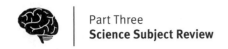

Socialization, Attitudes, and Behavior

High-Yield

Socialization is the process of developing and spreading norms, customs, and beliefs. **Norms** are what determine the boundaries of acceptable behavior within society. Agents of socialization include family, peers, school, religious affiliation, and other groups that promote socialization.

Stigma is the extreme disapproval or dislike of a person or group based on perceived differences from the rest of society. **Deviance** refers to any violation of norms, rules, or expectations within a society. **Conformity** is changing beliefs or behaviors in order to fit into a group or society. **Compliance** occurs when individuals change their behavior based on the requests of others. Methods of gaining compliance include the foot-in-the-door technique, door-in-the-face technique, lowball technique, and that's-not-all technique, among others. **Obedience** is a change in behavior based on a command from someone seen as an authority figure.

Attitudes are tendencies toward expressions of positive or negative feelings or toward evaluations of something. Attitudes have affective, behavioral, and cognitive components. The **functional attitudes theory** states that four functional areas of attitudes serve individuals in life: knowledge, ego expression, adaptability, and ego defense. The **learning theory** states that attitudes are developed through forms of learning: direct contact, direct interaction, direct instruction, and conditioning. The **elaboration likelihood model** states that attitudes are formed and changed through different routes of information processing based on the degree of elaboration (**central route processing**, **peripheral route processing**). The **social cognitive theory** states that attitudes are formed through observation of behavior, personal factors, and environment.

SOCIAL INTERACTION

Elements of Social Interactions

High-Yield

A **status** is a position in society used to classify individuals.

- An **ascribed status** is involuntarily assigned to an individual based on race, ethnicity, gender, family background, and so on.
- An **achieved status** is voluntarily earned by an individual.
- A **master status** is that by which an individual is primarily identified.

A **role** is a set of beliefs, values, and norms that define the expectations of a certain status in a social situation.

- **Role performance** refers to carrying out the behaviors of a given role.
- A **role partner** is another individual who helps define a specific role within the relationship.
- A **role set** contains all of the different roles associated with a status.
- **Role conflict** occurs when one has difficulty in satisfying the requirements of multiple roles simultaneously.
- **Role strain** occurs when one has difficulty satisfying multiple requirements of the same role simultaneously.

Groups are made up of two or more individuals with similar characteristics that share a sense of unity.

- A **peer group** is a self-selected group formed around similar interests, ages, and statuses.
- A **family group** is the group into which an individual is born, adopted, or married.
- An **in-group** is one with which an individual identifies.
- An **out-group** is a group with which an individual does not identify.
- A **reference group** is a group to which an individual compares himself or herself.

Primary groups are those that contain strong, emotional bonds. **Secondary groups** are often temporary. They contain fewer emotional bonds and weaker bonds overall.

Gemeinschaft (**community**) is a group unified by feelings of togetherness due to shared beliefs, ancestry, or geography. *Gesellschaft* (**society**) is a group unified by mutual self-interests in achieving a goal. **Groupthink** occurs when members begin to conform to one another's views and ignore outside perspectives. A **network** is an observable pattern of social relationships among individuals or groups. **Organizations** are bodies of people with a structure and culture designed to achieve specific goals. They exist outside of each individual's membership within the organization.

Self-Presentation

Various models have been proposed for how we express emotion in social situations. The **basic model** states that there are universal emotions along with corresponding expressions that can be understood across cultures. The **social construction model** states that emotions are solely based on the situational context of social interactions. **Display rules** are unspoken rules that govern the expression of emotion. A **cultural syndrome** is a shared set of beliefs, norms, values, and behaviors organized around a central theme, as is found among people sharing the same language and geography.

Impression management refers to the maintenance of a public image, which is accomplished through various strategies. **Self-disclosure** is sharing factual information. **Managing appearances** refers to using props, appearance, emotional expression, or associations to create a positive image. **Ingratiation** is using flattery or conformity to win over someone else. **Aligning actions** is the use of excuses to account for questionable behavior. **Alter-casting** is imposing an identity onto another person.

The **dramaturgical approach** says that individuals create images of themselves in the same way that actors perform a role in front of an audience. The **front stage** is where the individual is seen by the audience and strives to preserve his/her desired image. The **back stage** is where the individual is not in front of an audience and is free to act outside of his/her desired image.

Communication includes both verbal and nonverbal elements. **Verbal communication** is the conveyance of information through spoken, written, or signed words. **Nonverbal communication** is the conveyance of information by means other than the use of words, such as body language, prosody, facial expressions, and gestures. **Animal communication** takes place not only between nonhuman animals but between humans and other animals as well. Animals use body language, rudimentary facial expressions, visual displays, scents, and vocalizations to communicate.

SOCIAL THINKING

Interpersonal attraction is what makes people like each other. It is influenced by multiple factors: physical attractiveness, which is increased with symmetry and proportions close to the **golden ratio**; similarity of attitudes, intelligence, education, height, age, religion, appearance, and socioeconomic status; **self-disclosure**, which includes sharing fears, thoughts, and goals with another person and being met with empathy and nonjudgment; **reciprocity**, in which we like people who we think like us; and **proximity**, or being physically close to someone.

Attachment is an emotional bond to another person and usually refers to the bond between a child and a caregiver. There are four types of attachment.

- **Secure attachment** requires a consistent caregiver; the child shows strong preference for the caregiver.
- **Avoidant attachment** occurs when a caregiver has little or no response to a distressed, crying child; the child shows no preference for the caregiver compared to strangers.
- **Ambivalent attachment** occurs when a caregiver has an inconsistent response to a child's distress, sometimes responding appropriately, sometimes neglectful; the child becomes distressed when the caregiver leaves and is ambivalent when he or she returns.
- **Disorganized attachment** occurs when a caregiver is erratic or abusive; the child shows no clear pattern of behavior in response to the caregiver's absence or presence.

Social support is the perception or reality that one is cared for by a social network. **Emotional support** includes listening to, affirming, and empathizing with someone's feelings. **Esteem support** affirms the qualities and skills of the person. **Material support** is providing physical or monetary resources to aid a person. **Informational support** is providing useful information to a person. **Network support** is providing a sense of belonging to a person.

A **mating system** describes the way in which a group is organized in terms of sexual behavior. **Monogamy** consists of exclusive mating relationships. **Polygamy** consists of one member of a sex having multiple exclusive relationships with members of the opposite sex. **Promiscuity** allows a member of one sex to mate with any member of the opposite sex without exclusivity. **Mate choice** is the selection of a mate based on attraction and traits.

Altruism is a form of helping behavior in which the person's intent is to benefit someone else at some personal cost. **Inclusive fitness** is a measure of an organism's success in the population. This is based on the number of offspring, the success in supporting offspring, and the ability of the offspring to support others.

Social perception or **social cognition** is the way by which we generate impressions about people in our social environment. It contains a **perceiver**, a **target**, and the **situation** or social context of the scenario.

Implicit personality theory states that people make assumptions about how different types of people, their traits, and their behavior are related. The **primacy effect** refers to when first impressions are more important than subsequent impressions. In contrast, the **recency effect** is when the most recent information we have about an individual is most important in forming our impressions.

A **reliance on central traits** is the tendency to organize the perception of others based on traits and personal characteristics that matter to the perceiver. The **halo effect** is when judgments of an individual's character can be affected by the overall impression of the individual. The **just-world hypothesis** is the tendency of individuals to believe that good things happen to good people and that bad things happen to bad people. **Self-serving bias** refers to the fact that individuals view their own successes as being based on internal factors while viewing failures as being based on external factors.

Attribution theory focuses on the tendency for individuals to infer the causes of other people's behavior. **Dispositional (internal)** causes are those that relate to the features of the person whose behavior is being considered. **Situational (external)** causes are related to features of the surroundings or social context. **Fundamental attribution error** is the bias toward making dispositional attributions rather than situational attributions in regard to the actions of others. **Attribute substitution** occurs when individuals must make judgments that are complex but, instead, substitute a simpler solution or heuristic. Attributions are highly influenced by the culture in which one resides.

Stereotypes occur when attitudes and impressions are made based on limited and superficial information about a person or a group of individuals. Stereotypes can lead to expectations, which can create conditions that lead to confirmation of the stereotype, a process referred to as **self-fulfilling prophecy. Stereotype threat** is concern or anxiety about confirming a negative stereotype about one's social group.

Prejudice is defined as an irrational positive or negative attitude toward a person, group, or thing prior to an actual experience. **Ethnocentrism** refers to the practice of making judgments about other cultures based on the values and beliefs of one's own culture. **Cultural relativism** refers to the recognition that social groups and cultures should be studied on their own terms.

Discrimination is when prejudicial attitudes cause individuals of a particular group to be treated differently from others. **Individual discrimination** refers to one person discriminating against a particular person or group. **Institutional discrimination** refers to the discrimination against a particular person or group by an entire institution.

SOCIAL STRUCTURE AND DEMOGRAPHICS

High-Yield

Theoretical approaches provide frameworks for the interactions we observe within society. **Functionalism** focuses on the function of each component of society and how those components fit together. **Manifest functions** are deliberate actions that serve to help a given system. In contrast, **latent functions** are unexpected, unintended, or unrecognized positive consequences of manifest functions.

Conflict theory focuses on how power differentials are created and how these differentials contribute to the maintenance of social order. **Symbolic interactionism** is the study of the ways individuals interact through a shared understanding of words, gestures, and other symbols. **Social constructionism** explores the ways in which individuals and groups make decisions to agree upon a given social reality. **Rational choice theory** states that individuals make decisions that maximize potential benefit and minimize potential harm; **exchange theory** applies rational choice theory within social groups.

Social institutions are well-established social structures that dictate certain patterns of behavior or relationships and are accepted as a fundamental part of culture. Common social institutions include the family, education, religion, government and the economy, and health and medicine.

There are four key ethical tenets of American medicine.

- **Beneficence** refers to acting in the patient's best interest.
- **Nonmaleficence** refers to avoiding treatments for which the risk is larger than the benefit.
- **Respect for autonomy** refers to respecting patients' rights to make decisions about their own health care.
- **Justice** refers to treating similar patients similarly and distributing health care resources fairly.

Culture encompasses the lifestyle of a group of people and includes both material and symbolic elements. **Material culture** includes the physical items one associates with a given group, such as artwork, emblems, clothing, jewelry, foods, buildings, and tools. **Symbolic culture** includes the ideas associated with a cultural group. There is evidence that culture flows from evolutionary principles and that culture can also influence evolution.

Cultural lag is the idea that material culture changes more quickly than symbolic culture. A **cultural barrier** is a social difference that impedes interaction. A **value** is what a person deems important in life, while a **belief** is something a person considers to be true.

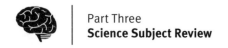
A **ritual** is a formalized ceremonial behavior in which members of a group or community regularly engage. It is governed by specific rules, including appropriate behavior and a predetermined order of events. **Norms** are societal rules that define the boundaries of acceptable behavior.

Demographics refer to the statistics of populations and are the mathematical applications of sociology. One can analyze hundreds of demographic variables; some of the most common are age, gender, race and ethnicity, sexual orientation, and immigration status.

Ageism is prejudice or discrimination on the basis of a person's age. **Gender** is the set of behavioral, cultural, or psychological traits typically associated with a biological sex. **Gender inequality** is the intentional or unintentional empowerment of one gender to the detriment of the other. **Race** is a social construct based on phenotypic differences among groups of people; these may be either real or perceived differences. **Ethnicity** is also a social construct that sorts people by cultural factors, including language, nationality, religion, and other factors. **Symbolic ethnicity** is recognition of an ethnic identity that is relevant only on special occasions or in specific circumstances and does not specifically impact everyday life. **Sexual orientation** can be defined by one's sexual interest toward members of the same, opposite, or both sexes.

A **fertility rate** is the average number of children born to a woman during her lifetime in a population. A **birthrate** is relative to a population size over time, usually measured as the number of births per 1,000 people per year. A **mortality rate** is the average number of deaths per population size over time, usually measured as the number of deaths per 1,000 people per year. **Demographic transition**, as shown in Figure 8.3, is a model used to represent drops in birthrates and death rates as a result of industrialization.

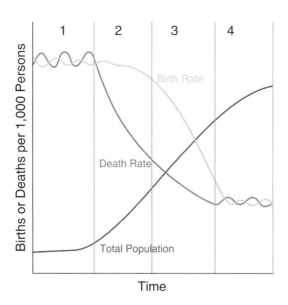

Figure 8.3. Demographic Transition

Social movements are organized either to promote (**proactive**) or to resist (**reactive**) change. **Globalization** is the process of integrating a global economy with free trade and tapping of foreign labor markets. **Urbanization** refers to the process of dense areas of population creating a pull for migration, in other words, creating cities.

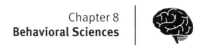

SOCIAL STRATIFICATION

Social stratification is based on **socioeconomic status** (**SES**), which depends on ascribed status and achieved status. **Ascribed status** is involuntary and derives from clearly identifiable characteristics, such as age, gender, and skin color. In contrast, **achieved status** is acquired through direct, individual efforts. A **social class** is a category of people with shared socioeconomic characteristics. The three main social classes are upper, middle, and lower classes. Members of each of these groups have similar lifestyles, job opportunities, attitudes, and behaviors.

Prestige is the respect and importance tied to specific occupations or associations, while **power** is the capacity to influence people through real or perceived rewards and punishments. Power often depends on the unequal distribution of valued resources. Power differentials create social inequality. *Anomie* is a state of normlessness. Anomic conditions erode social solidarity by means of excessive individualism, social inequality, and isolation.

Social capital is the investment people make in their society in return for economic or collective rewards. Social networks, either situational or positional, are one of the most powerful forms of social capital and can be achieved through establishing strong and weak social ties. **Meritocracy** refers to a society in which advancement up the social ladder is based on intellectual talent and achievement. **Social mobility** allows one to acquire higher-level employment opportunities by achieving required credentials and experience. Social mobility can occur in either a positive upward direction or a negative downward direction depending on whether one is promoted or demoted in status.

Poverty is a socioeconomic condition. In the United States, the poverty line is determined by the government's calculation of the minimum income requirements for families to acquire the minimum necessities of life. **Social reproduction** refers to the passing on of social inequality, especially poverty, from one generation to the next. There are two forms of poverty. **Absolute poverty** is when people do not have enough resources to acquire basic life necessities, such as shelter, food, clothing, and water. **Relative poverty** is when one is poor in comparison to a larger population. **Social exclusion** is a sense of powerlessness due to alienation from society.

Spatial inequality is a form of social stratification across territories and their populations. It can occur along residential, environmental, and global lines. Urban areas tend to have more diverse economic opportunities and more ability for social mobility than rural areas. Urban areas also tend to have more low-income racial and ethnic minority neighborhoods than rural areas. Formation of higher-income suburbs is a common occurrence and is due in part to the limited mobility of lower-income groups in urban centers. **Environmental injustice** refers to an uneven distribution of environmental hazards in communities. Lower-income neighborhoods may lack the social and political power to prevent the placement of environmental hazards in their neighborhoods. **Globalization** has led to further inequalities in space, food and water, energy, housing, and education as the production of goods shifts to cheaper and cheaper labor markets. This has led to significant economic hardship in industrializing nations.

Incidence is calculated as the number of new cases of a disease per population at risk in a given period of time: for example, new cases per 1,000 at-risk people per year. **Prevalence** is calculated as the number of cases of a disease per population in a given period of time: for example, cases per 1,000 people per year. **Morbidity** is the burden or degree of illness associated with a given disease. **Mortality** refers to deaths caused by a given disease.

Health is dependent on geographic, social, and economic factors. The **second sickness** refers to an exacerbation of health outcomes caused by social injustice. Poverty is associated with worse health outcomes, including decreased life expectancy, higher rates of life-shortening diseases, higher rates of suicide and homicide, and higher infant mortality rates.

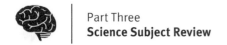
8.5 Behavioral Sciences Worked Examples

The following steps will walk you through the following passage using the Kaplan Passage Strategy.

PREVIEW FOR DIFFICULTY

Start by quickly glancing through the passage. Note the italicized words "dopamine hypothesis" in the first paragraph and additional general information in the second paragraph. The third paragraph has an abundance of acronyms and the fourth begins with "researchers conducted [a study]," which all lead to data in a figure. This passage appears to follow a pattern commonly seen on the MCAT: introduction to a concept, then new information, a hypothesis, and an experiment. Use your comfort with the content required and your prior experience with similar passages to guide your triaging decision.

CHOOSE YOUR APPROACH

Although this passage has three informational paragraphs, the presence of the experiment and accompanying data makes this an experimental passage. As such, **Interrogation** should be chosen. With this choice in mind, remember to read the informational paragraphs for context to help interpret the experimental results.

READ AND DISTILL

P1: We're introduced to the "classic" dopamine hypothesis and how D_2 receptors are associated with the positive symptoms of schizophrenia.

P2: We know the second paragraph will build off of the first because of the word "evolved." While reading, look for the new elements of the hypothesis. We're told that the D_2 receptor blockers mentioned in the first paragraph, which helped alleviate some positive symptoms, aren't working for the negative symptoms. The evolution is in the last sentence with the introduction of another receptor (D_1) and region of the brain (PFC).

P3: The third paragraph is where things get complicated. Notice all of the abbreviations! Because we're not sure that any questions are going to require detailed knowledge, it's best to be quick now and reread later if necessary. It's important to note that this paragraph is building a connection between the PFC and the subcortical regions (the connection being MC DA). It indicates that the VTA and VST are subcortical and that they are connected by ML DA. Further, we're told that there are glutamatergic neurons involved in the regulation of the ML/MC DA neurons.

P4: Notice the purpose of the experiment in the first sentence, signaled by the phrase "to investigate . . ." The study's purpose is to look more into the effect of glutamate on schizophrenia. Although the study uses ketamine, we're not told much about the intended effects of it. We'd expect to see a connection between NMDA and glutamate or dopamine or GABA, but nothing is given. We are told that dopamine is measured in the subcortical region.

F1: Interrogation of Figure 1 should focus on identifying the key trends in the data. Begin by identify the different sample groups as the independent variable (IV). All groups other than control were given ketamine. The dependent variable (DV) is dopamine concentration. There's a trend: healthy individuals have the lowest dopamine, and active schizophrenics have the highest. At this point, we should be thinking: ↑ ketamine, ↓ NMDA (because ketamine is an antagonist), ↑ dopamine (subcortical), ↑ positive symptoms of schizophrenia.

PASSAGE I: BIOLOGICAL BASIS OF BEHAVIOR

The classic *dopamine hypothesis* is the most well studied and longest standing of the schizophrenia hypotheses. The hypothesis is centered on the mesolimbic pathway of the brain—specifically, D_2 receptors located in the subcortical region of the brain. These receptors are strongly associated with the positive symptoms of schizophrenia (e.g., hallucinations and delusions). The treatment of schizophrenic patients with certain antipsychotic medications, which block D_2 receptors, alleviates some symptoms. Furthermore, dopamine-enhancing drugs have been shown to have psychotogenic effects, thus establishing the connection between dopamine and schizophrenia.

The classic dopamine hypothesis has evolved to explain the enduring symptoms (e.g., apathy and antisocial behavior) and cognitive symptoms (e.g., memory loss and attention deficits) of schizophrenia. These functional deficits were only marginally treatable with D_2 antagonists. Hypostimulation of D_1 receptors in the prefrontal cortex (PFC) has been implicated in the negative symptoms of schizophrenia.

Research also suggests an association between the PFC and the subcortical region of the brain, including the ventral tegmental area (VTA) and the ventral striatum (VST). Mesolimbic dopaminergic (ML DA) neurons and mesocortical dopaminergic (MC DA) neurons of the VTA project to the VST and PFC, respectively. Glutamatergic neurons from the PFC project to the VTA and upregulate the MC DA neurons. At the same time, other glutamatergic neurons indirectly downregulate ML DA neurons through an intermediate GABAergic neuron.

Researchers conducted an imaging study to investigate the influence of glutamate on schizophrenia. Ketamine, a potential *N*-methyl-*D*-aspartate (NMDA) antagonist, was administered to four groups of patients: active schizophrenics, schizophrenics in remission (no psychotic episode within six months), abusers of psychostimulants, and healthy subjects. Dopamine levels were measured in the subcortical region. The results of the study are illustrated in Figure 1.

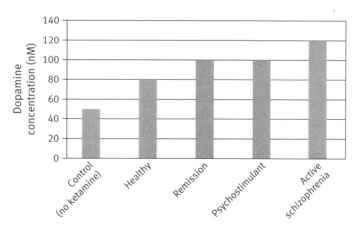

Figure 1. Dopamine measurements in various individuals treated with 0.5 mg ketamine per pound of body weight

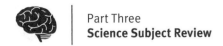

KEY CONCEPT

Mechanism of neurotransmitter function

1. Ecopipam, an antipsychotic drug, is administered to a healthy patient who, following treatment, begins hallucinating. Which of the following could correctly characterize the function of ecopipam?

   A. It increases the activity of MC DA neurons.
   B. It increases the activity of ML DA neurons.
   C. It acts as a D_2 receptor antagonist.
   D. It acts as an NMDA receptor agonist.

① Type the question

The question stem is long, describing a drug that wasn't mentioned in the passage, ecopipam. However, we see hallucination, which was mentioned, so it's likely that this question is passage based. Answer choices are short, mentioning neurons and agonists/antagonists, but have no clear pattern.

② Rephrase the question stem

The question asks you to consider the description of hallucination in the passage and link it to a possible mechanism with the new drug. When Rephrased, the question asks, *What is the mechanism of action of an antipsychotic on inducing hallucination according to the passage?*

③ Investigate potential solutions

The first paragraph implies that hyperstimulation of subcortical D_2 receptors is a possible cause of hallucinations. The correct answer will likely address this fact and should serve as your general prediction. Take a look at the answer choices, and eliminate those that are not aligned with the cause of hallucination.

④ Match your prediction to an answer choice

(A) discusses MC DA neurons. These neurons project to the PFC, which is largely filled with D_1 receptors, not D_2 receptors. Because only D_2 receptors are linked to the positive symptoms of schizophrenia, **(A)** is not correct.

(B) mentions ML DA neurons, which project to the VST (part of the subcortical region). Upregulation of these neurons would increase dopamine concentration in the subcortical region, increasing the likelihood of hallucinations. Therefore, **(B)** is likely the correct answer.

(C) may be tempting because it directly mentions D_2 receptors. However, it states that ecopipam is a D_2 receptor *antagonist*. Because antagonists decrease receptor activity, ecopipam would reduce hallucinations. So **(C)** is not the correct answer.

(D) states that ecopipam is an NMDA receptor agonist. According to Figure 1, ketamine, an NMDA antagonist, increases dopamine concentration in the subcortical region. Therefore, if ecopipam were an NMDA receptor agonist, it would decrease dopamine concentration in the subcortical region. A decrease in dopamine concentration would reduce the prevalence of hallucinations, so **(D)** also is incorrect.

2. Patients with the high-activity allele coding for the enzyme catechol-*O*-methyltransferase (COMT) exhibit negative symptoms of schizophrenia. Which of the following best explains this discovery?

   A. COMT converts *L*-dopamine to dopamine in the PFC.
   B. COMT converts plasma dopamine to dopamine sulfate.
   C. COMT oxidizes dopamine to dopamine-melanin.
   D. COMT deactivates dopamine through methylation.

❶ Type the question

No specific information is provided about the high-activity allele of COMT except that it causes the negative symptoms of schizophrenia. The answer choices all describe the possible functions of COMT.

❷ Rephrase the question stem

The question asks you to consider the description of negative symptoms in the passage and link it to a possible mechanism of COMT. When Rephrased, the question asks, *What is the mechanism of action behind negative symptoms of schizophrenia according to the passage?*

❸ Investigate potential solutions

The second paragraph elaborates on the negative symptoms of schizophrenia. Specifically, this paragraph states that negative symptoms result from hypostimulation of D_1 receptors in the PFC, and this idea should form the basis of a general prediction.

❹ Match your prediction to an answer choice

(**A**) states that COMT causes the conversion of *L*-dopamine to dopamine in the PFC, thereby increasing dopamine levels. However, negative symptoms arise from hypostimulation of D_1 receptors, not *hyper*stimulation. So (**A**) is eliminated.

(**B**) states that COMT converts plasma dopamine to dopamine sulfate. Plasma dopamine is in the blood, not the brain, so this conversion would not cause the negative symptoms and is not correct.

(**C**) states that COMT converts dopamine to dopamine-melanin. Melanin is the compound that determines skin color. The more melanin present, the darker the skin becomes. Because this function has nothing to do with the brain, (**C**) cannot be correct.

Finally, (**D**) describes a mechanism that is plausible and would result in hypostimulation of D_1 receptors. Hence, (**D**) is correct.

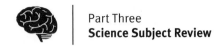
KEY CONCEPT

Neurotransmitter function

> 3. Which of the following would lead to both positive and negative symptoms of schizophrenia?
>
>   **A.** Administration of a sufficient amount of ketamine
>   **B.** Administration of acamprosate, a GABA receptor agonist
>   **C.** Administration of talipexole, a D_2 receptor agonist
>   **D.** Administration of a benzazepine derivative, a D_1 receptor antagonist

① Type the question

A quick glance at the answer choices reveals the names of different drugs and their functions. Because knowledge of the drugs is not pertinent, focus on the function as it relates to passage information regarding negative and positive symptoms of schizophrenia.

② Rephrase the question stem

This question is sufficiently succinct and does not require rephrasing, particularly since the answer choices do not help formulate the task. However, make sure you note that the correct answer fulfills *both* negative and positive symptoms.

③ Investigate potential solutions

The positive and negative symptoms of schizophrenia are discussed in paragraphs 1 and 2, respectively. The positive symptoms of schizophrenia arise from hyperstimulation of D_2 receptors in the subcortical region of the brain, whereas the negative symptoms of schizophrenia come about from the hypostimulation of D_1 receptors in the PFC. The correct answer fulfills both conditions. Keep an eye out for wrong answers that may fulfill one condition but not the other.

④ Match your prediction to an answer choice

(A) states that ketamine fulfills both conditions. After looking closely at paragraph 3, it is possible to determine the role of NMDA receptors (and the associated neurotransmitter, glutamate) in schizophrenia. ML DA neurons project to the VST (subcortical region) and are indirectly inhibited by glutamate, whereas the MC DA neurons project to the PFC and are upregulated by glutamate. Limiting the activity of the NMDA receptors would lead to disinhibition of the ML DA neurons (causing hyperstimulation of the D_2 receptors) and inhibition of the MC DA neurons (causing hypostimulation of the D_1 receptors). Therefore, ketamine administration would produce the desired result, and **(A)** is correct.

(B) proposes a GABA receptor agonist. GABA inhibits ML DA neuronal activity. Because ML DA neurons secrete dopamine into the subcortical region, inhibiting them would result in less dopamine in this region. Less dopamine in the subcortical region will translate into less psychotic episodes because D_2 receptors will be less stimulated and is therefore incorrect.

(C) suggests a D_2 receptor agonist. Although this effect would lead to increased dopamine release in the subcortical region, it does not explain the absence of dopamine in the PFC, which makes it incorrect.

(D) is wrong for the same reason that (C) is wrong. A D_1 receptor antagonist will decrease dopaminergic activity in the PFC. However, this effect does not explain the hyperstimulation of D_2 necessary for positive symptoms to occur.

---

4. The dopamine hypothesis is useful for the clinical treatment of schizophrenia. However, some researchers believe the name is misleading. Why might they think this?

    A. GABA neurons act as a deactivating system to keep subcortical dopamine levels low.
    B. Glutamatergic neurons are located upstream of the dopaminergic neurons.
    C. Multiple types of dopaminergic receptors exist, making the name ambiguous.
    D. Psychostimulants exacerbate the positive symptoms of schizophrenia.

KEY CONCEPT

Neurotransmitter function

---

1 Type the question

The question poses an issue with the name of the *dopamine hypothesis* and asks you why this name might be misleading. In addition, there is no clear pattern in the answer choices. Together these issues can make a tough question to reason through, so this question might be a good candidate for triaging.

2 Rephrase the question stem

The question indicates that the name *dopamine hypothesis* is misleading. It can be inferred that the dopamine hypothesis is either an oversimplification or an incorrect characterization of the origin of schizophrenia. When Rephrased, the question says, *Why is the dopamine hypothesis incorrect or overgeneralized?*

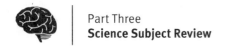
③ Investigate potential solutions

Paragraphs 3 and 4 investigate the other neurotransmitters involved in schizophrenia, so these are a good place to start when searching for a prediction. After taking a closer look at paragraph 3, it is clear that glutamate is a key player in schizophrenia. Its presence causes upregulation of MC DA neurons and indirectly causes downregulation of ML DA neurons. In all likelihood, the correct answer includes a reference to glutamate or the associated NMDA receptors and should form the basis of a prediction.

④ Match your prediction to an answer choice

(B) matches the prediction that the correct answer would mention glutamate. In addition, it is true that glutamatergic neurons are located upstream of the dopaminergic neurons. Researchers might argue that it would almost make sense to rename the hypothesis as the glutamate hypothesis. **(B)** is the correct answer.

(A) mentions GABAergic neurons, which downregulate ML DA neurons. This is only a small piece of the puzzle and does not explain why the dopamine hypothesis is a misleading title.

(C) states that multiple dopaminergic receptors exist. Although ambiguity might be a cause for concern, "the dopamine hypothesis of schizophrenia" is fairly clear. This is not the best explanation based on the provided passage information.

(D) brings up psychostimulants. This answer choice is out of scope and therefore does not answer the question.

> 5. Which of the following individuals would experience the most pronounced negative symptoms after treatment with ketamine?
>
>   A. Active psychostimulant abusers
>   B. Healthy individuals
>   C. Schizophrenics in remission
>   D. Not possible to determine

① Type the question

The answer choices are the different groups included in Figure 1.

② Rephrase the question stem

The question stem is focused on the negative symptoms associated with schizophrenia. When Rephrased, the question asks, *Which group in Figure 1 has the most negative symptoms after ketamine?*

③ Investigate potential solutions

Recall that the negative symptoms are linked to hypostimulation of the D_1 receptors of the PFC. Note that Figure 1 illustrates the change in dopamine concentration in the *subcortical region* after ketamine administration. No data are provided about the relative impact of ketamine on the D_1 receptors of the PFC. Because no data are available about ketamine's impact on the PFC, determining which group will experience the most pronounced negative symptoms is impossible.

④ Match your prediction to an answer choice

The prediction is met with a match. It is impossible to determine which group will experience the most pronounced negative symptoms, therefore (**D**) is correct.

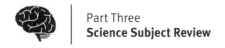

BEHAVIORAL SCIENCES PASSAGE II: MEMORY

Long-term memory storage is ultimately the result of strengthened synaptic connections. The process of long-term memory formation uses cytoplasmic polyadenylation element binding (CPEB) proteins that, remarkably, resemble prions in that they act as a template for promoting the local formation of other CPEB proteins. These proteins, once formed, stack together to form oligomers. The presence of stacked CPEB proteins in the axon terminal strengthens the synaptic connection and helps maintain memory. Regulation of these proteins, however, presents a biological problem: too much oligomerization can lead to the formation of too many memories. Although this might initially seem desirable, it is important to consider that forgetting nonessential memories strengthens the recall of important ones.

Searching for a mechanism of regulation, researchers studied *Drosophila*. The CPEB protein in *Drosophila* is Orb2, which exists in A and B isoforms. Orb2A is far less common but shows more prion-like activity. The researchers observed that Orb2A binds with Tob, another protein that seems to regulate Orb2A levels. They hypothesized that Tob stabilized Orb2A, which is usually labile. Tests confirmed that increasing Tob reduced Orb2A decay by a factor of two, and neuronal stimulation was shown to increase Tob-Orb2A binding. The other Orb2 protein, Orb2B, is far more common but requires an Orb2A "seed" to promote oligomerization. Once the seed is formed, Orb2B can continue to stack with itself. This mechanism is demonstrated in Figure 1.

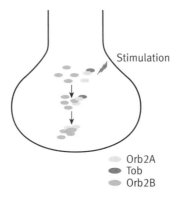

Figure 1. Tob-Orb2A binding leads to Orb2B oligomerization

To test the behavioral effects of the Tob-Orb2A complex, researchers examined courtship behavior, a well-documented application of long-term memory, in *Drosophila*. Typically, a male fly will display courtship behavior toward a newly introduced female, but as time passes, this behavior is prone to extinction if the female is unreceptive. Using RNA interference techniques, researchers suppressed Tob production and found that Tob-deficient flies continued to try to mate with unreceptive females after repeated exposure.

Finding the mechanism for the timing of long-term memory formation proved more difficult, but researchers relied on the discovery that the protein phosphatase (PP2A) is contained in the Orb2A-Tob complex. PP2A is an enzyme that removes phosphates from Orb2A. When dephosphorylation was chemically blocked, this destabilized Tob but stabilized Orb2A and caused an overall reduction in Tob-Orb2A binding. Researchers hypothesized that the primary function of PP2A is to remove phosphates from Orb2A and destabilize it when the synapse is unstimulated, thus preventing oligomerization. Stimulation promotes Tob binding, which stabilizes Orb2A and forms the seed required for the more abundant Orb2B to continue oligomerization.

1. The results of the study in the passage suggest that the Tob-Orb2A complex is a mechanism for which of the following?

    A. Neuroplasticity
    B. Synaptic pruning
    C. Spreading activation
    D. Potentiation

2. If Orb2B stacking did not require an Orb2A seed, which of the following effects is most likely to be observed?

    A. Increased efficiency of and a higher success rate for elaborative rehearsal
    B. An increase in the ratio of automatic processing to effortful processing
    C. An increased necessity for maintenance rehearsal in forming new pathways
    D. Stronger and more efficient semantic networks throughout the cortex

3. Hyperthymesia is a neurological condition that results in an exceptionally strong autobiographical memory; individuals with the condition are able to recall an abnormally large number of their life experiences. Which of the following describe(s) the type(s) of memory affected by this condition?

    I.   Implicit
    II. Episodic
    III. Declarative

    A. I only
    B. II only
    C. I and III only
    D. II and III only

4. Based on the study cited in the passage, which of the following can most reasonably be concluded regarding courtship behavior in *Drosophila*?

    A. Tob-resistant male flies are less responsive than normal flies to negative reinforcement cues from females.
    B. Without the ability to differentiate receptive from unreceptive females, courtship behavior is prone to instinctive drift.
    C. Lacking Tob to regulate long-term memory formation, male flies exhibit the spontaneous recovery of extinct behaviors.
    D. The Tob-Orb2A complex in male *Drosophila* aids in their learning to discriminate between similar stimuli.

5. Suppose that it was discovered that, during binding, Tob recruits LimK, a kinase that phosphorylates Orb2A. What effect would this have on the researcher's conclusions?

    A. They would be weakened because phosphorylation destabilizes Tob, making it less likely for an Orb2B seed.
    B. They would be strengthened because the finding shows how Orb2A conformation changes can cause Orb2B stacking.
    C. They would be strengthened because the finding provides a potential mechanism by which Tob can stabilize Orb2A.
    D. These findings are superfluous and would have no effect because PP2A already performs this function in the axon.

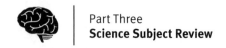

MCAT EXPERTISE

Memory is a high-yield topic in the Psychological, Social, and Biological Foundations of Behavior section of the MCAT. Make sure to know the basics of all four memory processes: encoding, short term, long term, and retrieval. Also be sure to know the common failures of these systems.

USING THE KAPLAN METHOD

Preview the passage: At a glance, the passage is fairly dense and descriptive. It includes a diagram but no experimental data.

Choose your approach: Outline

Read and Distill:

P1: Sets up the context for how CPEB oligomerization is linked with memory formation and how it must be carefully regulated.
  Outline: CPEB protein stacking helps long-term memory formation

P2: *Drosophila* as model for studying CPEB, which is called Orb2. There's a complex pathway involving three different proteins, Orb2A, Orb2B, and Tob.
  Outline: Mech: stimulation → Tob binds Orb2A → prevents decay; Orb2B requires seed

F1: Diagram of mechanism described in P2
  Outline: Mechanism diagram

P3: Male flies remember unreceptive females, so the researchers knock out Tob and find that these flies keep courting unreceptive females.
  Outline: Tob-deficient male flies forget female unreceptiveness

P4: Researchers interested in the timing aspect for memory formation. So they inhibited dephosphorylation of Orb2A, resulting in unstable Orb2A-Tob complex, which prevented formation of memory.
  Outline: Timing: PP2A removes phosphates from Orb2A, causing degradation until the neuron is stimulated

> 1. The results of the study in the passage suggest that the Tob-Orb2A complex is a mechanism for which of the following?
>
>   A. Neuroplasticity
>   B. Synaptic pruning
>   C. Spreading activation
>   D. Potentiation

❶ Type the question

A quick glance at the question shows that it's passage based and is testing knowledge of memory vocabulary.

❷ Rephrase the question stem

What type of memory is involved with the Tob-Orb2A complex?

❸ Investigate potential solutions

Start with an analysis of the Tob-Orb2A complex. According to the passage, the Tob-Orb2A complex is a mechanism for long-term memory that helps strengthen the connections between synapses, which serves as a general prediction.

❹ Match your prediction to an answer choice

Start with (**A**); neuroplasticity describes the ability of the brain to mold its function to adapt to changes in general. So neuroplasticity is too broad to be explained by the mechanism described by the passage and is incorrect.

(**B**) is the process of removing synaptic connections over time. This is nearly opposite and is therefore incorrect.

(**C**) is the process by which nodes that are close together in a semantic network stimulate each other. This process sounds relevant but refers to a process that occurs once the memories are already formed and is therefore incorrect.

Finally, (**D**) is the process by which synaptic activation is strengthened through repeated stimulation, turning a short-term memory into a long-term one. Choose (**D**) with confidence.

TAKEAWAYS

Sometimes the studies described get quite technical; if so, your goal should be to focus on the procedure and the results. Questions focus on the application of our psychology and sociology content knowledge to the overall structure of the experiments in the passages.

THINGS TO WATCH OUT FOR

Memory and learning are both subjects that contain quite a bit of vocabulary. Expect questions that test critical thinking also to require keeping terminology straight.

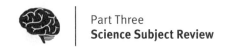

> **2.** If Orb2B stacking did not require an Orb2A seed, which of the following effects is most likely to be observed?
>
> **A.** Increased efficiency of and a higher success rate for elaborative rehearsal
> **B.** An increase in the ratio of automatic processing to effortful processing
> **C.** An increased necessity for maintenance rehearsal in forming new pathways
> **D.** Stronger and more efficient semantic networks throughout the cortex

① Type the question

This question is another passage-based question, with no clear pattern in the answer choices. Although this one could be saved for later, the 2A/2B interaction was discussed succinctly in the passage. So a little bit of passage research should be enough to answer this question quickly.

② Rephrase the question stem

What would happen if Orb2A wasn't required for Orb2B stacking?

③ Investigate potential solutions

Paragraph 2 mentions Orb2B explicitly, and paragraph 1 describes the overall relationship between the oligomers involved and long-term memory. Orb2B can oligomerize with itself once it attaches to an Orb2A seed. The passage also mentions that Orb2B is quite common in the axon terminal. So, if Orb2B was allowed to oligomerize more freely, synaptic connections would be stronger in general and long-term memories would be far easier to form, perhaps even pathologically so. This observation serves as a specific prediction.

④ Match your prediction to an answer choice

(A) seems to match, after consideration of memory vocabulary. Elaboration is the kind of rehearsal that links new concepts to preexisting memories. If Orb2B is able to stack freely, this synaptic connection should be far less effortful. **(A)** matches the prediction and is correct.

(B) describes automatic and effortful processing, which are important concepts in encoding. Synaptic connection strength shouldn't affect the way in which information is obtained, and **(B)** is therefore incorrect.

(C), like **(A)**, describes rehearsal. However, **(C)** mentions maintenance. This type of rehearsal is simply a way to keep information in short-term memory and prevent it from being forgotten. Short-term memory does not rely on synaptic connection strength and is, therefore, incorrect.

(D) is tempting but extreme. The expectation is that long-term memories form more easily, but this does not necessarily have any bearing on how those memories are organized. **(D)** is incorrect.

TAKEAWAYS

Questions that ask for a modification of a study are relatively common. Attempt these only after obtaining points from more straightforward questions.

3. Hyperthymesia is a neurological condition that results in an exceptionally strong autobiographical memory; individuals with the condition are able to recall an abnormally large number of their life experiences. Which of the following describe(s) the type(s) of memory affected by this condition?

   I. Implicit

   II. Episodic

   III. Declarative

A. I only

B. II only

C. I and III only

D. II and III only

① Type the question

This question is a Roman numeral question, and it is the third question in a row that rewards vocabulary knowledge. It's also a pseudodiscrete question, so it can be done right away.

② Rephrase the question stem

What type(s) of memory is/are involved in the recall of life experience?

③ Investigate potential solutions

The stem describes hyperthymesia, so little research should be necessary. Hyperthymesia is described as causing an overload of life experience memory. This condition might immediately bring to mind the concept of episodic memory, which is a choice, and so "episodic memory" is a great prediction. Keep in mind, though, that the diagram of the different types of memory is a branching tree, so more than one answer may be correct here.

TAKEAWAYS

Predicting is a helpful tool in Roman numeral questions, but keep an open mind because more than one statement can be correct.

④ Match your prediction to an answer choice

Based on our prediction, Roman numeral II should be a part of the correct answer, which eliminates (**A**) and (**C**). Neither of the remaining choices includes Roman numeral I, so we need to consider only whether III should be included. Declarative memory is the part of long-term memory that is conscious, and it includes both episodic and semantic memory. Roman numeral III should therefore be part of our answer, so (**D**) is correct.

KEY CONCEPT

It's important to keep straight the different kinds of memory and the ways in which psychologists classify each.

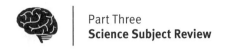
> **4.** Based on the study cited in the passage, which of the following can most reasonably be concluded regarding courtship behavior in *Drosophila*?
>
> **A.** Tob-resistant male flies are less responsive than normal flies to negative reinforcement cues from females.
>
> **B.** Without the ability to differentiate receptive from unreceptive females, courtship behavior is prone to instinctive drift.
>
> **C.** Lacking Tob to regulate long-term memory formation, male flies exhibit the spontaneous recovery of extinct behaviors.
>
> **D.** The Tob-Orb2A complex in male *Drosophila* aides in their learning to discriminate between similar stimuli.

① Type the question

This question is asking for an inference that can be drawn from the passage, and the question stem indicates exactly where to go. So approach this question immediately.

② Rephrase the question stem

What must be true regarding Drosophila *courtship behavior?*

③ Investigate potential solutions

The study in question is presented in paragraph 3, so review the procedure and results there. According to the passage, male flies that lacked Tob were not able to learn which females were unreceptive, so the males continued to try to mate even after being rejected. The study supports the ideas presented earlier in the passage, that a lack of the Tob-Orb2A complex prevents long-term memory formation. So this idea should form the basis of a prediction.

④ Match your prediction to an answer choice

(A) mentions negative reinforcement, which refers to an increase in behavior resulting from the removal of an unwanted stimulus. If anything, the female flies are signaling that they would like the males to decrease courtship behavior, so **(A)** seems unlikely.

(B) mentions instinctive drift, which is another learning phenomenon in which an animal learning a complicated behavior reverts to a more natural one. No such complicated behavior is described in the study.

(C) makes sense only if the males' courtship behavior became extinct; that is, the males learned not to pursue unresponsive females in the first place. This is not supported by the study, so **(C)** can likely be eliminated.

TAKEAWAYS

Whenever a passage presents the results of a study without a conclusion, expect to formulate that conclusion on your own. As you Distill that portion of the passage, take a moment to summarize the results so that you can be ready for such a question.

By elimination, **(D)** must be correct. It discusses discrimination, which is a phenomenon by which an organism can differentiate between two similar but distinct stimuli. Here, the similar stimuli are the receptive and unreceptive females. Because male flies are usually able to remember the difference and exhibit courtship behavior only toward receptive females (whereas Tob-deficient males are not), it stands to reason that Tob is at least partly responsible for the difference.

5. Suppose that it was discovered that, during binding, Tob recruits LimK, a kinase that phosphorylates Orb2A. What effect would this have on the researcher's conclusions?

   A. They would be weakened because phosphorylation destabilizes Tob, making it less likely for an Orb2B seed.

   B. They would be strengthened because the finding shows how Orb2A conformation changes can cause Orb2B stacking.

   C. They would be strengthened because the finding provides a potential mechanism by which Tob can stabilize Orb2A.

   D. These findings are superfluous and would have no effect because PP2A already performs this function in the axon.

① Type the question

This question requires the incorporation of new information with the passage information, phrased in a similar manner as a CARS Strengthen–Weaken Reasoning Beyond the Text question. As these questions can be challenging, it might be wise to save this question for after you've completed the other ones.

② Rephrase the question stem

Tob allows for phosphorylation of Orb2A during binding. What is the effect on the passage argument?

③ Investigate potential solutions

The question stem mentions phosphorylation, a process discussed in paragraph 4. It's likely that we'll need to understand the role of phosphorus, so start with some research. PP2A removes phosphorus from Orb2A, and when this was blocked, Orb2A was stabilized. If during binding Tob causes phosphorus to be added to dephosphorylated Orb2A, this provides an answer to the question of *how* binding strengthens Orb2A. Armed with this prediction, look for a match.

④ Match your prediction to an answer choice

(A) and **(D)** are eliminated immediately because the process mentioned in the question stem helps to qualify a previously unexplained portion of the hypothesis. Of the rest, **(C)** matches the prediction perfectly.

THINGS TO WATCH OUT FOR

Always beware of extreme answer choices for questions that ask you to make conclusions based on a study. Choices that mention "proof" or "causes" are likely to be incorrect.

TAKEAWAYS

When answer choices are grouped as they are here, even a general prediction can eliminate half of the answer choices.

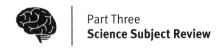
8.6   Behavioral Sciences on Your Own

BEHAVIORAL SCIENCES PASSAGE III (QUESTIONS 1–6)

Throughout the day, humans experience innumerable sensory stimuli. These stimuli originate from a variety of sources and are usually categorized based on the five traditional human senses of sight, smell, hearing, taste, and touch. Psychologists sort stimuli based on their physical constituents, which are referred to as stimulus modalities. These modalities match up fairly closely with the five senses but are slightly more general. Some stimulus modalities are light, sound, temperature, taste, smell, and pressure. These modalities also are called *proximal stimuli*, which refers to the fact that they directly stimulate the sensory organs of the body, such as the eyes, nociceptors, or the bones of the inner ear. *Distal stimuli*, by contrast, are the external source of a sensory input and thus do not directly interact with the sensory organs of the body.

The proximal stimulus initiates neural processing. For the eye, the modality is the electromagnetic radiation (in the visible spectrum) that reflects from an object and makes its way to the retina. From the neural information, the brain (re-)creates an image of the object. The process is analogous for the other sensory modalities, for instance, the sound of a barking dog and the perception of a dog or the scent of a rose and the perception thereof. The brain takes proximal stimuli and transforms them into what we detect as our world.

There are hundreds of proximal stimuli running through the brain at any given time. How can humans take all of this information and organize it into something meaningful and useful? One theory is gestaltism, which is explained as the tendency of humans to integrate pieces of information into meaningful wholes. For example, someone looking at a bookshelf would see a shelf full of books, as a whole, before noticing that there were individual books, or that the books had different titles, or that the books were made of paper, or that they were arranged in a certain way. Gestalt theorists attempt to understand how top-down processing affects perception. To account for the seemingly innate organization that occurs in the human brain, Gestalt theorists devised the principles of grouping. These principles are organized into six categories: proximity, similarity, closure, good continuation, common fate, and good form.

Another organizational principle that influences human perception is the idea of *perceptual sets*. Also shaped by top-down processing, the concept of perceptual sets implies that stimuli may be perceived in different ways depending on the perceiver. For instance, people may be exceptionally sensitive to the sound of their name, especially if they are waiting for it to be called. The thinker may even shape his or her perceptions so that reality correlates more closely to expectations. For instance, people waiting to hear their name may be more apt to mistakenly identify a similar sounding name as their own.

1. Suppose that an observer can discriminate between a 50 cd light and a 55 cd light but not a 50 cd light and a 54 cd light. Assuming the same setup, what is the faintest intensity of light that can be discriminated from a 300 cd light?

   A. 270 cd
   B. 305 cd
   C. 330 cd
   D. 355 cd

2. Which of the following statements would best support the idea of perceptive sets?

   A. A mother reserves judgment for her child's performance at a musical contest until the judges have returned their decision.
   B. A sports fan cheers for the other team when the team makes a skillful play, even if it results in his or her own team losing points.
   C. A mother advocates for her child in a competition but reminds the child to be a good sport whether winning or losing.
   D. A sports fan perceives the referees in a game to be against his or her team when the referees make any calls that hurt the team.

3. Which of the following CANNOT be considered a proximal stimulus?

   A. Light bouncing off of a flower and into the eye
   B. Small, volatile molecules released by a flower
   C. A shoe sitting on the floor
   D. The sound waves created by a bee's wings

4. Which of the following most accurately describes the body's reaction to a bee sting?

   A. An efferent action potential arrives at a relay neuron, which sends an afferent action potential to the effector muscle, after which the signal arrives and is interpreted at the brain.
   B. An afferent action potential arrives at a relay neuron, which sends an efferent action potential to the effector muscle, after which the signal arrives and is interpreted at the brain.
   C. An afferent action potential arrives at a relay neuron, which sends a signal to the brain, which then interprets the signal and sends an efferent action potential to the effector muscle.
   D. An efferent action potential arrives at a relay neuron, which sends a signal to the brain, which then interprets the signal and sends an afferent action potential to the effector muscle.

5. Phantosmia is a disorder characterized by olfactory hallucinations in the absence of any physical odors. Which of the following is most likely to cause phantosmia?

   A. An odor molecule stimulating the wrong kind of chemoreceptor
   B. Seizures occurring in a patient's occipital lobe of his or her brain
   C. Temporal lobe atrophy caused by Alzheimer's disease
   D. Parietal lobe activation caused by schizophrenia

6. Some children's games involve searching for a known character amid other similarly dressed characters and similarly colored objects. The thought process involved in this type of game could best be considered:

   A. top-down processing with multimodal stimuli.
   B. bottom-up processing with unimodal stimuli.
   C. top-down processing with unimodal stimuli.
   D. bottom-up processing with multimodal stimuli.

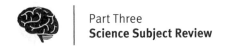

Behavioral Sciences Practice Passage Explanations

1. (A)

The just-noticeable difference (JND) for the discrimination of light (in this particular setup) can be determined from the question stem. According to Weber's law, the just-noticeable difference is calculated as a ratio. From the given information, the JND is $\frac{5}{50}$ or $\frac{1}{10}$ of the intensity of the light. Using this information, it can be predicted that the observer would be able to differentiate between a 300 cd light and another light as long as the intensities vary by 10 percent. The question asks for the *faintest*, which matches **(A)**. A 270 cd light could be differentiated from a $(270 \times 1.1) = 297$ cd light, so the observer would be able to differentiate between the two.

2. (D)

Perceptive sets are the expectations that affect one's perception. It may result in the organization and processing of information so that perceptions match one's expectations or motivations. This is the essential attribute that must be found in the correct answer. In **(A)**, **(B)**, and **(C)**, the perception isn't being modified in this way. **(D)**, however, has the sports fan's perceptions being changed because of the fan's commitment to the team and is the correct response.

3. (C)

Proximal stimuli are the physical stimuli that directly stimulate the sensory organs. This question asks which answer is not a proximal stimulus, so the correct answer will be unlike the others. **(A)** was discussed in the passage as an example of a proximal stimulus, so it is eliminated. **(B)** could be a little confusing, but these criteria all point toward an odorant and an example of a proximal stimulus. **(D)** is stimulus that will travel to the sensory system and be converted into an action potential, and thus it could be a proximal stimulus. This leaves **(C)** because the shoe itself constitutes a distal stimulus—something in the environment that is detected but is not directly interacting with sensory neurons. For reference, the proximal stimulus associated with the shoe might be the light reflecting off the shoe and entering the retina, or the volatile molecules released by the shoe that act as odorants.

4. (B)

When the body experiences a stimulus that elicits a reflex arc, there is a specific order for how the signal travels through the system. The afferent neuron takes the signal from the sensory organ to the central nervous system. In reflex loops, this signal is taken in by a relay neuron and then sent directly back out through an efferent neuron to the effector muscle to try and move the body away from the painful stimulus. Not until after this signal and reflex have happened does the brain realize the stimulus or the action at all, or **(B)**.

5. (C)

Looking at the answers shows that three have to do with different parts of the brain, whereas the other looks at a mix-up at the chemoreceptor. **(A)** can be eliminated because the question stem states that there is an absence of odor, thus no mix-up could occur because there is no odor molecule to stimulate the chemoreceptor. From there, this question is a matter of remembering which area of the brain is responsible for interpreting scent. The answer to that question is the temporal lobe, and phantosmia can be caused by Alzheimer's disease when it atrophies the temporal lobe, or **(C)**.

6. (C)

Examining the answer choices reveals that this question is looking for the modality of the sensory stimulus and how the children's game is being processed. The question states that the child will be looking for something amid a field of other objects. This means the child already has an idea of what he or she is looking for and is parsing a larger image looking for a specific thing. This means that the child is using top-down processing, which eliminates **(B)** and **(D)**. The modality of the stimulus has to do with what senses are being used. In this case, light is collected and vision is being used exclusively—implying a unimodal stimulus and **(C)**.

CHAPTER 9

Biochemistry

The MCAT tests introductory biochemistry as a portion of both the Chemical and Physical Foundations of Biological Systems and the Biological and Biochemical Foundations of Living Systems sections. Each of these sections is approximately 25 percent biochemistry. The information tested is material likely to be covered in an introductory biochemistry course for those studying the life sciences. Therefore, it is important that you take your preparation for biochemistry very seriously because a significant portion of your score will depend on biochemistry. That being said, the biochemistry tested in each section is likely to be in different contexts. This chapter explores how the MCAT tests your knowledge of biochemistry in both the Chemical and Physical Foundations of Biological Systems and the Biological and Biochemical Foundations of Living Systems sections.

9.1   Reading the Passage

When glancing at a biochemistry passage for the first time, you will likely notice images, data, and/or chemical equations. The images may represent a cellular structure, a biochemical experiment, or a graph representing experimental data. Because biochemistry shares many topics with biology and chemistry, images alone may not provide sufficient information to determine the specific topic. However, biochemistry passages and images are usually easily distinguished from their physics counterparts.

PASSAGE TYPES

Biochemistry passages can be either experiment or information passages. However, the experiment passages in biochemistry are much different from those found in the other sciences. In biochemistry, experiment passages may be related to a biological process. Data may be represented visually as a change in structure of a cell or tissue or as a graph, rather than as raw numerical data points. Questions on these passages are likely to assess your ability to analyze visual evidence. Experiment passages require the test taker to put together all of the information presented in order to to answer the questions. Although the passage presentations are similar in both sections, the scope of the information tested is different.

Chemical and Physical Foundations of Biological Systems

Passages in the Chemical and Physical Foundations of Biological Systems section are likely accompanied by chemical equations. In addition, those biochemistry passages are likely to fall more within the context of chemistry, both organic and inorganic (general) chemistry. Success

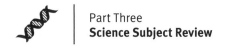

on biochemistry passages in this section will rely on your ability to connect the concepts in biochemistry, organic chemistry, and general chemistry and apply these connections to biological situations. Biochemistry passages in this section are more likely to reflect changes that occur at the molecular and tissue levels. (See Table 9.1.)

- Experiment passages in this section may include organic synthesis pathways and molecular structures.
  - Experimental results are likely summarized in the form of a graph, chart, or other visual representation of data.
  - Experiment passages require integration of biochemistry concepts at the molecular level.
- Information passages in biochemistry also present information. However, understanding this information requires a fundamental understanding of biology, even though this is not in the Biological and Biochemical Foundations of Living Systems section.
  - These passages integrate multiple subject areas.
  - Connections between topics in the passage may be present but not explicitly stated. The test taker will have to make these connections to understand the passage fully.

Overall, biochemistry passages in this section are a perfect opportunity for the test maker to present questions and passages that require a thorough understanding in the areas of general chemistry, organic chemistry, biochemistry, and biology. The divisions between these sciences are blurred on the MCAT, such that a single passage with questions is likely to test multiple areas, with individual questions requiring knowledge in multiple subjects.

Biological and Biochemical Foundations of Living Systems

Biochemistry passages in this section are likely to focus on biology and less on the details of organic and general chemistry. Although knowledge of the fundamentals of chemistry are required, the biochemistry passages in this section are more likely to explore how the biochemistry of an organism affects the organism and its physiology as a whole. (See Table 9.1.)

- Experiment passages in this section feature an experiment, but you are less likely to have a passage with an organic synthesis pathway.
  - The data may be less numerical, but you have to analyze figures and data to understand how a process influences the overall physiology of the organism.
- Information passages also focus more on the biological side of biochemistry.
  - Expect that information passages that appear to be more biology in scope may also be accompanied by questions regarding biochemistry concepts.

	Chemical and Physical Foundations of Biological Systems	Biology and Biochemical Foundations of Living Systems
Experiment passages	Incorporate an organic chemistry synthesis or general chemistry concepts. Experiment is likely to focus on biochemistry at the molecular, cellular, or tissue level rather than on the organism as a whole.	Heavy in biological concepts, often physiology. Experiment is likely to focus on how a biochemical process affects the organism as a whole.
Information passages	Is a combination of concepts from general chemistry, organic chemistry, and biochemistry, and a grasp of these subject areas is required in order to determine the goal of the passage.	Also heavy in biological concepts, passages may be defined as both biochemistry and biology, with little distinction between the two.
Scope	From the molecular to the tissue level.	From the molecular level to the entire organism.
Images	May involve molecular structures, chemical equations, graphs and charts representing data, and illustrations of biochemical processes at the molecular and cellular levels.	Less likely to involve molecular structures, but physiological pathways may predominate. Chemical equations represent physiology. Illustrations focus on biochemical processes at the level of the organism.

Table 9.1. Biochemistry in Its Different Sections

READING AND DISTILLING THE PASSAGE

Regardless of the section, biochemistry passages are approached in the same way, using the Kaplan Method. Read the passage quickly and efficiently; apply the Distill method best suited to the kind of information being conveyed.

- **Preview** for difficulty
  - The structure of biochemistry passages depends somewhat on the passage type and the section. Passages in the Chemical and Physical Foundations of Biological Systems section are more likely to be accompanied by molecular structures and organic synthesis pathways, whereas passages in the Biology and Biochemical Foundations of Living Systems section are more likely to be accompanied by images of organisms or cells.
  - Determine whether the passage is *experimental* or *informational.*
  - Note the location of the paragraphs and any figures, such as charts, graphs, tables, or diagrams.
  - Data are more likely to be represented graphically or visually rather than numerically.
  - Decide whether this passage is one to do now or later.

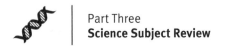

- **Choose** your approach
  - ○ Using information from the Preview step, Choose an appropriate Distill approach for the passage (Interrogate, Outline, or Highlight).
  - ○ **Interrogation** should be chosen for experiment passages.
  - ○ **Outlining** should be chosen for information passages that are dense or detail heavy.
  - ○ **Highlighting** should be chosen for information passages that are light on details.

- **Read and Distill** key themes
  - ○ While reading the passage, your aim is to distill the major takeaway of each paragraph and identify testable information using one of the following approaches.
  - ○ **Interrogate:** Thoroughly examine the experiment passage by identifying the key components of experimental design and interrogating *why* specific procedures were done and *how* they connect to the overall purpose of the experiment.
  - ○ **Outline:** Create a brief label for each paragraph that summarizes the contents of the paragraph and allows you to return quickly to the passage when demanded by a question.
  - ○ **Highlight:** Highlight one to three terms per paragraph that can pull your attention back to testable information when demanded by a question.
  - ○ For paragraphs that describe a pathway or series of relationships without an accompanying figure, sketching your own figure (with shorthand symbols and notation) often pays off in the questions.

9.2   Answering the Questions

Like other sciences tested on the MCAT, there are four types of biochemistry questions:

- **Discrete questions**
    - Questions are not connected to a passage.
    - Often require you to recall or apply a basic concept, such as a theory or a process.
    - Questions likely focus on single topics or the integration of two topics.

- **Questions that stand alone from the passage**
    - Questions that accompany a passage but do not require information or data from the passage to identify the correct answer.
    - More likely to require application of a basic concept, theory, or process to a situation presented in the question stem.

- **Questions that require data from the passage**
    - Questions that require a piece of data or information from the passage but do not require the goal of the passage.
    - Likely to focus on data analysis or an evaluation of an experimental procedure.
    - May focus on the information section of the passage and require you to identify a detail presented.
    - Questions are less likely to involve a calculation on a biochemistry passage.

- **Questions that require the goal of the passage**
    - Questions that require the goal of the passage or a fundamental grasp of the passage as a whole.
    - Likely to focus on the results and a discussion of the results of an experiment.
    - May assess your ability to analyze data or evaluate an experimental design from a broad perspective, such as predicting how changes to the experiment may impact results.
    - May require you to evaluate the results of an experiment and apply those results to the information presented earlier in the passage.
    - Most likely related to your ability to understand biochemistry on the tissue or organismal level.

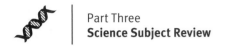
ATTACKING THE QUESTIONS

Biochemistry questions on the MCAT are likely to target multiple skills, including statistical data analysis and research design. Given that biochemistry is one of the most tested topics on Test Day, some passages and questions will probably cover concepts related to biochemistry research. However, questions like this can also be answered using a systematic approach. We have already introduced the Kaplan Method to approach questions. Now we will focus on how to use that strategy to your advantage on biochemistry questions.

- **Type** the question
  - Read the question; peek at the answer choices, but do not read them too closely.
  - Assess the topic and degree of difficulty and decide whether to work the question now or later.
  - Identify the level of time involvement: is this question likely to take a tremendous amount of time to identify the answer? If so, skip it and come back after you do the other questions in the passage set.
  - Good questions to do now for biochemistry are those that stand alone from the passage because these are generally quick and easy points.
- **Rephrase** the question stem
  - Rephrase the question, focusing on the task(s) to be accomplished.
  - Simplify the phrasing of the original question stem.
  - Translate the question into a specific set of tasks to be accomplished using the passage and your background knowledge.
  - Biochemistry passages are less likely to involve math but are more likely to involve reasoning and analysis.
- **Investigate** potential solutions
  - Complete the task(s) identified in your Rephrase step.
  - Tasks in biochemistry are likely to involve analyzing data in graph or chart form, analyzing information in the passage, or identifying how a biochemical process affects the organism or another process.
  - Many of the questions require you to apply your knowledge of other subject areas, such as biology, organic chemistry, and/or general chemistry, to biochemical concepts.
  - Carry out your plan, going back to the passage and locating required information, analyzing the data, or determining the results and impact of a biochemical process.
  - Predict what you can about the answer.
  - Be flexible if your initial approach fails.
- **Match** your prediction to an answer choice
  - Search the answer choices for a response that is synonymous with your prediction, or eliminate answers that are not correct.
  - Select an answer and move on.
  - If you cannot find a match to your prediction, eliminate wrong answers, select a response from the remaining choices, and move on.
  - Some questions give you graphics in the answer choices instead of words. When approaching a set of answer choices like this, be sure to eliminate ones that simply are not possible or sensible in the context of the question.

Biochemistry

9.3   Getting the Edge in Biochemistry

Getting a high score on Test Day requires a very solid foundation in biochemistry because this subject area is heavily tested. However, it is important to develop a grasp of biochemistry in the context of the other sciences, especially biology, organic chemistry, and general chemistry. Many of the passages you encounter on Test Day require you to make connections between the other sciences and biochemistry. In addition, biochemical processes do not occur in isolation. Many of the passages and questions focus on how changes at the molecular level result in changes in the entire organism's physiology.

On Test Day, biochemistry passages will feature a variety of figures, including graphs, charts, molecular structures, chemical equations, and visual representations of biochemical concepts. Be prepared to analyze a variety of different images because you will be repeatedly asked to do so on Test Day.

9.4   Preparing for the MCAT: Biochemistry

The following presents the biochemistry content you are likely to see on Test Day. This is one of the most important subjects on the MCAT, so be sure to familiarize yourself with all of the content. The High-Yield badges point out the topics that are tested most frequently.

AMINO ACIDS, PEPTIDES, AND PROTEINS

High-Yield

Amino acids have four groups attached to a central (α) carbon: an amino group, a carboxylic acid group, a hydrogen atom, and an **R-group** that determines chemistry and function of that amino acid. Twenty amino acids appear in the proteins of eukaryotic organisms.

The stereochemistry of the α-carbon is L- for all chiral amino acids in eukaryotes, although D-amino acids exist in prokaryotes. All chiral amino acids except **cysteine** have S- configuration, and all amino acids are chiral except **glycine**, which has a hydrogen atom as its R-group.

Side chains can be polar or nonpolar, aromatic or nonaromatic, charged or uncharged. Amino acids with long alkyl chains are hydrophobic, and those with charges are hydrophilic. Many others fall somewhere in between.

- **Nonpolar, nonaromatic:** glycine, alanine, valine, leucine, isoleucine, methionine, proline
- **Aromatic:** tryptophan, phenylalanine, tyrosine
- **Polar:** serine, threonine, asparagine, glutamine, cysteine
- **Negatively charged (acidic):** aspartate, glutamate
- **Positively charged (basic):** lysine, arginine, histidine

Amino acids are **amphoteric**, meaning they can accept or donate protons. The **pK_a** of a group is the pH at which half of the species is deprotonated; $[HA] = [A^-]$. Amino acids exist in different forms at different pH values. At a low (acidic) pH, the amino acid is fully protonated. At a pH near the pI (isoelectric point) of the amino acid, the amino acid is a neutral **zwitterion**. At a high (alkaline) pH, the amino acid is fully deprotonated.

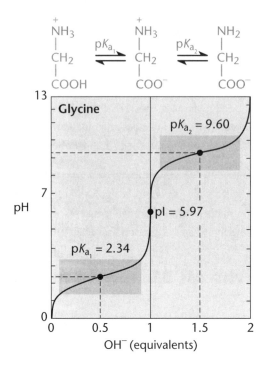

Figure 9.1. Titration Curve for Glycine

The **isoelectric point (pI)** of an amino acid without a charged side chain can be calculated by averaging the two pK_a values. On the titration curve of an amino acid (see Figure 9.1), the curve is nearly flat at the pK_a values of the amino acid and nearly vertical at the pI of the amino acid. Amino acids with charged side chains have an additional pK_a value; their pI is calculated by averaging the two pK_a values that correspond to protonation and deprotonation of the zwitterion. Amino acids without charged side chains have a pI around 6, acidic amino acids have a pI well below 6, and basic amino acids have a pI well above 6.

Dipeptides have two amino acid residues; tripeptides have three. Oligopeptides have a "few" amino acid residues (< 20); polypeptides have "many" (> 20). Forming a peptide bond is a **condensation** or **dehydration reaction** (releasing one molecule of water). The nucleophilic amino group of one amino acid attacks the electrophilic carbonyl group of another amino acid, resulting in amide bonds that are rigid because of resonance. Breaking a peptide bond is a **hydrolysis** reaction.

- **Primary structure** is the linear sequence of amino acids in a peptide and is stabilized by peptide bonds.
- **Secondary structure** is the local structure of neighboring amino acids due to hydrogen bonding between amino groups and nonadjacent carboxyl groups. There are several forms of secondary structure: **α-helices** are clockwise coils around a central axis, **β-pleated sheets** are rippled strands that can be parallel or antiparallel, and **proline** can interrupt secondary structure because of its rigid cyclic structure.
- **Tertiary structure** is the three-dimensional shape of a single polypeptide chain. It is stabilized by hydrophobic interactions, acid-base interactions (salt bridges), hydrogen bonding, and disulfide bonds. **Hydrophobic interactions** push hydrophobic R-groups to the interior of a protein, which increases entropy of the surrounding water molecules and creates a negative Gibbs free energy. **Disulfide bonds** occur when two **cysteine** molecules are oxidized and create a covalent bond to form **cystine**.
- **Quaternary structure** is the interaction among peptides in proteins that contain multiple subunits.

Proteins with covalently attached molecules are termed **conjugated proteins**. The attached molecule is a **prosthetic group** and may be a metal ion, vitamin, lipid, carbohydrate, or nucleic acid. Both heat and increasing solute concentration can lead to loss of three-dimensional protein structure (secondary, tertiary, and quaternary), which is termed **denaturation**.

ENZYMES

Enzymes as Biological Catalysts

Enzymes are biological catalysts that remain unchanged by the reactions they catalyze and that are reusable. Enzymes lower the activation energy necessary for biological reactions. Enzymes do not alter the free energy (ΔG) or enthalpy (ΔH) change that accompanies the reaction, neither do they not the final equilibrium position; rather, they change the rate (kinetics) at which equilibrium is reached. Each enzyme catalyzes a single reaction or type of reaction with high specificity.

- **Oxidoreductases** catalyze oxidation-reduction reactions that involve the transfer of electrons.
- **Transferases** move a functional group from one molecule to another molecule.
- **Hydrolases** catalyze cleavage with the addition of water.
- **Lyases** catalyze cleavage without the addition of water and without the transfer of electrons. The reverse reaction (synthesis) is often more important biologically.
- **Isomerases** catalyze the interconversion of isomers.
- **Ligases** are responsible for joining two large biomolecules, often of the same type.

Enzyme Mechanics and Kinetics

Enzymes act by stabilizing the transition state, providing a favorable microenvironment, or bonding with the substrate molecules. Enzymes have an **active site**, which is the site of catalysis. Binding to the active site is explained by the **lock and key theory** or the **induced fit model**. The lock and key theory hypothesizes that the enzyme and substrate are exactly complementary, while the induced fit model hypothesizes that the enzyme and substrate undergo conformational changes to interact fully. Some enzymes require metal cation **cofactors** or small organic **coenzymes** to be active.

Enzymes experience **saturation kinetics**: as substrate concentration increases, the reaction rate does as well until a maximum value is reached. **Michaelis-Menten** and **Lineweaver-Burk** plots represent this relationship as a hyperbola and line, respectively. Enzymes can be compared on the basis of their K_m and v_{max} values. **Cooperative enzymes** display a sigmoidal curve because of the change in activity with substrate binding.

Enzyme Activity

Temperature and pH affect an enzyme's activity in vivo; changes in temperature and pH can result in denaturing of the enzyme and loss of activity due to loss of secondary, tertiary, or, if present, quaternary structure. In vitro, salinity can impact the action of enzymes.

Enzyme pathways are highly regulated and subject to inhibition and activation. **Feedback inhibition** is a regulatory mechanism whereby the catalytic activity of an enzyme is inhibited by the presence of high levels of a product later in the same pathway.

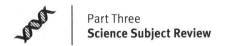

- **Reversible inhibition** is characterized by the ability to replace the inhibitor with a compound of greater affinity or to remove the inhibitor using mild laboratory treatment. There are four main types of reversible inhibition (see Table 9.2).
- **Competitive inhibition** results when the inhibitor is similar to the substrate and binds at the active site. Competitive inhibition can be overcome by adding more substrate; v_{max} remains unchanged, but K_m increases.
- **Noncompetitive inhibition** results when the inhibitor binds with equal affinity to the enzyme and the enzyme–substrate complex. v_{max} is decreased, K_m is unchanged.
- **Mixed inhibition** results when the inhibitor binds with unequal affinity to the enzyme and the enzyme-substrate complex. In this situation, v_{max} is decreased and K_m is increased or decreased depending on if the inhibitor has higher affinity for the enzyme or enzyme-substrate complex.
- **Uncompetitive inhibition** results when the inhibitor binds only with the enzyme-substrate complex; K_m and v_{max} both decrease.
- **Irreversible inhibition** alters the enzyme in such a way that the active site is unavailable for a prolonged duration or permanently; new enzyme molecules must be synthesized for the reaction to occur again.

	Competitive	Noncompetitive	Mixed	Uncompetitive
Binding site	Active site	Allosteric site	Allosteric site	Enzyme-substrate complex
Impact on K_m	Increases	Unchanged	Increases or Decreases	Decreases
Impact on v_{max}	Unchanged	Decreases	Decreases	Decreases

Table 9.2. Comparison of Reversible Inhibitors

Regulatory enzymes can experience activation as well as inhibition. **Allosteric** sites can be occupied by activators, which increase either affinity or enzymatic turnover. **Phosphorylation** (covalent modification with phosphate) or **glycosylation** (covalent modification with carbohydrate) can alter the activity or selectivity of enzymes. **Zymogens** are secreted in an inactive form and are activated by cleavage.

NONENZYMATIC CELLULAR FUNCTIONS OF PROTEINS

Structural proteins compose the cytoskeleton, anchoring proteins and much of the extracellular matrix, and are generally fibrous in nature. The most common structural proteins are **collagen, elastin, keratin, actin**, and **tubulin. Motor proteins** have one or more heads capable of force generation through a conformational change. They have catalytic activity, acting as ATPases to power movement. Muscle contraction, vesicle movement within cells, and cell motility are the most common applications of motor proteins. Common examples include **myosin, kinesin**, and **dynein. Binding proteins** bind a specific substrate, either to sequester it in the body or hold its concentration at steady state.

Cell adhesion molecules (CAM) allow cells to bind to other cells or surfaces. **Cadherins** are calcium-dependent glycoproteins that hold similar cells together. **Integrins** have two membrane-spanning chains and permit cells to adhere to proteins in the extracellular matrix. Some also have signaling capabilities. **Selectins** allow cells to adhere to carbohydrates on the surfaces of other cells and are most commonly used in the immune system.

Antibodies (or **immunoglobulins, Ig**) are used by the immune system to target a specific **antigen**, which may be a protein on the surface of a pathogen (invading organism) or a toxin. Immunoglobulins contain a constant region and a variable region; the variable region is responsible for antigen binding. Two identical heavy chains and two identical light chains form a single antibody; they are held together by disulfide linkages and noncovalent interactions.

Biosignaling

Ion channels can be used for regulating ion flow into or out of a cell. There are three main types of ion channels. **Ungated channels** are always open. **Voltage-gated channels** are open within a range of membrane potentials. **Ligand-gated channels** open in the presence of a specific binding substance, usually a hormone or neurotransmitter.

Enzyme-linked receptors participate in cell signaling through extracellular ligand binding and initiation of second messenger cascades.

G protein-coupled receptors have a membrane-bound protein associated with a trimeric **G protein**. They also initiate second messenger systems. First, ligand binding engages the G protein. Next, GDP is replaced with GTP and the α subunit dissociates from the β and γ subunits. Then, the activated α subunit alters the activity of **adenylate cyclase** or **phospholipase C**. Finally, GTP is dephosphorylated to GDP and the α subunit rebinds to the β and γ subunits.

Protein Isolation and Analysis

High-Yield

Electrophoresis uses a gel matrix to observe the migration of proteins in response to an electric field. **Native PAGE** maintains the protein's shape, but results are difficult to compare because the mass-to-charge ratio differs for each protein. **SDS-PAGE** denatures the proteins and masks the native charge so that comparison of size is more accurate, but the functional protein cannot be recaptured from the gel. **Isoelectric focusing** separates proteins by their **isoelectric point** (**pI**); the protein migrates toward an electrode until it reaches a region of the gel where pH = pI of the protein.

Chromatography separates protein mixtures on the basis of their affinity for a **stationary phase** or a **mobile phase**.

- **Column chromatography** uses beads of a polar compound, like silica or alumina (stationary phase), with a nonpolar solvent (mobile phase).
- **Ion-exchange chromatography** uses a charged column and a variably saline eluent.
- **Size-exclusion chromatography** relies on porous beads. Larger molecules elute first because they are not trapped in the small pores.
- **Affinity chromatography** uses a bound receptor or ligand and an eluent with free ligand or a receptor for the protein of interest.

Protein structure is primarily determined through **X-ray crystallography** after the protein is isolated, although NMR can also be used. Amino acid composition can be determined by simple hydrolysis. However, amino acid sequencing requires sequential degradation, such as the **Edman degradation**. Activity levels for enzymatic samples are determined by following the process of a known reaction, often accompanied by a color change. Protein concentration is also determined colorimetrically, either by UV spectroscopy or through a color change reaction.

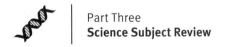

CARBOHYDRATE STRUCTURE AND FUNCTION

Carbohydrates are organized by their number of carbon atoms and functional groups. Common names are also frequently used when referring to sugars, such as glucose, fructose, and galactose. Three-carbon sugars are trioses, four-carbon sugars are tetroses, and so on. Sugars with aldehydes as their most oxidized group are **aldoses**; sugars with ketones as their most oxidized group are **ketoses**.

The nomenclature of all sugars is based on the D- and L-forms of glyceraldehyde. Sugars with the highest-numbered chiral carbon with the −OH group on the right (in a Fischer projection) are D-sugars; those with the −OH on the left are L-sugars. The D- and L-forms of the same sugar are **enantiomers**. **Diastereomers** are nonsuperimposable configurations of molecules with similar connectivity. They differ at least one—but not all—chiral carbons. These also include epimers and anomers. **Epimers** are a subtype of diastereomers that differ at exactly one chiral carbon. **Anomers** are a subtype of epimers that differ at the anomeric carbon.

Cyclization describes the ring formation of carbohydrates from their straight-chain forms. When rings form, the anomeric carbon can take on either an α- or a β-conformation. The **anomeric carbon** acts as the new chiral center formed in ring closure; it was the carbon containing the carbonyl in the straight-chain form. **α-anomers** have the −OH on the anomeric carbon *trans* to the free −CH$_2$OH group, while **β-anomers** have the −OH on the anomeric carbon *cis* to the free −CH$_2$OH group. **Haworth projections** provide a good way to represent three-dimensional structure. Cyclic compounds can undergo **mutarotation**, in which they shift from one anomeric form to another with the straight-chain form as an intermediate.

Monosaccharides are single carbohydrate units, with glucose as the most commonly observed monomer. They can undergo three main reactions: oxidation-reduction, esterification, and glycoside formation.

- Sugars that can be oxidized are reducing agents (**reducing sugars**) themselves and can be detected by reacting with **Tollens'** or **Benedict's reagents**. Sugars with an −H replacing an −OH group are termed **deoxy sugars**.
- Sugars can react with carboxylic acids and their derivatives, forming esters (**esterification**). **Phosphorylation** is a similar reaction in which a phosphate ester is formed by transferring a phosphate group from ATP onto a sugar.
- **Glycoside formation** is the basis for building complex carbohydrates and requires the anomeric carbon to link to another sugar.

Complex carbohydrates include disaccharides and polysaccharides. Disaccharides form as result of glycosidic bonding between two monosaccharide subunits; polysaccharides form by repeated monosaccharide or polysaccharide glycosidic bonding. Common disaccharides include **sucrose** (glucose-α-1,2-fructose), **lactose** (galactose-β-1,4-glucose), and **maltose** (glucose-α-1,4-glucose). Polysaccharides play various roles. **Cellulose** is the main structural component for plant cell walls and is a main source of fiber in the human diet. **Starches** (**amylose** and **amylopectin**) function as a main energy storage form for plants. **Glycogen** functions as a main energy storage form for animals.

LIPIDS

Structural Lipids

Lipids are insoluble in water and are soluble in nonpolar organic solvents. **Phospholipids** are amphipathic and form the bilayer of biological membranes (see Figure 9.2). They contain a hydrophilic (polar) head group and hydrophobic (nonpolar) tails. The head group is attached by a **phosphodiester linkage** and, because it interacts with the environment, determines the function of the phospholipid. The **saturation** of the fatty acid tails determines the fluidity of the membrane; saturated fatty acids are less fluid than unsaturated ones. Fatty acids form most of the structural thickness of the phospholipid bilayer. **Glycerophospholipids** are phospholipids that contain a glycerol backbone.

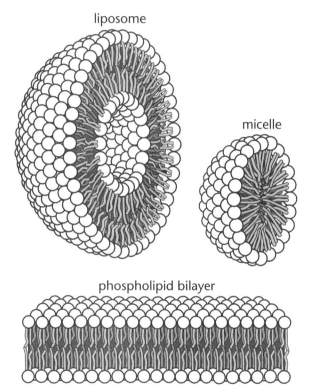

Figure 9.2. Membrane Lipids Form Various Structures in Aqueous Solutions

Sphingolipids contain a sphingosine or sphingoid backbone. Many (but not all) sphingolipids are also phospholipids, containing a phosphodiester bond; these are termed **sphingophospholipids**. **Sphingomyelins** are the major class of sphingophospholipids and contain a phosphatidylcholine or phosphatidylethanolamine head group. They are a major component of the myelin sheath. **Glycosphingolipids** are attached to sugar moieties instead of a phosphate group. **Cerebrosides** have one sugar connected to sphingosine; **globosides** have two or more. **Gangliosides** contain oligosaccharides with at least one terminal *N*-**acetylneuraminic acid** (**NANA**; also called **sialic acid**).

Waxes contain long-chain fatty acids esterified to long-chain alcohols. They are used as protection against evaporation and parasites in plants and animals.

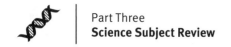

Signaling Lipids

Terpenes are odiferous steroid precursors made from **isoprene**, a five-carbon molecule. One terpene unit (a **monoterpene**) contains two isoprene units. **Terpenoids** are derived from terpenes via oxygenation or backbone rearrangement. They have similar odorous characteristics.

Steroids contain three cyclohexane rings and one cyclopentane ring. Their oxidation state and functional groups may vary. **Steroid hormones** have high-affinity receptors, work at low concentrations, and affect gene expression and metabolism. **Cholesterol** is a steroid important to membrane fluidity and stability; it serves as a precursor to a host of other molecules.

Prostaglandins are autocrine- and paracrine-signaling molecules that regulate cAMP levels. They have powerful effects on smooth muscle contraction, body temperature, the sleep-wake cycle, fever, and pain.

The fat-soluble vitamins include vitamins A, D, E, and K.

- **Vitamin A (carotene)** is metabolized to **retinal** for vision and to **retinoic acid** for gene expression in epithelial development.
- **Vitamin D (cholecalciferol)** is metabolized to **calcitriol** in the kidneys. It regulates calcium and phosphorus homeostasis in the intestines (increasing calcium and phosphate absorption), promoting bone formation. A deficiency of vitamin D causes **rickets**.
- **Vitamin E (tocopherols)** act as biological antioxidants. Their aromatic rings destroy free radicals, preventing oxidative damage.
- **Vitamin K (phylloquinone** and **menaquinones)** is important for formation of prothrombin, a clotting factor. It performs post-translational modifications on a number of proteins, creating calcium-binding sites.

Energy Storage

Triacylglycerols (triglycerides) are the preferred method of storing energy for long-term use. They contain one glycerol attached to three fatty acids by ester bonds. The fatty acids usually vary within the same triacylglycerol. The carbon atoms in lipids are more reduced than carbohydrates, giving twice as much energy per gram during oxidation. Triacylglycerols are very hydrophobic, so they are not hydrated by body water and do not carry additional water weight. Animal cells specifically used for storage of large triacylglycerol deposits are called **adipocytes**.

Free fatty acids are unesterified fatty acids that travel in the bloodstream. Salts of free fatty acids are **soaps** and can be synthesized in saponification. **Saponification** is the ester hydrolysis of triacylglycerols using a strong base, like sodium or potassium hydroxide. Soaps act as surfactants, forming micelles. A **micelle** can dissolve a lipid-soluble molecule in its fatty acid core and washes away with water because of its shell of carboxylate head groups.

DNA

DNA Structure and Organization

High-Yield

Deoxyribonucleic acid (DNA) is a macromolecule that stores genetic information in all living organisms. **Nucleosides** contain a five-carbon sugar bonded to a nitrogenous base; **nucleotides** are nucleosides with one to three phosphate groups added. Nucleotides are abbreviated by letter: **adenine (A)**, **cytosine (C)**, **guanine (G)**, **thymine (T)**, and **uracil (U)**.

DNA is organized according to the **Watson-Crick model**. The backbone is composed of alternating sugar and phosphate groups and is always read **5′** to **3′**. There are two strands with **antiparallel** polarity, wound into a **double helix**. **Purines** (A and G) always pair with **pyrimidines** (C, U, and T). In DNA, A pairs with T (via two hydrogen bonds) and C pairs with G (via three hydrogen bonds). RNA does not contain thymine but contains uracil instead; thus, in RNA, A pairs with U (via two hydrogen bonds). **Chargaff's rules** state that purines and pyrimidines are equal in number in a DNA molecule. Because of base pairing, the amount of adenine equals the amount of thymine and the amount of cytosine equals the amount of guanine.

DNA strands can be pulled apart (**denatured**) and brought back together (**reannealed**). Heat, alkaline pH, and chemicals like formaldehyde and urea can cause denaturation of DNA; removal of these conditions may result in reannealing of the strands.

DNA is organized into 46 chromosomes in human cells. In eukaryotes, DNA is wound around **histone proteins** (H2A, H2B, H3, and H4) to form **nucleosomes**, which may be stabilized by another histone protein (H1). As a whole, DNA and its associated histones make up **chromatin** in the nucleus. **Heterochromatin** is dense, transcriptionally silent DNA that appears dark under light microscopy. **Euchromatin** is less dense, transcriptionally active DNA that appears light under light microscopy.

Telomeres are the ends of chromosomes. They contain a high GC content to prevent unraveling of the DNA. During replication, telomeres are slightly shortened, although this can be (partially) reversed by the enzyme telomerase. **Centromeres** are located in the middle of chromosomes and hold sister chromatids together until they are separated during anaphase in mitosis. They also contain a high GC content to maintain a strong bond between chromatids.

DNA Replication

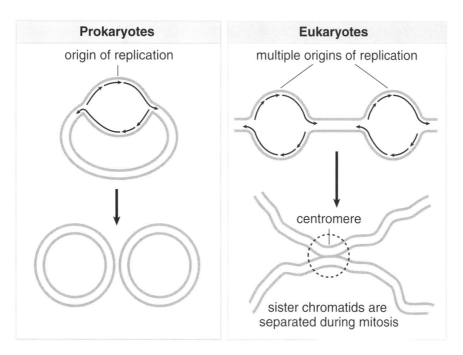

Figure 9.3. DNA Replication in Prokaryotes and Eukaryotes

The **replisome** (**replication complex**) is a set of specialized proteins that assist the DNA polymerases. To replicate DNA, it is first unwound at an **origin of replication** by **helicases**. This produces two **replication forks** on either side of the origin. Prokaryotes have a circular chromosome that contains only one origin of replication. Eukaryotes have linear chromosomes that contain many origins of replication. DNA replication is **semiconservative**: one old **parent strand** and one new **daughter strand** is incorporated into each of the two new DNA molecules. (See Figure 9.3.)

Unwound strands are kept from reannealing or being degraded by **single-stranded DNA-binding proteins**. **Super-coiling** causes torsional strain on the DNA molecule, which can be released by **DNA topoisomerases** that create nicks in the DNA molecule. DNA cannot be synthesized without an adjacent nucleotide to hook onto, so a small RNA primer is put down by **primase**.

DNA polymerase III (in prokaryotes) or **DNA polymerase** α, δ, and ε (in eukaryotes) can then synthesize a new strand of DNA; they read the template DNA 3' to 5' and synthesize the new strand 5' to 3'. The **leading strand** requires only one primer and can then be synthesized continuously in its entirety. The **lagging strand** requires many primers and is synthesized in discrete sections called **Okazaki fragments**.

RNA primers can later be removed by **DNA polymerase I** (in prokaryotes) or **RNase H** (in eukaryotes) and can be filled in with DNA by DNA polymerase I (in prokaryotes) or DNA polymerase δ (in eukaryotes). **DNA ligase** can then fuse the DNA strands together to create one complete molecule. (See Figure 9.4.)

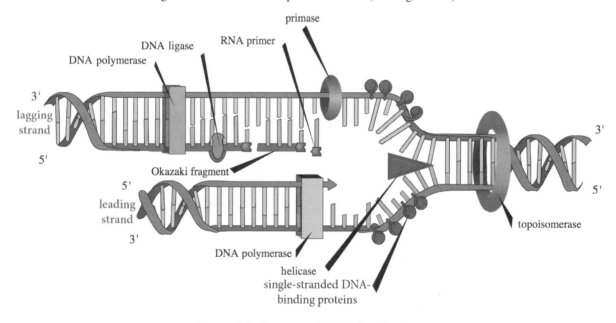

Figure 9.4. Enzymes of DNA Replication

DNA Repair

Oncogenes develop from mutations of **proto-oncogenes** and promote cell cycling. They may lead to **cancer**, which is defined by unchecked cell proliferation with the ability to spread by local invasion or **metastasize** (migrate to distant sites via the bloodstream or lymphatic system). **Tumor suppressor genes** code for proteins that reduce cell cycling or promote DNA repair; mutations of tumor suppressor genes can also lead to cancer.

During replication, DNA polymerase **proofreads** its work and excises incorrectly matched bases. The daughter strand is identified by its lack of methylation and corrected accordingly. **Mismatch repair** also occurs during the G_2 phase of the cell cycle, using the genes *MSH2* and *MLH1*. **Nucleotide excision repair** fixes helix-deforming lesions of DNA (such as thymine dimers) via a cut-and-patch process that requires an **excision endonuclease**. **Base excision repair** fixes nondeforming lesions of the DNA helix (such as cytosine deamination) by removing the base, leaving an **apurinic/apyrimidinic (AP) site**. An **AP endonuclease** then removes the damaged sequence, which can be filled in with the correct bases.

Recombinant DNA and Biotechnology

Recombinant DNA is DNA composed of nucleotides from two different sources. **DNA cloning** introduces a fragment of DNA into a **vector plasmid**. **A restriction enzyme (restriction endonuclease)** cuts both the plasmid and the fragment, which are left with **sticky ends**. Once the fragment binds to the plasmid, it can be introduced into a bacterial cell and permitted to replicate, generating many copies of the fragment of interest. Vectors contain an origin of replication, the fragment of interest, and at least one gene for antibiotic resistance (to permit for selection of that colony after replication). Once replicated, the bacterial cells can be used to create a protein of interest, or they can be lysed to allow for isolation of the fragment of interest from the vector.

DNA libraries are large collections of known DNA sequences. **Genomic libraries** contain large fragments of DNA, including both coding and noncoding regions of the genome. They cannot be used to make recombinant proteins or for gene therapy. **cDNA libraries (expression libraries)** contain smaller fragments of DNA and include only the exons of genes expressed by the sample tissue. They can be used to make recombinant proteins or for gene therapy.

Hybridization is the joining of complementary base pair sequences. **Polymerase chain reaction (PCR)** is an automated process by which millions of copies of a DNA sequence can be created from a very small sample by hybridization.

DNA molecules can be separated by size using **agarose gel electrophoresis**. **Southern blotting** can be used to detect the presence and quantity of various DNA strands in a sample. After electrophoresis, the sample is transferred to a membrane that can be **probed** with single-stranded DNA molecules to look for a sequence of interest.

DNA sequencing uses **dideoxyribonucleotides**, which terminate the DNA chain because they lack a $3' -OH$ group. The resulting fragments can be separated by gel electrophoresis, and the sequence can be read directly from the gel.

Gene therapy is a method of curing genetic deficiencies by introducing a functional gene with a viral vector. **Transgenic mice** are created by integrating a gene of interest into the germ line or embryonic stem cells of a developing mouse. Organisms that contain cells from two different lineages (such as mice formed by integration of transgenic embryonic stem cells into a normal mouse blastocyst) are called **chimeras**. Transgenic mice can be mated to select for the transgene. Transgenic organisms are created through the introduction of a gene of interest, whereas **knockout organisms** are created by deleting a gene of interest. Biotechnology brings up a number of safety and ethical issues, including pathogen resistance and the ethics of choosing individuals for specific traits.

THE CENTRAL DOGMA OF GENETICS

The Genetic Code and Transcription

The **central dogma** states that DNA is transcribed to RNA, which is translated to protein. Every three nucleotide bases codes for an amino acid, and a degenerate code allows multiple codons to encode for the same amino acid. AUG is the initiation (start) codon, and UAA, UGA, and UAG are all termination (stop) codons. Redundancy and the **wobble** factor at the third nucleotide base in the codon allow mutations to occur without affecting the protein formed.

Point mutations can cause **silent** mutations with no effect on protein synthesis, **nonsense** (**truncation**) mutations that produce a premature stop codon, or **missense** mutations that produce a codon that codes for a different amino acid. **Frameshift mutations** result from nucleotide addition or deletion, and they change the reading frame of subsequent codons.

RNA is structurally similar to DNA except RNA has ribose sugar instead of deoxyribose and uracil in place of thymine; RNA is also single stranded, unlike double-stranded DNA. The three types of RNA have separate jobs in transcription. **Messenger RNA (mRNA)** carries the message from DNA in the nucleus via transcription of the gene; it travels into the cytoplasm to be translated. **Transfer RNA (tRNA)** brings in amino acids and recognizes the codon on the mRNA using the tRNA's anticodon. **Ribosomal RNA (rRNA)** makes up the ribosome and is enzymatically active.

During **transcription, helicase** unwinds the DNA double helix, and **RNA polymerase II** binds to the **TATA box** within the **promoter** region of the gene (25 base pairs upstream from first transcribed base). Then **hnRNA** is synthesized from the DNA template (antisense) strand. Once the new strand is completed, it undergoes several post-transcriptional modifications. A 7-methylguanylate triphosphate cap is added to the 5′ end, and a polyadenosyl (poly-A) tail is added to the 3′ end. The transcript is also spliced by snRNA and snRNPs in the **spliceosome**; introns are removed in a **lariat** structure, and exons are ligated together. Prokaryotic cells can increase the variability of gene products from one transcript through **polycistronic genes** (in which starting transcription in different sites within the gene leads to different gene products). Eukaryotic cells can increase variability of gene products through **alternative splicing** (combining different exons in a modular fashion to acquire different gene products).

Translation

There are three stages of **translation** (protein synthesis), which primarily occur at the ribosome. (See Figure 9.5.)

- **Initiation** in prokaryotes occurs when the 30S ribosome attaches to the **Shine-Dalgarno sequence** and scans for a start codon; it lays down *N*-formylmethionine in the P site of the ribosome. Initiation in eukaryotes occurs when the 40S ribosome attaches to the 5′ cap and scans for a start codon; it lays down methionine in the P site of the ribosome.

- **Elongation** involves the addition of a new aminoacyl-tRNA into the A site of the ribosome and transfer of the growing polypeptide chain from the tRNA in the P site to the tRNA in the A site. The now uncharged tRNA pauses in the E site before exiting the ribosome.

- **Termination** occurs when the codon in the A site is a stop codon; a **release factor** places a water molecule onto the polypeptide chain and thus releases the protein. Post-translational modifications include folding by **chaperones**, formation of a protein's quaternary structure, cleavage of proteins or signal sequences, and covalent addition of other biomolecules (phosphorylation, carboxylation, glycosylation, prenylation).

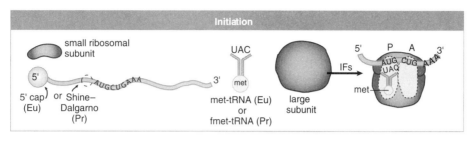

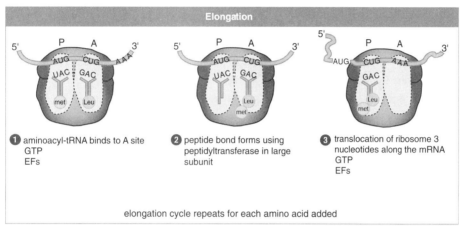

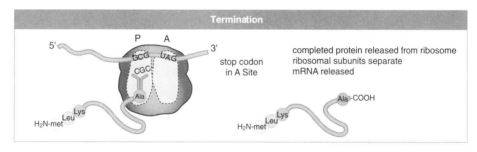

Figure 9.5. Steps in Translation

Control of Gene Expression in Prokaryotes

The **Jacob-Monod model** of repressors and activators explains that **operons** are inducible or repressible clusters of genes transcribed as a single mRNA. **Inducible systems** (such as the *lac* operon) are bonded to a **repressor** under normal conditions; they can be turned on by an **inducer** pulling the repressor from the **operator site**. **Repressible systems** (such as the *trp* operon) are transcribed under normal conditions; they can be turned off by a corepressor coupling with the repressor and the binding of this complex to the operator site.

Control of Gene Expression in Eukaryotes

Transcription factors search for promoter and enhancer regions in the DNA. **Promoters** are within 25 base pairs of the transcription start site, while **enhancers** are more than 25 base pairs away from the transcription start site. Modification of chromatin structure affects the ability of transcriptional enzymes to access the DNA through histone acetylation (increases accessibility) or DNA methylation (decreases accessibility).

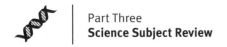

BIOLOGICAL MEMBRANES

`High-Yield`

The **fluid mosaic model** accounts for the presence of lipids, proteins, and carbohydrates in a dynamic, semisolid plasma membrane that surrounds cells. The plasma membrane contains proteins embedded within the **phospholipid bilayer**. Lipids move freely in the plane of the membrane and can assemble into **lipid rafts**. **Flippases** are specific membrane proteins that maintain the bidirectional transport of lipids between the layers of the phospholipid bilayer in cells. Proteins and carbohydrates may also move within the membrane but are slowed by their relatively large size.

Lipids are the primary membrane component, both by mass and mole fraction. **Triacylglycerols** and **free fatty acids** act as phospholipid precursors and are found in low levels in the membrane. **Glycerophospholipids** replace one fatty acid with a phosphate group, which is often linked to other hydrophilic groups. **Cholesterol** is present in large amounts and contributes to membrane fluidity and stability. **Waxes** are present in very small amounts, if at all; they are most prevalent in plants and function in waterproofing and defense.

Proteins located within the cell membrane act as transporters, cell adhesion molecules, and enzymes. **Transmembrane proteins** can have one or more hydrophobic domains and are most likely to function as receptors or channels. **Embedded proteins** are most likely part of a catalytic complex or involved in cellular communication. **Membrane-associated proteins** may act as recognition molecules or enzymes.

Carbohydrates can form a protective **glycoprotein coat** and also function in cell recognition. Extracellular ligands can bind to membrane receptors, which function as channels or enzymes in second messenger pathways. Cell-cell junctions regulate transport intracellularly and intercellularly. **Gap junctions** allow for the rapid exchange of ions and other small molecules between adjacent cells. **Tight junctions** prevent **paracellular** transport but do not provide intercellular transport. **Desmosomes** and **hemidesmosomes** anchor layers of epithelial tissue together.

Concentration gradients help to determine appropriate membrane transport mechanisms in cells. (See Table 9.3.) **Osmotic pressure**, a **colligative property**, is the pressure applied to a pure solvent to prevent osmosis and is used to express the concentration of the solution.

- **Passive transport** does not require energy because the molecule is moving down its concentration gradient or from an area with higher concentration to an area with lower concentration.
- **Endocytosis** and **exocytosis** are methods of engulfing material into cells or releasing material to the exterior of cells, both via the cell membrane.
- **Pinocytosis** is the ingestion of liquid into the cell in vesicles formed from the cell membrane, and **phagocytosis** is the ingestion of larger, solid molecules.

	Simple Diffusion	Osmosis	Facilitated Diffusion	Active Transport
Concentration gradient of solute	High → Low	Low → High	High → Low	Low → High
Membrane protein required	No	No	Yes	Yes
Energy required	No—this is a passive process	No—this is a passive process	No—this is a passive process	Yes—this is an active process; requires energy
Example molecule(s) transported	Small, nonpolar (O_2, CO_2)	H_2O	Polar molecules (glucose) or ions (Na^+, Cl^-)	Polar molecules or ions (Na^+, Cl^-, K^+)

Table 9.3. Membrane Transport Processes

The composition of cell membranes is fairly consistent; however, some cells contain specialized membranes. For instance in nerves, a **membrane potential** is maintained by the sodium-potassium pump and leak channels. The electrical potential created by one ion can be calculated using the **Nernst equation**, while the resting potential of a membrane at physiological temperature can be calculated using the **Goldman-Hodgkin-Katz voltage equation**, which is derived from the Nernst equation. Membranes have multiple functions and therefore may differ in permeability, conductivity, and composition.

CARBOHYDRATE METABOLISM

GLUT 2 has a high K_m and is found in the liver (for glucose storage) and pancreatic β-islet cells (as part of the glucose sensor). **GLUT 4** has a low K_m and is found in adipose tissue and muscle and is stimulated by insulin.

Glycolysis

`High-Yield`

Glycolysis occurs in the cytoplasm of all cells and does not require oxygen. It yields 2 ATP per molecule of glucose.

- **Glucokinase** converts glucose to glucose 6-phosphate. It is present in the pancreatic β-islet cells as part of the glucose sensor and is responsive to insulin in the liver. **Hexokinase** converts glucose to glucose 6-phosphate in peripheral tissues.
- **Phosphofructokinase-1** (**PFK-1**) phosphorylates fructose 6-phosphate to fructose 1,6-bisphosphate in the rate-limiting step of glycolysis. PFK-1 is activated by AMP and fructose 2,6-bisphosphate (F2,6-BP) and is inhibited by ATP and citrate. **Phosphofructokinase-2** (**PFK-2**), which produces the F2,6-BP that activates PFK-1, is activated by insulin and inhibited by glucagon.
- **Glyceraldehyde-3-phosphate dehydrogenase** produces NADH, which can feed into the electron transport chain.
- **3-phosphoglycerate kinase** and **pyruvate kinase** each perform **substrate-level phosphorylation**, placing an inorganic phosphate (P_i) onto ADP to form ATP.

Glucokinase/hexokinase, PFK-1, and pyruvate kinase catalyze irreversible reactions. The NADH produced in glycolysis is oxidized by the mitochondrial electron transport chain when oxygen is present. If oxygen or mitochondria are absent, the NADH produced in glycolysis is oxidized by cytoplasmic **lactate dehydrogenase**. This occurs, for example, in red blood cells, skeletal muscle (during short, intense bursts of exercise), and any cell deprived of oxygen.

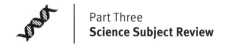

Glycogenesis and Glycogenolysis

Pyruvate dehydrogenase refers to a complex of enzymes that convert pyruvate to acetyl-CoA. It is stimulated by insulin and inhibited by acetyl-CoA. **Glycogenesis** (glycogen synthesis) is the production of glycogen using two main enzymes: glycogen synthase and branching enzyme. **Glycogen synthase** creates α-1,4 glycosidic links between glucose molecules when activated by insulin in liver and muscle; **branching enzyme** moves a block of oligoglucose from one chain and adds it to the growing glycogen as a new branch using an α-1,6 glycosidic link. **Glycogenolysis** is the breakdown of glycogen using two main enzymes: glycogen phosphorylase and debranching enzyme. **Glycogen phosphorylase** removes single glucose 1-phosphate molecules by breaking α-1,4 glycosidic links. In the liver, it is activated by glucagon to prevent low blood sugar; in exercising skeletal muscle, it is activated by epinephrine and AMP to provide glucose for the muscle itself. **Debranching enzyme** moves a block of oligoglucose from one branch and connects it to the chain using an α-1,4 glycosidic link and removes the branch-point, which is connected via an α-1,6 glycosidic link, releasing a free glucose molecule.

Gluconeogenesis occurs in both the cytoplasm and mitochondria, predominantly in the liver. Most of gluconeogenesis is simply the reverse of glycolysis, using the same enzymes. The three irreversible steps of glycolysis must be bypassed by different enzymes.

- First, **pyruvate carboxylase** converts pyruvate into oxaloacetate, which is converted to phosphoenolpyruvate by **phosphoenolpyruvate carboxykinase** (**PEPCK**). Together, these two enzymes bypass pyruvate kinase. Pyruvate carboxylase is activated by acetyl-CoA from β-oxidation; PEPCK is activated by glucagon and cortisol.
- Next, **fructose 1,6-bisphosphatase** converts fructose 1,6-bisphosphate to fructose 6-phosphate, bypassing phosphofructokinase-1. This is the rate-limiting step of gluconeogenesis. It is activated by ATP directly and by glucagon indirectly (via decreased levels of fructose 2,6-bisphosphate). It is inhibited by AMP directly and insulin indirectly (via increased levels of fructose 2,6-bisphosphate).
- Last, **glucose 6-phosphatase** converts glucose 6-phosphate to free glucose, bypassing glucokinase. It is found only in the endoplasmic reticulum of the liver.

The Pentose Phosphate Pathway and Acetyl-CoA

The **pentose phosphate pathway** (**PPP**), also known as the **hexose monophosphate** (**HMP**) **shunt**, occurs in the cytoplasm of most cells, generating **NADPH** and sugars for biosynthesis (derived from ribulose 5-phosphate). The rate-limiting enzyme is **glucose 6-phosphate dehydrogenase**, which is activated by NADP+ and insulin and which is inhibited by NADPH.

Acetyl-CoA contains a high-energy thioester bond that can be used to drive other reactions when hydrolysis occurs. **Pyruvate dehydrogenase complex** is a five-enzyme complex in the mitochondrial matrix that forms—and is also inhibited by—acetyl-CoA and NADH. **Pyruvate dehydrogenase** (PDH) oxidizes pyruvate. **Dihydrolipoyl transacetylase** oxidizes the remaining two-carbon molecule using lipoic acid and transfers the resulting acetyl group to CoA, forming acetyl-CoA. **Dihydrolipoyl dehydrogenase** uses FAD to reoxidize lipoic acid, forming $FADH_2$. This $FADH_2$ can later transfer electrons to NAD^+, forming NADH that can feed into the electron transport chain. **Pyruvate dehydrogenase kinase** phosphorylates PDH when ATP or acetyl-CoA levels are high, turning it off. **Pyruvate dehydrogenase phosphatase** dephosphorylates PDH when ADP levels are high, turning it on.

Acetyl-CoA can be formed from fatty acids, which enter the mitochondria using carriers. The fatty acid couples with CoA in the cytosol to form fatty acyl-CoA, which moves to the intermembrane space. The acyl group is transferred to carnitine to form acyl-carnitine, which crosses the inner membrane. The acyl group is transferred to a mitochondrial CoA to re-form fatty acyl-CoA, which can undergo β-oxidation to form acetyl-CoA. Acetyl-CoA can also be formed from the carbon skeletons of ketogenic amino acids, ketone bodies, and alcohol.

REACTIONS OF THE CITRIC ACID CYCLE

The **citric acid cycle**, as shown in Figure 9.6, takes place in the mitochondrial matrix. Its main purpose is to oxidize carbons in intermediates to CO_2 and generate high-energy electron carriers (NADH and $FADH_2$) and GTP.

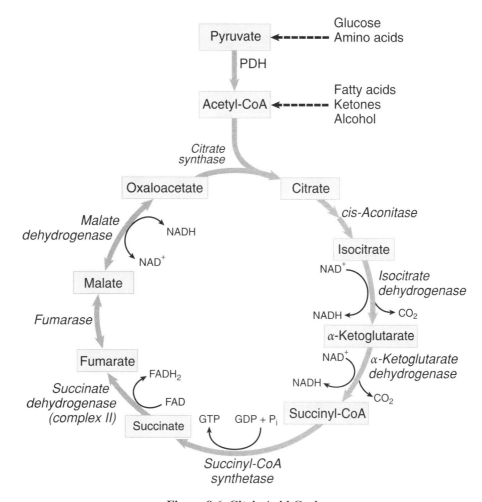

Figure 9.6 Citric Acid Cycle

THE ELECTRON TRANSPORT CHAIN

The **electron transport chain** (ETC) takes place on the matrix-facing surface of the inner mitochondrial membrane (see Figure 9.7). NADH donates electrons to the chain, which are passed from one complex to the next. As the ETC progresses, reduction potentials increase until oxygen, which has the highest reduction potential, receives the electrons.

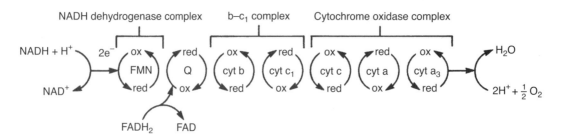

Figure 9.7. Electron Transport Chain

- **Complex I** (**NADH-CoQ oxidoreductase**) uses an iron-sulfur cluster to transfer electrons from NADH to flavin mononucleotide (FMN) and then to **coenzyme Q** (**CoQ**), forming $CoQH_2$. Four protons are translocated by Complex I.
- **Complex II** (**succinate-CoQ oxidoreductase**) uses an iron-sulfur cluster to transfer electrons from succinate to FAD and then to CoQ, forming $CoQH_2$. No proton pumping occurs at Complex II.
- **Complex III** (**$CoQH_2$-cytochrome *c* oxidoreductase**) uses an iron-sulfur cluster to transfer electrons from $CoQH_2$ to heme, forming cytochrome *c* as part of the **Q cycle**. Four protons are translocated by Complex III.
- **Complex IV** (**cytochrome *c* oxidase**) uses cytochromes and Cu^{2+} to transfer electrons in the form of hydride ions (H^-) from cytochrome *c* to oxygen, forming water. Two protons are translocated by Complex IV.

NADH cannot cross the inner mitochondrial membrane. Therefore, one of two available shuttle mechanisms to transfer electrons in the mitochondrial matrix must be used. In the **glycerol 3-phosphate shuttle**, electrons are transferred from NADH to dihydroxyacetone phosphate (DHAP), forming glycerol 3-phosphate. These electrons can then be transferred to mitochondrial FAD, forming $FADH_2$. In the **malate-aspartate shuttle**, electrons are transferred from NADH to oxaloacetate, forming malate. Malate can then cross the inner mitochondrial membrane and transfer the electrons to mitochondrial NAD^+, forming NADH.

OXIDATIVE PHOSPHORYLATION

`High-Yield ◀◀`

The **proton-motive force** is the electrochemical gradient generated by the electron transport chain across the inner mitochondrial membrane. The intermembrane space has a higher concentration of protons than the matrix; this gradient stores energy, which can be used to form ATP via **chemiosmotic coupling**. **ATP synthase** generates ATP from ADP and an inorganic phosphate (P_i). The **F_0 portion** is an ion channel, allowing protons to flow down the gradient from the intermembrane space to the matrix. The **F_1 portion** uses the energy released by the gradient to phosphorylate ADP into ATP.

The following is a summary of the energy yield of the various carbohydrate metabolism processes:

- Glycolysis generates 2 NADH and 2 ATP.
- Pyruvate dehydrogenase generates 1 NADH per molecule of pyruvate. Because each glucose forms two molecules of pyruvate, this complex produces a net of 2 NADH.
- The citric acid cycle generates 3 NADH, 1 $FADH_2$, and 1 GTP (6 NADH, 2 $FADH_2$, and 2 GTP per molecule of glucose).
- Each NADH yields 2.5 ATP; 10 NADH form 25 ATP.
- Each $FADH_2$ yields 1.5 ATP; 2 $FADH_2$ form 3 ATP.

- GTP is converted to ATP.
- 2 ATP from glycolysis + 2 ATP (GTP) from the citric acid cycle + 25 ATP from NADH + 3 ATP from $FADH_2$ = 32 ATP per molecule of glucose (optimal). Inefficiencies of the system and variability between cells make 30–32 ATP/glucose, which is the commonly accepted range for energy yield.

LIPID DIGESTION AND ABSORPTION

Mechanical digestion of lipids occurs primarily in the mouth and stomach. In contrast, chemical digestion of lipids occurs in the small intestine and is facilitated by **bile**, **pancreatic lipase**, **colipase**, and **cholesterol esterase**. Digested lipids may form **micelles** for absorption or be absorbed directly. Short-chain fatty acids are absorbed across the intestine into the blood, whereas long-chain fatty acids are absorbed as micelles and assembled into **chylomicrons** for release into the lymphatic system. **Hormone-sensitive lipase** mobilizes lipids from adipocytes, **while lipoprotein lipase** mobilizes lipids from lipoproteins.

Chylomicrons transport dietary triacylglycerol molecules and are transported via the lymphatic system. **VLDL** transports newly synthesized triacylglycerol molecules from the liver to peripheral tissues in the bloodstream. **LDL** primarily transports cholesterol for use by tissues, while **HDL** is involved in the reverse transport of cholesterol. **Apoproteins** control interactions between lipoproteins. (See Figure 9.8.)

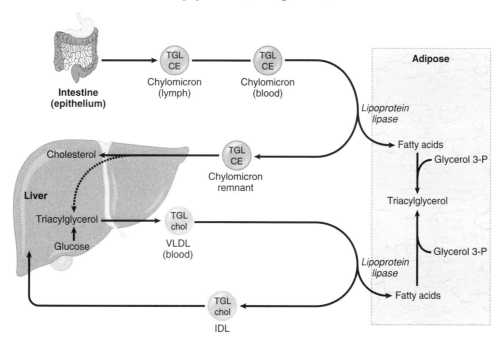

Figure 9.8. Lipid Transport in Lipoproteins
TGL = triacylglycerol; CE = cholesterylesters; chol = cholesterol

Cholesterol may be obtained through dietary sources or through de novo synthesis in the liver via **HMG-CoA reductase**. **LCAT** catalyzes the formation of cholesteryl esters for transport with HDL. **CETP** catalyzes the transition of IDL to LDL by transferring cholesteryl esters from HDL.

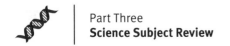
Fatty acids are carboxylic acids, typically with a single long chain, although they can be branched. **Saturated fatty acids** have no double bonds between carbons. **Unsaturated fatty acids** have one or more double bonds. Fatty acids are synthesized in the cytoplasm from acetyl-CoA transported out of the mitochondria. Synthesis includes five steps: activation, bond formation, reduction, dehydration, and a second reduction. These steps are repeated eight times to form **palmitic acid**, the only fatty acid that humans can synthesize.

Fatty acid oxidation occurs in the mitochondria following transport by the carnitine shuttle; β-**oxidation** uses cycles of oxidation, hydration, oxidation, and cleavage. Branched and unsaturated fatty acids require special enzymes. Unsaturated fatty acids use **isomerase** and **reductase** during cleavage.

KETONE AND PROTEIN CATABOLISM

Ketone bodies form (**ketogenesis**) during a prolonged starvation state due to excess acetyl-CoA in the liver. **Ketolysis** regenerates acetyl-CoA for use as an energy source in peripheral tissues. The brain can derive up to two-thirds of its energy from ketone bodies during prolonged starvation.

Protein digestion occurs primarily in the small intestine. Catabolism of cellular proteins occurs only under conditions of starvation. Carbon skeletons of amino acids are used for energy, through either gluconeogenesis or ketone body formation. Amino groups are fed into the **urea cycle** for excretion. The fate of a side chain depends on its chemistry.

BIOENERGETICS AND REGULATION OF METABOLISM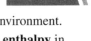

Biological systems are considered **open** when both matter and energy can be exchanged with the environment. They are considered closed when only energy can be exchanged with the environment. Changes in **enthalpy** in a closed biological system are equal to changes in **internal energy**, which is equal to **heat exchange** within the environment. No work is performed in a closed biological system because pressure and volume remain constant. **Entropy** is a measure of energy dispersion in a system. Of note, physiological concentrations are usually much less than standard concentrations.

ATP is a midlevel energy molecule containing high-energy phosphate bonds that are stabilized upon hydrolysis by resonance, ionization, and loss of charge repulsion. ATP provides energy through **hydrolysis** and **coupling** to energetically unfavorable reactions, or as a phosphate donor.

Biological **oxidation** and **reduction** reactions can be broken down into component **half-reactions**. Half-reactions provide useful information about stoichiometry and thermodynamics. Many oxidation-reduction reactions involve an electron carrier to transport high-energy electrons. **Electron carriers** may be soluble or membrane bound.

Equilibrium is an undesirable state for most biochemical reactions because organisms need to harness free energy to survive. In the **postprandial/well-fed** (**absorptive**) state, insulin secretion is high and anabolic metabolism prevails. In the short-term **postabsorptive** (**fasting**) state, insulin secretion decreases while glucagon and catecholamine secretion increases. Prolonged fasting (**starvation**) dramatically increases glucagon and catecholamine secretion. (See Table 9.4.)

- **Insulin** and **glucagon** have opposing activities during most aspects of metabolism. Insulin causes a decrease in blood glucose levels by increasing cellular uptake, and it increases the rate of anabolic metabolism.
- **Glucocorticoids** increase blood glucose in response to stress by mobilizing fat stores and inhibiting glucose uptake. Insulin is secreted by pancreatic β-cells in response to high blood glucose levels, while glucagon is secreted by pancreatic α-cells due to low glucose and high amino acid levels.
- **Glucocorticoids** increase blood glucose in response to stress by mobilizing fat stores and inhibiting glucose uptake. They increase the impact of glucagon and catecholamines.
- **Catecholamines** promote glycogenolysis and increase basal metabolic rate through sympathetic nervous system activity.
- **Thyroid hormones** modulate other metabolic hormones and have a direct impact on basal metabolic rate.

Organ	Well-Fed	Fasting
Liver	Glucose and amino acids	Fatty acids
Resting skeletal muscle	Glucose	Fatty acids, ketones
Cardiac muscle	Fatty acids	Fatty acids, ketones
Adipose tissue	Glucose	Fatty acids
Brain	Glucose	Glucose (ketones in prolonged fast)
Red blood cells	Glucose	Glucose

Table 9.4. Preferred Fuels in the Well-Fed and Fasting States for Specific Tissues

Metabolic rates can be measured using **calorimetry**, **respirometry**, consumption tracking, or measurement of blood concentrations of substrates and hormones. The composition of fuel that is actively consumed by the body is estimated by the **respiratory quotient** (**RQ**). Body mass regulation is multifactorial with consumption and activity as modifiable factors. The hormones **leptin**, **ghrelin**, and **orexin**, as well as their receptors, play a role in body mass. Long-term changes in body mass result from changes in lipid storage. Changes in consumption or activity must surpass a **threshold** to cause weight change. The threshold is lower for weight gain than for weight loss.

9.5 Biochemistry Worked Examples

The following steps will walk you through the following passage using the Kaplan Passage Strategy.

PREVIEW FOR DIFFICULTY

Start by quickly glancing at the passage. Note "mitochondrial" in the first sentence and in the figure caption. By glancing at the first few nouns and verbs of each paragraph, you can see that you are dealing with mitochondrial *regulation*. The figure shows three ion carriers, so it's likely that the passage is going to describe each of them. There doesn't appear to be experimental data, so this is likely an information passage.

CHOOSE YOUR APPROACH

Information passages tend to describe a topic that is tangentially related to, but slightly beyond the scope of, required MCAT content. These can be intimidating because of the new information. Rest assured, though, that the MCAT tests basic science and critical thinking! Given that this is an information passage, **Outlining** should be chosen.

READ AND DISTILL

P1: This paragraph introduces calcium's role in mitochondrial function. Increases in calcium levels stimulate several enzymes. There's also a contrast keyword ("however") right in the middle, indicating a shift. As it turns out, too much calcium can be damaging. There's also a mention of heart attacks at the end; this could be insignificant or could be part of a theme.
Outline: Calcium affects mitochondrial activity

P2: The second paragraph starts with "several proteins" and then introduces only one: mCU. At this point, you might take a quick look at the other paragraphs. "Another protein" is mentioned in the third paragraph and potentially yet another in the last paragraph. A glance at the figure confirms that these are the three ion carriers. The figure summarizes the movement of ions, so it might be a useful reference. Details are given about mCU, but those details will still be there if we get asked a question about mCU. So there is no need to write them all down.
Outline: mCU moves calcium into matrix

P3: The third paragraph talks about another protein, NCX, and the details of its function. Again there's no sense in getting bogged down by the details—just note the details that stand out. Interestingly, NCX is found in the plasma membrane of *cardiac* myocytes.
Outline: NCX antiporter: 3 Na^+ for 1 Ca^{2+}

P4: The final paragraph mentions the last ion carrier, and this time it's only indirectly related to calcium. There's also a note at the end of the paragraph, which might be a key piece of information for a question.
Outline: NHE antiporter: 1 Na^+ for 1 H^+

F1: The figure provides a succinct overview of the ion carriers. This could be a useful first stop when asked a question about ion movement.
Outline: Ion carriers in inner mitochondrial membrane

PASSAGE I: OXIDATIVE PHOSPHORYLATION

Mitochondrial function is heavily regulated by calcium ions. When cytosolic Ca^{2+} levels increase, that increase is transmitted to the mitochondria, where Ca^{2+} stimulates the activity of α-ketoglutarate dehydrogenase, isocitrate dehydrogenase, and pyruvate dehydrogenase. Excessive mitochondrial Ca^{2+}, however, can trigger mitochondrial release of cytochrome c. Derangements of mitochondrial Ca^{2+} are believed to play a role in damage to the heart muscle that results from the changes in blood flow that occur in heart attacks.

Several proteins are involved in regulating mitochondrial calcium levels. One of these is the *mitochondrial calcium uniporter* (mCU). mCU, which has low affinity for Ca^{2+} but a high capacity, allows passive transport of Ca^{2+} into the mitochondrial matrix. This occurs because there is a large voltage gradient across the inner mitochondrial membrane (approximately -200 mV on the matrix side).

Another protein that regulates mitochondrial Ca^{2+} is the *sodium-calcium exchanger* (NCX). This antiport protein is found both in the inner mitochondrial membrane and in the plasma membrane of cardiac myocytes. In its normal "forward" mode, NCX removes one Ca^{2+} ion from the mitochondrial matrix and allows three Na^+ to enter. In its "reverse" mode, NCX brings one Ca^{2+} ion into the matrix and removes three Na^+.

The flow of sodium ions across the inner mitochondrial membrane is intimately linked to the flow of protons by the *sodium-proton exchanger* (NHE), which can also run in reverse. Therefore, the flow of calcium also affects the flow of protons across the inner mitochondrial membrane, as depicted schematically in Figure 1. Note that because of pores in the outer mitochondrial membrane, ion concentrations in the intermembrane space are essentially identical with those in the cytosol.

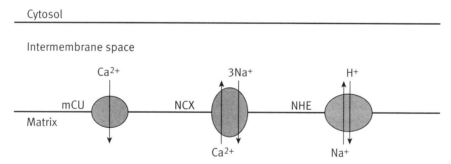

Figure 1. Ion carriers in the inner mitochondrial membrane

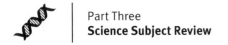

KEY CONCEPT

Membrane potential
Oxidative phosphorylation

---

1. Based on information in the passage, which of the following is the most likely explanation for why the forward mode of NCX transports three Na^+ ions into the matrix for every one Ca^{2+} ion it transports out?

   A. As a result, the antiporter does not consume ATP.
   B. NCX evolved from the Na^+/K^+ ATPase.
   C. It reduces the tendency of Ca^{2+} to reenter the matrix.
   D. It enhances ATP synthase's ability to produce ATP.

❶ Type the question

The words *most likely* in the question stem are a sign that we are expected to reason out the answer to this question. This question wants to know the reason why NCX exhibits a 3:1 charge ratio. When we see a *why* question, we should always ask ourselves two questions about the correct answer: Is it true? Is it relevant? If the answer to either question is no, we can eliminate that answer choice. Answer choices are short, with no obvious pattern.

❷ Rephrase the question stem

As the question mentions a transporter that is not a part of content background, this question does require passage information. When Rephrased it asks, *Why does NCX transport 3 Na^+ out for 1 Ca^{2+} in?*

❸ Investigate potential solutions

As the question stem notes, NCX normally ejects one Ca^{2+} ion for every three Na^+ ions that enter the matrix. The net result of this is that each time NCX operates in the forward mode, it moves a charge into the matrix.

Paragraph 2 of the passage states that there is large gradient across the inner mitochondrial membrane, with the matrix side at -200 mV; this drives the passive flow of Ca^{2+} into the matrix through the mCU.

By combining these two facts, we can predict that each time the NCX fires in its forward mode, the inner mitochondrial membrane is depolarized: the gradient becomes smaller. Our correct answer should deal, in some way, with this decrease in the membrane potential.

④ Match your prediction to an answer choice

(A) is true, but it is irrelevant; the question asks why NCX works the way it does.

(B) says that NCX evolved from the sodium-potassium pump. This might sound tempting—after all, the sodium-potassium pump moves three Na^+ ions out of the cell to move two K^+ ions into the cell. It's a stretch, though, to reach the conclusion that NCX evolved from it, as this is unsupported by the passage. **(B)** is incorrect.

(C) fits the bill. If we're ejecting Ca^{2+} from the matrix, we don't want it to just reenter the matrix again. Depolarizing the membrane would reduce the tendency of Ca^{2+} to enter the matrix via the mCU, which would prevent that from happening. **(C)** is the correct answer.

(D), on the other hand, is simply false. The chemiosmotic hypothesis states that ATP synthesis depends on the existence of a gradient across the inner mitochondrial membrane. Depolarizing that membrane would tend to reduce ATP synthase's ability to make ATP, not increase it, and is incorrect.

---

2. Based on information in the passage, mCU most likely has:

   A. a relatively high K_m value and a relatively high v_{max}.
   B. a relatively high K_m value and a relatively low v_{max}.
   C. a relatively low K_m value and a relatively high v_{max}.
   D. a relatively low K_m value and a relatively low v_{max}.

KEY CONCEPT

Enzyme kinetics

---

① Type the question

The question asks for information regarding the kinetics of mCU from the passage. There is a 2×2 pattern in the answer choices, varying between high/low K_m and v_{max}.

② Rephrase the question stem

This question requires you to connect information about mCU and apply it to kinetics. When Rephrased it asks, *Does mCU have high or low K_m and v_{max}?*

③ Investigate potential solutions

mCU is discussed in paragraph 2, where we're told that mCU has a low affinity for calcium ions but a high capacity. The passage doesn't tell us, though, how that correlates to K_m and v_{max}. So we'll need to pull those from memory.

Of the two, v_{max} is simpler, so let's start there. In enzyme kinetics, v_{max} is a measure of how fast an enzyme can convert its substrate to product. Because we're told that mCU has a high capacity, we can assume that it can carry out its function quickly, which means it should have a high value for v_{max}.

K_m represents the substrate concentration at which the enzyme's velocity is one-half of v_{max}. Because the passage says that mCU has a low affinity for calcium ions, that means it does not bind Ca^{2+} very well. We would expect that a relatively high concentration of Ca^{2+} would be needed to reach v_{max}, so K_m also should be relatively high.

TAKEAWAYS

When questions have multipart answers, you should start eliminating wrong answer choices as soon as you've figured out one part.

4 Match your prediction to an answer choice

Once we know that v_{max} should be relatively high, we can eliminate (**B**) and (**D**). The fact that K_m also should be relatively high eliminates the one remaining wrong answer (**C**), leaving (**A**) as the correct answer.

---

3. During a heart attack, cytosolic Ca^{2+} levels often increase. An increase in Ca^{2+} in the intermembrane space of mitochondria would most likely cause:

    A. increased ATP synthesis as a result of H^+ flow into the mitochondrial matrix.

    B. increased ATP synthesis as a result of H^+ flow out of the mitochondrial matrix.

    C. decreased ATP synthesis as a result of H^+ flow into the mitochondrial matrix.

    D. decreased ATP synthesis as a result of H^+ flow out of the mitochondrial matrix.

KEY CONCEPT

Electron transport chain
Oxidative phosphorylation

1 Type the question

This is a prediction based on a change in Ca^{2+} levels. The answers have a pattern, with increased or decreased ATP synthesis and with H^+ ions flowing into or out of the matrix.

2 Rephrase the question stem

We are given some additional information about an increase in Ca^{2+} levels in the cell and then asked to predict what would happen. When Rephrased it asks, *What would an increase in cytosolic Ca^{2+} do to ATP synthesis and H^+ movement?*

③ Investigate potential solutions

To answer this question, we need two pieces of information. First, we need to figure out what effect increased Ca^{2+} levels have in the intermembrane space. The answer to that question comes from Figure 1. The second piece of information is the effect of that flow on ATP synthesis. We need to pull that from our knowledge of the electron transport chain and oxidative phosphorylation.

According to Figure 1, the mCU brings Ca^{2+} in the intermembrane space into the matrix. When Ca^{2+} builds up in the matrix, NCX exchanges the extra calcium for sodium ions, so Na^+ accumulates in the matrix. According to paragraph 4, the NHE exchanges Na^+ for H^+. So when Ca^{2+} builds up in the intermembrane space, the net result is the flow of protons into the mitochondrial matrix.

Does that help or hurt ATP synthesis? According to the chemiosmotic hypothesis, ATP synthase uses the proton gradient across the inner mitochondrial membrane as the energy source for ATP synthesis and sends protons into the matrix to do so. (The electron transport chain uses the energy from the oxidation of NADH and $FADH_2$ to move protons into the intermembrane space.) The flow of protons as a result of calcium buildup is the same as the flow of protons in ATP synthesis. We can conclude that the two processes compete for the same pool of protons, so ATP synthesis should decline.

④ Match your prediction to an answer choice

Once we predict that protons should flow into the mitochondrial matrix, we can immediately eliminate (**B**) and (**D**). Knowledge of the chemiosmotic hypothesis allows us to confidently pick (**C**) as the correct answer.

MCAT EXPERTISE

Many MCAT questions have two-part answers. Once you predict half the answer, it's worth checking the answer choices. Sometimes, only one answer choice has that part correct!

Enzyme binding
Enzyme inhibition

4. A recently discovered protein in the intermembrane space of mitochondria in rat cardiac myocytes binds both Ca^{2+} and ATP synthase. A biochemist studying its function in isolated mitochondria found the following:

Intermembrane Ca^{2+}/ ATPase-binding protein concentration, μM	Intermembrane Ca^{2+} concentration, μM	ATP synthase activity (arbitrary units)
0.0	0.0	12.5
0.1	0.0	9.4
0.5	0.0	1.5
0.5	2.0	11.9

Which of the following conclusions regarding this protein is most reasonable?

A. When the protein binds Ca^{2+} ions, it binds to ATP synthase, increasing ATP synthase activity.

B. The protein, which normally binds ATP synthase, loses its ability to bind ATP synthase when it binds to calcium.

C. The protein has a higher affinity for calcium than it does for ATP synthase.

D. The protein is one of the calcium-activated dehydrogenases mentioned in the passage.

❶ Type the question

This question talks about a completely new experiment in the form of a table that is only tangentially related to the topic of the passage, making it a good candidate for triaging. A glance at the answer choices shows the correct answer must deal with the function of the protein that binds Ca^{2+} ions and ATP synthase.

❷ Rephrase the question stem

The question stem is asking you to draw the most reasonable conclusion among the four listed; there might be better ones, but those four are the only ones that matter on Test Day. When Rephrased it asks, *What answer choice is supported by the information in the table?*

❸ Investigate potential solutions

First, we need to examine the table and see how changes in the calcium and protein concentrations affect the activity of ATP synthase. The first trial is our control; with zero protein and zero calcium, ATP synthase has a relatively high activity. In the second and third trials, the biochemist increases the concentration of the ATP synthase–binding protein but leaves out calcium. What happens? ATP synthase activity drops, and the more protein we add, the more it drops. So we can reasonably conclude that the protein inhibits ATP synthase.

Look at the last trial, though. The biochemist adds a lot of calcium to the intermembrane space while also adding a lot of the protein. What happens now? ATP synthase activity is nearly normal! This suggests that calcium acts as an antagonist to this protein, preventing it from inhibiting ATP synthase activity. This understanding will formulate a great prediction as we work through the answer choices.

④ Match your prediction to an answer choice

Scanning the answers shows that only one—(**B**)—agrees with our analysis. The new binding protein cannot bind to ATP synthase in the presence of calcium.

(**A**) might be tempting because ATP synthase activity does rise when calcium is added in the fourth trial. However, it doesn't explain why ATP synthase activity decreases when the protein is added in the absence of calcium.

We don't have enough information to decide adequately about (**C**). We know that 2.0 µM of calcium ions is enough to restore ATP synthase activity more or less completely. For all we know, though, that could be an enormous excess. Moreover, we can't be sure what the protein's affinity for ATP synthase is; even when we add 0.5 µM of protein, that's not enough to inhibit ATP synthase completely.

(**D**) suffers from the same problem as (**A**). Although that might be a reasonable inference from the last two trials, it doesn't explain the overall data. Even worse, the dehydrogenases mentioned in the passage are part of the Krebs cycle, which takes place in the mitochondrial matrix. The question stem clearly states that this protein was discovered in the intermembrane space, not the matrix.

THINGS TO WATCH OUT FOR

When a question asks *Which of the following is most likely?* remember that you're limited to the four choices in the answer question. Don't waste time trying to come up with the best possible conclusion!

KEY CONCEPT

Krebs cycle
Electron transport chain
Oxidative phosphorylation

---

5. A biochemist studying mCU has two samples of mitochondria. To one, the biochemist adds enough ruthenium red, a known mCU inhibitor, to inhibit mCU completely. Both samples are given radiolabeled glucose. The biochemist could most reasonably predict that the ruthenium red sample, compared to the control, would:

    A. exhibit complete cessation of ATP synthesis.
    B. have increased production of radiolabeled carbon dioxide.
    C. exhibit a long-term decrease in ATP synthesis.
    D. have increased production of radiolabeled ATP.

① Type the question

We're given details of an experiment in the question stem. Two of the answers deal with decreases in ATP synthesis, whereas the other two deal with the radiolabeled carbon.

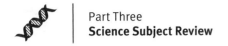
② Rephrase the question stem

We have information in the form of details of a new experiment, and then the question asks what the researcher could predict. When Rephrased it asks, *What happens to mitochondrial function when mCU is inhibited?*

③ Investigate potential solutions

The first step here is to figure out what effect completely inhibiting mCU would have on the mitochondrion. That information is in paragraph 2, which says that mCU transports calcium into the matrix. However, what effect does that have on the mitochondrion? To answer that question, we need to look at paragraph 1, which says that Ca^{2+} ions upregulate the activity of dehydrogenases in the Krebs cycle.

So now we need to consider how the Krebs cycle feeds into ATP synthesis in oxidative phosphorylation. That information is not in the passage, so it'll need to come from our knowledge of aerobic respiration. We may also need to use our knowledge of how ATP synthase makes ATP.

If we inhibit mCU completely, that would reduce Ca^{2+} levels in the mitochondrial matrix. According to paragraph 1, that would reduce flux through the Krebs cycle, which would mean less NADH and $FADH_2$ would be produced. If we have less NADH and $FADH_2$, that necessarily means that we have less substrate available for the electron transport chain. Therefore we would expect a decrease in ATP synthesis, which will form our prediction.

④ Match your prediction to an answer choice

After scanning the answer choices, we can eliminate two answers immediately. **(B)** can't be the answer because it would require increased flux through the Krebs cycle. **(D)** also doesn't work: not only would it require ATP synthesis, but the carbons from glucose are not directly incorporated into ATP during ATP synthesis.

That leaves two choices: **(A)**, which says that ATP synthesis stops completely, and **(C)**, which says it decreases. To decide which is correct, we need to look at paragraph 1, which says that Ca^{2+} stimulates enzymes in the Krebs cycle. *Stimulates* means that calcium increases their activity but is not required for their activity. Thus, we can predict that a lack of calcium should slow down these enzymes, not shut them down. ATP synthesis should therefore decrease, not stop, so the correct answer is **(C)**.

MCAT EXPERTISE

For Test Day, you are responsible for understanding ATP synthesis at the level of detail presented in an introductory biochemistry course, which would include the fact that carbons from glucose are not directly incorporated into ATP. You are not required, however, to know how adenosine and other nucleotides are actually synthesized.

TAKEAWAYS

When answer choices cover two (or more) different topics, you may need to consider multiple issues to determine the correct answer.

This chapter continues on the next page. ▶ ▶ ▶

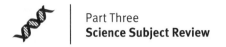

BIOCHEMISTRY PASSAGE II: METABOLIC REGULATION

In humans, the enzyme *isocitrate dehydrogenase* (IDH) exists in multiple forms; one form, IDH1, is found in the cytosol, whereas two others, IDH2 and IDH3, are expressed in the mitochondria. IDH3 exists as a hetero-trimer of three subunits. In *Escherichia coli* (*E. coli*), a facultative anaerobe, only one IDH exists; it is a dimer of 416-subunit residues. The percentage of residues in *E. coli* IDH that are equivalent to those in any form of human IDH is less than 15 percent. Unlike all human IDH forms, *E. coli* IDH is inhibited by phosphorylation. Moreover, unlike most enzymes regulated by phosphorylation, *E. coli* IDH undergoes phosphorylation at its active site.

IDH phosphorylation is critical in *E. coli* because decreased IDH activity increases flow through the *glyoxylate cycle*, an alternative metabolic pathway shown schematically in Figure 1. The glyoxylate cycle, which also is found in plants, is used to bypass parts of the citric acid cycle when the organism is depending on fatty acids and/ or acetyl-CoA as its primary source of energy. In the glyoxylate cycle, *isocitrate lyase* converts isocitrate to gly-oxylate and succinate. *Malate synthase* then combines glyoxylate and a molecule of acetyl-CoA to form malate. Isocitrate lyase and malate synthase are not known to exist in humans, although recent evidence suggests that at least some vertebrates may produce them.

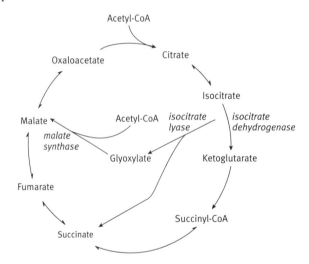

Figure 1. Glyoxylate cycle

To study IDH regulation, researchers cultured cells, as shown in Table 1, in media containing ^{31}P. After lysing the cells, SDS-PAGE was run on an aliquot from each sample. A western blot, which gives a spot (a positive result) when a protein capable of binding a particular antibody is present, was performed on samples 1–4 using an anti-body that detects *E. coli* IDH.

Sample	Cells used	Carbon Source used
1	*E. coli*	0.4% glucose
2	*E. coli*	0.4% sodium acetate
3	Human hepatocytes	0.4% glucose
4	Human hepatocytes	0.4% sodium acetate
5	*E. coli*	0.2% sodium acetate
6	*E. coli*	0.4% sodium acetate + 0.4% glucose

Table 1. Cell Cultures Used to Study IDH Activity

1. Which of the following most likely shows the result of the western blot experiment described in the passage? (Note: the numbers 1 through 4 correspond to the samples in Table 1.)

   A.

   1 2 3 4

   — — — —

   B.

   1 2 3 4

           — —
           — —
   — — — —

   C.

   1 2 3 4

   — —

   D.

   1 2 3 4

         —

2. In *E. coli*, which of the following would be expected to increase as a consequence of a drop in IDH activity?

   I.   Pyruvate kinase activity
   II. Acetyl-CoA levels
   III. CO_2 production

   A. I only
   B. II only
   C. I and III only
   D. I, II, and III

3. A biochemist decides to perform autoradiography, which can quantify the amount of a radioactive isotope present, on the samples described in Table 1. Based on information in the passage, he would predict that IDH from:

   A. only sample 1 would exhibit ^{31}P activity.
   B. only samples 2 and 5 would exhibit ^{31}P activity.
   C. only samples 2, 5, and 6 would exhibit ^{31}P activity.
   D. all the IDH samples would exhibit ^{31}P activity.

4. Based on information in the passage, which of the following is the most likely explanation for how phosphorylation inhibits IDH in *E. coli*?

   A. Phosphorylation causes allosteric changes to the active site that prevent isocitrate from binding.
   B. Phosphorylation causes electrostatic repulsion of the negatively charged isocitrate.
   C. Phosphorylation targets IDH for destruction by lysosomes.
   D. Phosphorylation results in the dissociation of the IDH dimer.

5. In humans, IDH3 is NAD^+ dependent, whereas IDH1 and IDH2 are dependent on $NADP^+$. Which of the following would be LEAST likely to be true?

   A. Expression of IDH1 is regulated by mechanisms that have no effect on IDH3 expression.
   B. The values of K_m and v_{max} for IDH1 and IDH2 are likely to differ significantly from those for IDH3.
   C. The gene for IDH1 and the gene for IDH3 are located on different chromosomes.
   D. In vitro, the equilibrium ratio of isocitrate to α-ketoglutarate using IDH1 equals the ratio for IDH3.

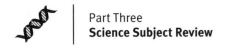

<table>
<tr><td>

KEY CONCEPT

Nonenzymatic protein function

</td></tr>
</table>

USING THE KAPLAN METHOD

Preview the passage: At a glance, the first few paragraphs indicate this is an information passage. The passage does include a figure and table. However, a closer look reveals that the table describes only the setup of an experiment rather than actual data.

Choose your approach: Outline

Read and Distill:

P1: Description of different isoforms of IDH in humans. Differences in IDH in *E. coli* comparing residues and regulation with phosphorylation.
Outline: IDH different in humans, *E. coli*

P2: Regulation of IDH in *E. coli* important since it affects Krebs alternate pathway, called glycoxylate cycle. Glycoxylate has enzymes not found in humans.
Outline: Glycoxylate cycle

F1: Diagram of glycoxylate cycle described in P2 and how it relates to Krebs cycle.
Outline: Glycoxylate cycle and Krebs cycle

P3: Experimental setup to study the regulation of IDH. Specifically, it looks to be analyzing changes in phosphorylation of IDH. Anticipate that questions will ask about predicting the results or will give you experimental results in the question stem and ask you to synthesize it with passage information.
Outline: IDH regulation experiment

T1: Table guides the setup of the experiment. It looks like the experimenters have cell type and carbon source both as independent variables, and when put together with the information in P3, they're going to measure the effect on phosphorylation of IDH.
Outline: Cell cultures used in IDH regulation experiment

1. Which of the following most likely shows the result of the western blot experiment described in the passage? (Note: the numbers 1 through 4 correspond to the samples in Table 1.)

    A.
    ```
    1   2   3   4



    _   _   _   _
    ```

    B.
    ```
    1   2   3   4


           _  _
            _ _
    _  _   _ _
    ```

    C.
    ```
    1   2   3   4



    _   _
    ```

    D.
    ```
    1   2   3   4



        _
    ```

① Type the question

A glance through this question shows that we have data in the form of gels as answer choices. Note that in every case, sample 2 gives a positive result.

② Rephrase the question stem

As expected, this question is asking you to predict the results of the experiment described in the last paragraph. When Rephrased it asks, *Which gel matches the western blot for samples 1–4?*

③ Investigate potential solutions

To answer this question, we need the brief description of how western blots work given in paragraph 3. We also need to know whether human IDH will respond to an antibody specific for *E. coli* IDH; to answer that question, we'll need information in paragraph 1. First, based on paragraph 3, a western blot produces a spot whenever there's a protein capable of binding to the antibody. In this case, we're using an antibody for *E. coli* IDH.

To answer the second question, we need to know if the human IDH will bind the antibody. According to paragraph 1, there's less than a 15 percent match between the sequences of *E. coli* IDH and human IDH. If there's that little similarity, it's reasonable to conclude that the antibody for *E. coli* IDH will not be able to bind human IDH. That means samples 3 and 4 should give no response.

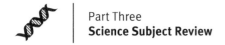

4 Match your prediction to an answer choice

If we look at the answer choices, we can immediately eliminate both **(A)** and **(B)**. They show spots for lanes 3 and 4, where there shouldn't be any.

That leaves us with two choices, **(C)** and **(D)**. To decide which one is correct, we need to ask: *Does* E. coli *always produce IDH?* The answer to this question is yes. Paragraph 1 tells us *E. coli* is a facultative anaerobe, which means it is capable of performing aerobic respiration if oxygen is present. To do that, it needs to have the enzymes of the Krebs cycle available. Both lanes 1 and 2 should thus yield a spot on a western blot, so the answer is **(C)**.

---

2. In *E. coli*, which of the following would be expected to increase as a consequence of a drop in IDH activity?

 I.   Pyruvate kinase activity
 II. Acetyl-CoA levels
 III. CO_2 production

 A. I only
 B. II only
 C. I and III only
 D. I, II, and III

---

1 Type the question

This is a Roman numeral question that asks about information in the passage and knowledge of metabolism. Use your familiarity with the content area to decide whether this question will take you a long time and hence may be worth triaging for later.

2 Rephrase the question stem

Which of these three things increases when IDH activity decreases?

3 Investigate potential solutions

To answer this question, we'll need to use Figure 1 and our knowledge of the Krebs cycle to figure out what happens when IDH activity drops. Take a strategic approach to Roman numeral questions, and attack the answer choice that appears twice. That way, you're left with just two answer choices to consider and may not have to analyze each Roman numeral.

④ Match your prediction to an answer choice

Since Roman numeral II appears twice, let's start there. According to the passage, when IDH activity drops, glyoxylate forms. Glyoxylate combines with acetyl-CoA to form oxaloacetate. So each time a molecule of isocitrate enters the glyoxylate cycle, a molecule of acetyl-CoA is consumed, not produced. Roman numeral II is incorrect, so eliminate (**B**) and (**D**).

Notice this means that Roman numeral I is automatically correct, and on Test Day, you shouldn't spend time analyzing why. However, in review, it's important to understand all aspects of the questions. According to Figure 1, if IDH doesn't convert isocitrate to α-ketoglutarate, it'll enter the glyoxylate cycle, where it'll be turned into glyoxylate and succinate. That means we bypass the formation of α-ketoglutarate and succinyl-CoA. This is important because both of those steps produce NADH, which is used to produce ATP. So less IDH activity means less ATP.

Pyruvate kinase, the last enzyme in glycolysis, produces ATP as it converts phospho-enolpyruvate (PEP) into pyruvate. Because ATP is a product of the reaction, Le Châtelier's Principle says that low levels of it should increase pyruvate kinase's activity. Item I is therefore true.

Look at item III; isocitrate has six carbons, but succinate has four carbons. So where do the other two carbons go in the Krebs cycle? To CO_2! Less IDH activity means less CO_2 is produced. So item III is false, making answer choice (**A**) correct.

---

3. A biochemist decides to perform autoradiography, which can quantify the amount of a radioactive isotope present, on the samples described in Table 1. Based on information in the passage, he would predict that IDH from:

   A. only sample 1 would exhibit ^{31}P activity.
   B. only samples 2 and 5 would exhibit ^{31}P activity.
   C. only samples 2, 5, and 6 would exhibit ^{31}P activity.
   D. all the IDH samples would exhibit ^{31}P activity.

KEY CONCEPT

Citric acid cycle

① Type the question

You might have been wondering why the passage mentioned ^{31}P but then didn't mention it again. Or you might have wondered why Table 1 includes six samples, whereas the western blot experiment used only the first four. The first thing that should come to your mind in such cases is *There's probably a question coming up on that!* The answer choices are referring to the samples described in the table.

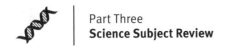
❷ Rephrase the question stem

Which IDH sample(s) will show incorporation of ^{31}P?

❸ Investigate potential solutions

To answer this question, we'll need to synthesize the information in the passage on IDH phosphorylation—which is in paragraphs 1 and 2—with our understanding of how organisms regulate metabolic pathways. Paragraph 2 states that IDH is phosphorylated when *E. coli* uses either fatty acids or acetyl-CoA as its primary fuel source. Paragraph 1 tells us that human IDH doesn't undergo phosphorylation. So we shouldn't expect any ^{31}P activity from samples 3 and 4.

What do the words *primary fuel source* mean? Practically speaking, it means that no glucose is available. So we would predict that *E. coli* will phosphorylate IDH in the absence of glucose. Looking at Table 1, that's samples 2 and 5.

❹ Match your prediction to an answer choice

(B) matches our prediction exactly and is the correct answer.

THINGS TO WATCH OUT FOR

Experiments with several trial groups are a great source of questions on Test Day.

(D) is wrong because human IDH is not regulated by phosphorylation. **(A)** doesn't work because sample 1 relies on glucose as its primary source. Similarly, **(C)** is wrong because sample 6 contains both acetate and glucose. Glucose is the preferred fuel source, and cells typically use glucose first when it's available.

KEY CONCEPT

Control of enzyme activity

4. Based on information in the passage, which of the following is the most likely explanation for how phosphorylation inhibits IDH in *E. coli*?

   A. Phosphorylation causes allosteric changes to the active site that prevent isocitrate from binding.

   B. Phosphorylation causes electrostatic repulsion of the negatively charged isocitrate.

   C. Phosphorylation targets IDH for destruction by lysosomes.

   D. Phosphorylation results in the dissociation of the IDH dimer.

① Type the question

This is a tough reasoning-style question, asking for an explanation for a phenomenon in the passage. The answer choices have no clear pattern, and thus this question might be a good candidate for triaging for later.

THINGS TO WATCH OUT FOR

On Test Day, if an MCAT passage notes that a particular phenomenon is unusual, pay attention to it. This is often a signal that you'll be tested on that concept!

② Rephrase the question stem

How does phosphorylation cause inhibition of IDH in E. coli?

③ Investigate potential solutions

To answer this question, we need to draw on our knowledge of enzyme function and inhibition. We'll also need to know what the passage tells us about phosphorylation of IDH in *E. coli*; that information is in paragraph 1. Enzyme inhibition means that the activity of the enzyme drops. Paragraph 1 tells us that in *E. coli*, IDH undergoes phosphorylation at its active site. That tells us that whatever happens, it must involve a change at the active site and should be a part of your prediction as you work through the answer choices.

④ Match your prediction to an answer choice

When cycling through the answer choices, notice that the only one that could plausibly involve the active site is **(B).** Therefore, it must be the correct response.

(A) is what we might predict if we didn't look at paragraph 1; most enzymes that are regulated by phosphorylation undergo allosteric changes. **(C)** can't be true because we're talking about *E. coli*, which is a bacterium, and bacteria don't have organelles such as lysosomes. **(D)** could be true. However, we're looking for the most likely explanation, and the passage doesn't give us any information that suggests that IDH must be dimerized to be active.

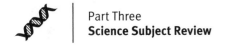
KEY CONCEPT

Principles of metabolic regulation

Enzyme activity

5. In humans, IDH3 is NAD$^+$ dependent, whereas IDH1 and IDH2 are dependent on NADP$^+$. Which of the following would be LEAST likely to be true?

    A. Expression of IDH1 is regulated by mechanisms that have no effect on IDH3 expression.

    B. The values of K_m and v_{max} for IDH1 and IDH2 are likely to differ significantly from those for IDH3.

    C. The gene for IDH1 and the gene for IDH3 are located on different chromosomes.

    D. In vitro, the equilibrium ratio of isocitrate to α-ketoglutarate using IDH1 equals the ratio for IDH3.

❶ Type the question

There is new information in the question stem, and you're asked to identify something that is LEAST likely to be true. There is no clear pattern in the answer choices. This is the type of question you would typically want to save for later.

❷ Rephrase the question stem

Questions that ask what is LEAST likely to be true are often more difficult because it's hard to predict what the correct answer will be. A good strategy might be to Rephrase as, *Given the cofactor dependence of different IDH isoforms, which of the following answers is supported?* Then eliminate the answers that are plausible.

❸ Investigate potential solutions

Our best bet will be to look at paragraph 1 to figure out what the passage tells us about IDH1, IDH2, and IDH3. We'll also need to use our knowledge of enzyme activity to answer this question. Paragraph 1 tells us that IDH1 is expressed in the cytosol, IDH3 is expressed in the mitochondria, and all three forms of IDH carry out the conversion of isocitrate to α-ketoglutarate. Because IDH3 uses NAD$^+$ while IDH1 and IDH2 use NADP$^+$, we can conclude that the mechanism used by IDH3 is different from the mechanism used by IDH1 and IDH2. (Note: we can't say if IDH1 and IDH2 have the same mechanism or not.)

At this point, it's useful to look through the answer choices one at a time. Because we're looking for the statement that is LEAST likely, anything that we can reasonably assume to be true can be eliminated; we want to select the answer that is either implausible or outright impossible.

4 Match your prediction to an answer choice

Let's start with (**A**). Can we think of a plausible scenario where IDH1 and IDH3 are regulated in different mechanisms? Absolutely. There's a great analogy in glucokinase and hexokinase. Both carry out the first step in glycolysis, but they are regulated in different ways. So (**A**) is likely to be true, and we can eliminate it.

(**B**) tests our understanding of enzyme kinetics. Should we expect IDH1 and IDH3 to have different values for v_{max}, the maximum velocity for the enzyme, and K_m, the substrate concentration at which it is half-saturated? Continuing our glucokinase/hexokinase discussion, absolutely. Glucokinase has a lower affinity for glucose than hexokinase and, therefore, different values for K_m and v_{max}. So it's reasonable to expect the same thing to be true here.

(**C**) is actually the easiest of the four; nothing in the passage gives us any reason to believe that IDH1 and IDH3 should have their genes on the same chromosome, so (**C**) is also likely to be true. Even the genes for the α and β subunits of hemoglobin are located on different chromosomes!

By process of elimination, that leaves (**D**). At first blush, this might seem to be true: enzymes speed up reactions, but they do not affect the equilibrium yield because K_{eq} depends only on the relative stability of the reactants and products. However, do IDH1 and IDH3 catalyze the same reaction? No! Because IDH1 depends on $NADP^+$ and IDH3 requires NAD^+, they don't. Thus they have two different expressions for K_{eq}, and we can't reasonably expect that the ratio of isocitrate to α-ketoglutarate is the same. Because (**D**) is likely to be *false*, it's the answer that earns us a point.

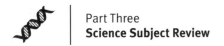

9.6 Biochemistry on Your Own

BIOCHEMISTRY PASSAGE III (QUESTIONS 1–5)

Peptide synthesis is a common target for antimicrobial compounds. Many such drugs, including chloramphenicol, work by directly inhibiting peptide bond synthesis. Another category, the macrolides, do not inhibit peptide bond formation but instead block the channel through which newly synthesized peptides exit the ribosome, the nascent peptide exit tunnel (NPET).

Macrolides are molecules with lactone rings containing 14 to 16 atoms and include erythromycin; a newer, more potent subclass called ketolides includes telithromycin. Macrolides were long thought to act like a "plug" in the NPET, blocking so much of the tunnel that peptides cannot pass through. More recent evidence, however, suggests this theory is incorrect.

First, neither drug completely inhibits protein synthesis. At least some proteins can exit the NPET and undergo complete translation, even in their presence. The likelihood of a protein being synthesized depends on its *N*-terminal sequence. Most sequences cause blockage of the NPET and an early end to protein synthesis, whereas some sequences permit complete synthesis of a protein. A sequence allowing full synthesis is shown in Figure 1; proteins with relatively homologous chains are also known to allow full synthesis. Moreover, a hybrid mRNA in which the sequence in Figure 1 precedes a chain that would normally be blocked also tends to be fully translated.

AUG	AGC	GAA	GCA	CUU	AAA	AUU	CUG	AAC	AAC	AUC	CGU
Met	Ser	Glu	Ala	Leu	Lys	Ile	Leu	Asn	Asn	Ile	Arg

Figure 1. A peptide sequence capable of escaping from a macrolide-bound NPET, along with its corresponding mRNA sequence

Second, telithromycin is actually less effective than erythromycin at inhibiting synthesis: cells exposed to telithromycin synthesize more proteins than do those exposed to erythromycin. Some proteins are fully expressed, whereas the synthesis of some ends after just a few residues; in such cases, the nascent peptide falls out of the ribosome before the ribosome ever reaches a stop codon. (The human genetic code is depicted in Figure 2.)

Second letter

	U	C	A	G	
U	UUU ⎤ Phe UUC ⎦ UUA ⎤ Leu UUG ⎦	UCU ⎤ UCC ⎥ Ser UCA ⎥ UCG ⎦	UAU ⎤ Tyr UAC ⎦ UAA Stop UAG Stop	UGU ⎤ Cys UGC ⎦ UGA Stop UGG Trp	U C A G
C	CUU ⎤ CUC ⎥ Leu CUA ⎥ CUG ⎦	CCU ⎤ CCC ⎥ Pro CCA ⎥ CCG ⎦	CAU ⎤ His CAC ⎦ CAA ⎤ Gln CAG ⎦	CGU ⎤ CGC ⎥ Arg CGA ⎥ CGG ⎦	U C A G
A	AUU ⎤ AUC ⎥ Ile AUA ⎦ AUG Met	ACU ⎤ ACC ⎥ Thr ACA ⎥ ACG ⎦	AAU ⎤ Asn AAC ⎦ AAA ⎤ Lys AAG ⎦	AGU ⎤ Ser AGC ⎦ AGA ⎤ Arg AGG ⎦	U C A G
G	GUU ⎤ GUC ⎥ Val GUA ⎥ GUG ⎦	GCU ⎤ GCC ⎥ Ala GCA ⎥ GCG ⎦	GAU ⎤ Asp GAC ⎦ GAA ⎤ Glu GAG ⎦	GGU ⎤ GGC ⎥ Gly GGA ⎥ GGG ⎦	U C A G

First letter (rows) / *Third letter* (columns)

Figure 2. The human genetic code for RNA molecules

1. A researcher cultures a bacterium sensitive to both erythromycin and telithromycin on three agar plates. Plate 1 has erythromycin, plate 2 has telithromycin, and plate 3 is a control. Based on information in the passage, the researcher would predict that the percentage of partially translated proteins would be:

   A. highest on plate 1 and lowest on plate 2.
   B. highest on plate 2 and lowest on plate 1.
   C. highest on plate 1 and lowest on plate 3.
   D. highest on plate 2 and lowest on plate 3.

2. Which of the following changes in the mRNA sequence shown in Figure 2 would most likely lead to the greatest inhibition in protein synthesis?

   A. Changing AGC to AGU in codon 2
   B. Changing GAA to GAG in codon 3
   C. Changing CUG to UUG in codon 8
   D. Changing AAC to AGC in codon 10

3. Based on information in the passage, which of the following changes is most likely to be observed in the first few minutes after erythromycin administration in a bacterium susceptible to it?

   A. A decrease in the concentration of charged tRNAs
   B. Covalent binding of 30S and 50S ribosomal subunits
   C. Mutations attaching the sequence in Figure 1 to other genes
   D. An increase in the concentration of peptidyl-tRNAs

4. The following graph shows protein synthesis in an *E. coli* cell culture in the absence of antibiotics.

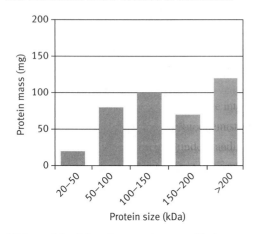

Which of the following graphs most likely represents the results obtained in the presence of telithromycin? (Note: peptides less than 20 kDa were not measured.)

A.

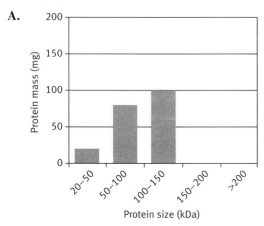

B.

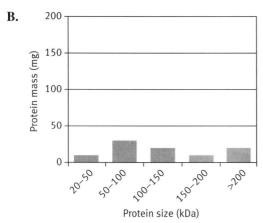

C.

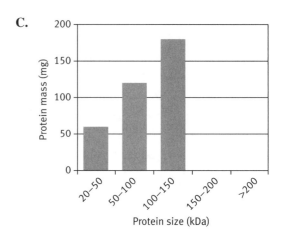

D.

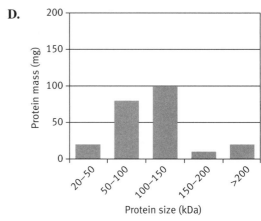

5. An *E. coli* cell is given methionine radiolabeled with ^{31}S. Five minutes later, which of the following is most likely to be true?

A. Most proteins synthesized in that five-minute period will express the radiolabel at their *N*-terminus.

B. Most proteins synthesized in that five-minute period will express the radiolabel but not at their *N*-terminus.

C. Most proteins synthesized in that five-minute period will express the radiolabel at both their *N*-terminus and their interior positions.

D. Both newly synthesized and already-existing proteins will exhibit the radiolabel.

This chapter continues on the next page. ▶ ▶ ▶

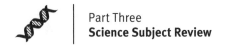

Biochemistry Practice Passage Explanations

1. (C)

The key to this question is a careful reading of the question stem and the passage. The question stem asks us which plate will have the highest and lowest percentages of partially translated proteins. Paragraph 2 tells us that telithromycin is more potent than erythromycin, so we might be led to predict that the order is plate 2 (telithromycin) > plate 1 (erythromycin) > plate 3 (control). That would lead us to **(D)**, which is a trap. Paragraph 3 tells us that although telithromycin is more potent as an antibiotic, it is actually worse at inhibiting synthesis than erythromycin is! So the correct answer is actually plate 1 > plate 2 > plate 3, which matches **(C)**.

2. (D)

Paragraph 3 states that the mRNA sequence shown in Figure 2 makes a peptide macrolide resistant; it can escape the tunnel even if erythromycin or telithromycin is bound. If we want the greatest increase in inhibition, we need a significant change in the sequence of that peptide. To answer this question, we'll need to use the genetic code in Figure 2 and look for a mutation that would lead to a different amino acid. By cycling through the choices, we find that the correct answer is **(D)**: AAC codes for asparagine, whereas AGC codes for serine.

In **(A)**, proximity to the start codon does not, by itself, increase the likelihood that a mutation would affect inhibition by macrolides. In **(B)**, the third nucleotide in the codon is in the wobble position, which tends to be the most likely nucleotide to result in a silent mutation when altered. **(C)** might look promising: it changes the first nucleotide in the codon. A look at the genetic code, though, shows us that this is one of the few cases where such a mutation is actually silent; both CUG and UUG code for leucine.

3. (D)

We're looking for a change likely to happen in the presence of erythromycin. According to paragraph 4, erythromycin can cause the nascent peptide to fall out of the ribosome. However, because this happens without a stop codon, the nascent peptide is not released from the tRNA. So we would expect a buildup of peptidyl-tRNA, or peptides still bound to tRNA molecules. This matches **(D)**.

In **(A)**, because protein synthesis decreases, we would not expect the concentration of charged tRNAs to drop; if anything, they would increase. In **(B)**, this would be true if erythromycin bound the two ribosomal subunits together, but nowhere does the passage imply this happens. In **(C)**, paragraph 4 states that this kind of mutation results in the expression of proteins that would normally be stopped by erythromycin. However, it is unlikely that such a mutation would happen spontaneously in the first few minutes after erythromycin administration.

4. (B)

The graph in the question stem represents the products of protein synthesis in normal *E. coli* cells. The graphs in the answer choices represent possible protein synthesis in *E. coli* after exposure to telithromycin. According to paragraph 3, the inhibition of synthesis is determined only by the nature of the *N*-terminal sequence of the peptide. Because we have no reason to believe that there is a specific correlation between *N*-terminal sequence and protein size, we would expect an overall decrease in protein synthesis at all molecular masses. This matches **(B)**.

(A) would be correct if the inhibition was based solely on molecular size (in this case, inhibiting synthesis of proteins >150 kDa in mass). In **(C)**, the total amount of protein produced is the same; according to paragraph 4, protein synthesis drops when macrolides are given. **(D)** shows partial inhibition, as the passage states, but only for proteins with high molecular weights; as with **(A)**, we have no reason to believe the inhibition is limited to certain molecular weights.

5. (B)

Where would we find radiolabeled methionine after five minutes? Every peptide chain begins with methionine; the only codon for Met also is the start codon. However, the majority of finished peptides do not have Met at their *N*-terminus. In most proteins, that initial Met, along with other N-terminal residues, are removed in post-translational processing. Among other things, that *N*-terminus sequence is often involved in signaling the destination of a protein (for example, whether it should end up in the cell membrane). There also is no mechanism for exchanging methionine in existing proteins, so the correct answer is (**B**).

In (**A**), most initial methionines are lost in post-translational processing. For (**C**), most proteins have internal methionines, but most of the initial methionines are removed. There is no mechanism in (**D**) for exchanging amino acids in existing proteins with new amino acids.

CHAPTER 10

Biology

MCAT test takers usually view biology as their strongest area; many students taking the MCAT are majoring in or have earned degrees in the biological sciences. However, the MCAT does not seek to test biological knowledge; it aims to test the scientific thinking and reasoning skills required for success in medical school. Although biology knowledge is important, how well you are able to use that knowledge is what earns points on Test Day.

When encountering an MCAT biology passage, many students try to apply the same strategies they used when studying for undergraduate biology courses, including reading the passage for understanding and focusing on the details in the passage. However, the MCAT is more like an open-book test. Memorizing details wastes time and doesn't necessarily result in correct answers. This chapter discusses the Kaplan approach to biology passages and questions.

10.1 Reading the Passage

One of the trademarks of MCAT biology passages is that the topic itself is familiar but the context is unfamiliar. For example, a passage on action potential transmission may discuss rare diseases associated with derangements in neural transmission. The job of the test taker is to apply what he or she already knows about the topic to new situations. The ability to use what you know in new ways is a significant part of succeeding as a medical student and as a physician.

One of the biggest movements in modern medicine is the practice of evidence-based medicine. What this means is that a physician uses current studies and information as a guide for diagnosis and treatment. Thus, the MCAT has shifted to test these skills by presenting information in the context of a study and asking questions about experimental design. Biology is tested in all three of the science sections of the MCAT but is most prevalently tested in the Biological and Biochemical Foundations of Living Systems section. Within this section, the areas tested include organic chemistry, biochemistry, and biology, with a small amount of general chemistry. Because experiments in chemistry do not typically involve control groups, population studies, or statistical analysis, you can expect that passages in biology will seek to test your skills in analyzing statistical data and evaluating the experiment design.

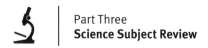

PASSAGE TYPES

The passage types related to biology on the MCAT are the same as in the other sciences. However, there are specific differences related to the field of biology. (See Table 10.1.)

Information Passages

- Contain prose similar to that found in a textbook.
- A typical passage might discuss a particular phenomenon such as a disease, describe its symptoms, and include a discussion about its pathophysiology (how a disease occurs), including genetics, environmental factors, and derangements at the molecular level.
- In addition to a recounting of information, these passages may also describe previous studies within this field, providing statistical data from a particular study.
- A very large amount of detail may be present. Note that the details are present and then move on. Avoid getting caught up in understanding every detail.

Experiment Passages

- Include one or more experiments and a description of the results in the form of a chart, graph, table, or diagram.
- Background information is generally presented to provide context.
- Experiments may be laboratory based or population based.

Remember, your goal is to get through a passage as quickly as possible but still read the passage critically enough to allow you to answer the questions. Be careful not to spend so much time digesting a passage that you run out of time when answering the questions. MCAT biology passages may contain a tremendous amount of information and data. However, it is important to remember that the passage will always be there to go back to, if needed.

	Information Passages	**Experiment Passages**
Scope	Discuss a particular phenomenon, disease, or study.	Discuss an experiment.
How to Read It	Read to get the gist of each paragraph; avoid getting caught up in the details.	Read to obtain the hypothesis, experimental design, and results.
Common Pitfalls	Spending too much time trying to understand and analyze the details	Spending too much time trying to understand the procedure and results before the questions ask for them

Table 10.1 Passage Types in Biology

READING AND DISTILLING THE PASSAGE

With the integration of a large number of possible topics and content areas, MCAT biology passages have the potential to be exceptionally detailed. Although the details are important, no points are awarded for one's ability to memorize and recall details. However, some sense of the details is required to answer the questions correctly. The key to a high score on Test Day is to find a balance between investing enough time in the passage to develop a solid understanding and reading quickly enough so that all of the questions may be answered in a timely manner. The most efficient way to do this is to read quickly—but critically—using the Kaplan Method.

- **Preview** for difficulty
  - Determine whether the passage is an *experiment* or an *information* passage.
  - Note the location of the paragraphs and any figures, such as charts, graphs, tables, or diagrams.
  - Determine the topic and the degree of difficulty.
  - Identify whether this passage will require a large time investment.
  - Decide whether this passage is one to do now or later.

- **Choose** your approach
  - Using information from the Preview step, Choose an appropriate Distill approach for the passage (Interrogate, Outline, or Highlight).
  - **Interrogation** should be chosen for experiment passages.
  - **Outlining** should be chosen for information passages that are dense or detail heavy.
  - **Highlighting** should be chosen for information passages that are light on details.

- **Read and Distill** key themes
  - While reading the passage, your aim is to distill the major takeaway of each paragraph and identify testable information using one of the following approaches.
  - **Interrogate**: Thoroughly examine the experiment passage by identifying the key components of experimental design and interrogating *why* specific procedures were done and *how* they connect to the overall purpose of the experiment.
  - **Outline**: Create a brief label for each paragraph that summarizes the contents of the paragraph, allowing you to return quickly to the passage when demanded by a question.
  - **Highlight**: Highlight one to three terms per paragraph that can pull your attention back to testable information when demanded by a question.

10.2 **Answering the Questions**

Like the other sciences, biology questions follow the four basic types of questions.

- **Discrete questions**
  - ○ Questions that are not based on a passage.
  - ○ Are preceded by a warning such as, "Questions 12–15 do not refer to a passage and are independent of each other."
  - ○ Most likely to ask a question about either a piece of information that you already know or a concept that requires you to apply your knowledge.

- **Questions that stand alone from the passage**
  - ○ Questions that accompany a passage but do not require information or data from the passage to identify the correct answer.
  - ○ More likely to require application of a basic concept, theory, or process to a situation presented in the question stem.

- **Questions that require data from the passage**
  - ○ Questions that require a piece of data or information from the passage but do not test the goal of the passage.
  - ○ These questions are likely to focus on data analysis or an evaluation of an experimental procedure.
  - ○ May focus on an informational section of the passage and require you to identify a detail presented.

- **Questions that require the goal of the passage**
  - ○ Questions that require the goal of the passage or a fundamental grasp of the passage as a whole.
  - ○ These questions are likely to focus on the results and a discussion of the results of an experiment.
  - ○ May assess your ability to analyze data or evaluate an experimental design but from a broader perspective, such as a change that could be made in the procedure that would affect the results in a particular way.
  - ○ May require you to evaluate the results of an experiment and apply those results to the information presented earlier in the passage.
  - ○ Likely to require the application of basic concepts and theories to understanding the passage as a whole.

ATTACKING THE QUESTIONS

MCAT biology covers a tremendous amount of topics. In addition, an understanding of several background concepts may be required to answer the question. Answering the questions quickly, efficiently, and correctly requires a solid passage outline and a systematic approach to ensure that the essential details are not missed.

- **Type** the question
  - Read the question; peek at the answer choices for patterns, but don't analyze closely.
  - Assess the topic and degree of difficulty.
  - Identify the level of time involvement: is this question likely to take a tremendous amount of time to identify the answer? If so, skip it and come back after you do the other questions in the passage set.
  - Good questions to do now in biology are ones that stand alone from the passage since they are generally quick and easy points.

- **Rephrase** the question stem
  - Rephrase the question, focusing on the task(s) to be accomplished.
  - Simplify the phrasing of the original question stem.
  - Translate the question into a specific set of tasks to be accomplished using the passage and your background knowledge.

- **Investigate** potential solutions
  - Complete the task(s) identified in your Rephrase step.
  - Analyze the data; evaluate the experimental design; locate the information required; and connect the information, data, and experimental design with the information you already know.
  - Predict what you can about the answer.
  - Be flexible if your initial approach fails.

- **Match** your prediction to an answer choice
  - Search the answer choices for a response that is synonymous with your prediction or eliminate answers that are not correct.
  - Incorrect answers often come in the form of answers that simply do not make sense. Critically read the answer choices and determine which answer choices do not make sense.
  - If a clear answer does not emerge, do your best to eliminate at least two answers and then guess between the remaining answers and move on. Don't get stuck!

10.3 **Getting the Edge in Biology**

Success on MCAT biology passages requires a quick but thorough reading of the passage. MCAT biology passages often cover a wide range of topics and include a large amount of detail. Learning to identify the location of a detail without investing time in interpreting that detail is an essential reading skill for Test Day success. This is often very difficult for students to learn how to do because it runs counter to how most students study for their undergraduate classes. However, the MCAT is not like the tests administered in undergraduate classes; it requires much more than memorization of concepts and details. The MCAT requires interpretation and evaluation of the concepts and details—but only when required by a question.

Answering questions on MCAT biology passages requires you to locate information quickly. In addition, the questions require you to think critically about both the question stem and the answer choices. Approaching the question stem and answer choices with confidence and a critical eye allows you to identify the correct question task and eliminate incorrect answer choices.

10.4 Preparing for the MCAT: Biology

The following presents the biology content you are likely to see on Test Day. The High-Yield badges point out the topics that are tested most frequently.

THE CELL

The **cell theory** has four basic tenets.

- All living things are composed of cells.
- The cell is the basic functional unit of life.
- Cells arise only from preexisting cells.
- Cells carry genetic information in the form of DNA. This genetic material is passed on from parent to daughter cell.

KEY CONCEPT

Viruses are not considered living things because they are acellular, cannot reproduce without the assistance of a host cell, and may contain RNA as their genetic material.

Eukaryotic Cells

`High-Yield`

Eukaryotes have membrane-bound organelles, have a nucleus, and may form multicellular organisms (see Figure 10.1). The cell membrane and membranes of organelles contain phospholipids, which organize to form hydrophilic interior and exterior surfaces with a hydrophobic core. The **cytosol** suspends the organelles and allows diffusion of molecules throughout the cell.

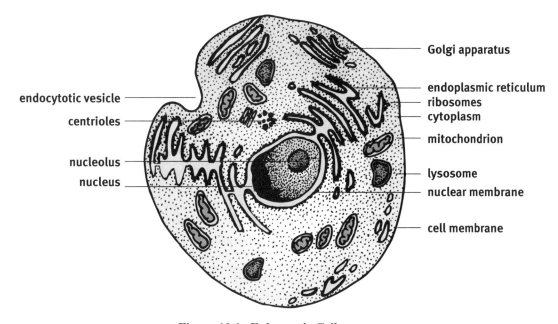

Figure 10.1. Eukaryotic Cell

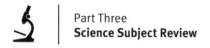
Each eukaryotic organelle serves a specific function.

- The **nucleus** contains DNA organized into **chromosomes**. It is surrounded by the **nuclear membrane** or **envelope**, a double membrane that contains **nuclear pores** for the two-way exchange of materials between the nucleus and cytosol. DNA is organized into coding regions called **genes**.
- The **nucleolus** is a subsection of the nucleus in which ribosomal RNA (rRNA) is synthesized.
- **Mitochondria** contain an outer and inner membrane. The **outer membrane** forms a barrier with the cytosol; the **inner membrane** is folded into **cristae** and contains enzymes for the electron transport chain. Between the membranes is the **intermembrane space**; inside the inner mitochondrial membrane is the mitochondrial **matrix**. Mitochondria can divide independently of the nucleus via binary fission; they can trigger **apoptosis** by releasing mitochondrial enzymes into the cytoplasm.
- **Lysosomes** contain hydrolytic enzymes that can break down substances ingested by endocytosis and cellular waste products. When these enzymes are released, **autolysis** of the cell can occur.
- The **endoplasmic reticulum** (**ER**) is a series of interconnected membranes and is continuous with the nuclear envelope. The **rough ER** (**RER**) is studded with ribosomes, which permit translation of proteins destined for secretion. The **smooth ER** (**SER**) is used for lipid synthesis and detoxification.
- The **Golgi apparatus** consists of stacked membrane-bound sacs in which cellular products can be modified, packaged, and directed to specific cellular locations.
- **Peroxisomes** contain hydrogen peroxide and can break down very long chain fatty acids via β-oxidation. They also participate in phospholipid synthesis and the pentose phosphate pathway.

The **cytoskeleton** provides stability and rigidity to the overall structure of the cell. It also provides transport pathways for molecules within the cell. (See Table 10.2.)

	Microfilaments	**Microtubules**	**Intermediate Filaments**
Structure	Solid polymers of actin protein	Hollow polymers of tubulin protein	Filaments of diverse proteins
Physical properties	Resistant to compression and fracture	Rigid; dynamic (undergo continual assembly and disassembly)	Resistant to tension
Function	1. Structural rigidity to cell 2. Actin filaments interact with myosin, generating contractile force in muscle	1. Create pathways for movement of motor proteins 2. Form cilia and flagella for cell locomotion	1. Integrity of cytoskeleton 2. Cell-to-cell adhesion
Role in cell division	Form cleavage furrow: actin filaments contract, pinching off cell	Form centrioles to create mitotic spindle: tubulin attaches to chromosomes, pulling them apart	N/A

Table 10.2. The Cytoskeleton

Epithelial tissues cover the body and line its cavities, protecting against pathogen invasion and desiccation. Some epithelial cells absorb or secrete substances, and some participate in sensation.

- In most organs, epithelial cells form the **parenchyma**, or the functional parts of the organ.
- Epithelial cells may be polarized, with one side facing a lumen or the outside world and the other side facing blood vessels and structural cells.
- Epithelia can be classified by the number of layers they contain. **Simple epithelia** have one layer. **Stratified epithelia** have many layers. **Pseudostratified epithelia** appear to have multiple layers because of differences in cell heights but actually have only one layer.
- Epithelia can be classified by the shapes of the cells they contain: **cuboidal cells** are cube shaped, **columnar cells** are long and narrow, and **squamous cells** are flat and scalelike.

Connective tissues support the body and provide a framework for epithelial cells.

- In most organs, connective tissues form the **stroma** or support structure by secreting materials to form an **extracellular matrix**.

Classification and Structure of Prokaryotic Cells

Prokaryotes do not contain membrane-bound organelles. Instead, they organize their genetic material in a single circular molecule of DNA concentrated in the nucleoid region.

There are three overarching domains of life; prokaryotes account for two of these.

- **Archaea** are often extremophiles, living in harsh environments (high temperature, high salinity, no light) and often using alternative sources of energy, like chemosynthesis. They have similarities to both eukaryotes (start translation with methionine, similar RNA polymerases, histones) and bacteria (single circular chromosome, divide by binary fission or budding).
- **Bacteria** have many similar structures to eukaryotes and have complex relationships with humans, including mutualistic symbiosis and pathogenesis.
- **Eukarya** is the only nonprokaryotic domain.

Bacteria can be classified by shape.
- Spherical bacteria are called **cocci**.
- Rod-shaped bacteria are called **bacilli**.
- Spiral-shaped bacteria are called **spirilla**.

Bacteria can be classified based on metabolic processes.
- **Obligate aerobes** require oxygen for metabolism.
- **Obligate anaerobes** cannot survive in oxygen-containing environments and can carry out only anaerobic metabolism.
- **Facultative anaerobes** can survive in environments with or without oxygen and toggle metabolic processes based on the environment.
- **Aerotolerant anaerobes** cannot use oxygen for metabolism but can survive in an oxygen-containing environment.

The cell wall and cell membrane of bacteria form the **envelope**. Together, they control the movement of solutes into and out of the cell. Bacteria can be classified by the color their cell walls turn during Gram staining with a crystal violet stain, followed by a counterstain with safranin. Gram-positive bacteria turn purple, while gram-negative bacteria turn pink-red. Gram-positive bacteria have a thick cell wall composed of **peptidoglycan** and **lipoteichoic acid**. Gram-negative bacteria have a thin cell wall composed of peptidoglycan and an outer membrane containing phospholipids and **lipopolysaccharides**.

Bacteria may have one, two, or many flagella that generate propulsion to move the bacterium toward food or away from immune cells. Moving in response to chemical stimuli is called **chemotaxis**. Bacterial flagella contain a filament composed of flagellin, a basal body that anchors and rotates the flagellum, and a hook that connects the two.

Genetics and Growth of Prokaryotic Cells

KEY CONCEPT

Prokaryotes carry out the electron transport chain using the cell membrane.

Prokaryotes multiply through **binary fission.** The chromosome replicates while the cell grows in size until the cell wall begins to grow inward along the midline of the cell and divides the parent cell into two identical daughter cells. In addition to the single circular chromosome in prokaryotes, extrachromosomal material can be carried in **plasmids.** Plasmids may contain antibiotic resistance genes or **virulence factors.** Plasmids that can integrate into the genome are called **episomes.**

Bacterial genetic recombination increases bacterial diversity.

- **Transformation** is the acquisition of genetic material from the environment, which can be integrated into the bacterial genome.
- **Conjugation** is the transfer of genetic material from one bacterium to another across a conjugation bridge. A plasmid can be transferred from F^+ cells to F^- cells. Alternatively, a portion of the genome can be transferred from an Hfr cell to a recipient.
- **Transduction** is the transfer of genetic material from one bacterium to another using a bacteriophage as a vector.
- **Transposons** are genetic elements that can insert into or remove themselves from the genome.

Bacterial growth follows a predictable pattern, as shown in Figure 10.2.

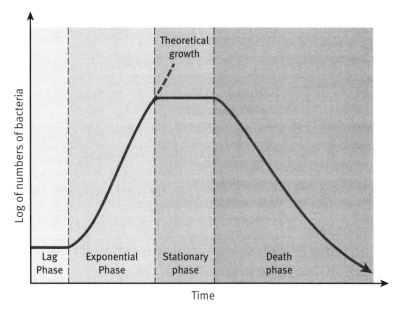

Figure 10.2. Bacterial Growth

Viruses and Subviral Particles

Viruses contain genetic material, a protein coat (**capsid**), and sometimes a lipid-containing envelope. Viruses are obligate intracellular parasites, meaning that they cannot survive and replicate outside of a **host cell.** Individual virus particles are called **virions.**

Bacteriophages are viruses that target bacteria. In addition to the other structures, they contain a **tail sheath**, which injects the genetic material into a bacterium, and **tail fibers**, which allow the bacteriophage to attach to the host cell. Viral genomes may be made of various nucleic acids:

- They may be composed of DNA or RNA and may be single or double stranded.
- Single-stranded RNA viruses may be **positive sense** (can be translated by the host cell) or **negative sense** (a complementary strand must be synthesized using **RNA replicase**, which can then be translated).
- **Retroviruses** contain a single-stranded RNA genome to which a complementary DNA strand is made using **reverse transcriptase.** The DNA strand can then be integrated into the genome.

Viruses infect cells by attaching to specific receptors. Viruses then either fuse with the cell's plasma membrane, being brought in by endocytosis, or inject their genome into the cell. The virus reproduces by replicating and translating genetic material using the host cell's ribosomes, tRNA, amino acids, and enzymes. Viral progeny are released through cell death, lysis, or **extrusion.**

Bacteriophages have two specific life cycles, as shown in Figure 10.3.

- In the **lytic cycle**, the bacteriophage produces massive numbers of new virions until the cell lyses. Bacteria in the lytic phase are termed **virulent**.
- In the **lysogenic cycle**, the virus integrates into the host genome as a provirus or prophage, which can then reproduce along with the cell. The provirus then leaves the genome in response to a stimulus at some later time and enters the lytic cycle.

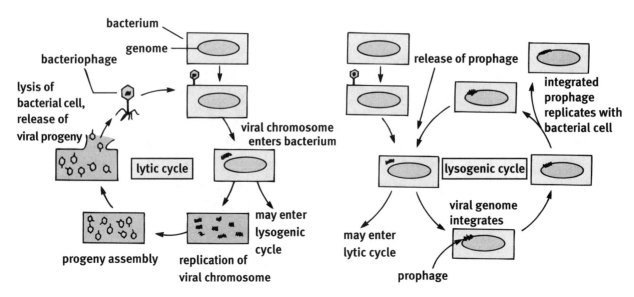

Figure 10.3. Bacteriophage Life Cycles

Prions are infectious proteins that trigger misfolding of other proteins, usually converting an α-helical structure to a β-pleated sheet. This decreases the solubility and degradability of the misfolded protein. **Viroids** are plant pathogens that are small circles of complementary RNA that can turn off genes, resulting in metabolic and structural derangements of the cell and—potentially—cell death.

REPRODUCTION

Mitosis and Meiosis

High-Yield

Diploid ($2n$) cells have two copies of each chromosome; **haploid** (n) cells have one copy. The cell cycle contains five stages. The G_1, S, and G_2 stages are collectively called **interphase**, during which the DNA is uncoiled in the form of **chromatin**.

- In the G_1 stage (**presynthetic gap**), cells create organelles for energy and protein production while also increasing their size. The **restriction point**, during which the DNA is checked for quality, must be passed for the cell to move into the S stage.
- In the **S** stage (**synthesis**), DNA is replicated. The strands of DNA, called **chromatids**, are held together at the centromere.
- In the G_2 stage (**postsynthetic gap**), there is further cell growth and replication of organelles in preparation for mitosis. Another quality checkpoint must be passed for the cell to enter into mitosis.
- In the **M** stage (**mitosis**), mitosis and cytokinesis occur.
- In the G_0 stage, the cell performs its function without any preparation for division.

Mitosis produces two genetically identical diploid daughter cells from a single cell and occurs in somatic cells. Mitosis has four phases.

- In **prophase**, the chromosomes condense, the nuclear membrane dissolves, nucleoli disappear, centrioles migrate to opposite sides of the cell, and the **spindle apparatus** begins to form. The **kinetochore** of each chromosome is contacted by a spindle fiber.
- In **metaphase**, chromosomes line up along the **metaphase plate** (**equatorial plate**).
- In **anaphase**, sister chromatids are separated and pulled to opposite poles.
- In **telophase**, the nuclear membrane reforms, spindle apparatus disappears, and cytosol and organelles are split between the two daughter cells through **cytokinesis**.

Cancer occurs when cell cycle control becomes deranged, allowing damaged cells to undergo mitosis without regard to quality or quantity of new cells produced. Cancerous cells may begin to produce factors that allow them to escape their site and invade or **metastasize** elsewhere.

Meiosis occurs in **gametocytes** (**germ cells**) and produces up to four nonidentical haploid sex cells (**gametes**). Meiosis has one round of replication and two rounds of division (the **reductional** and **equational** divisions). In **meiosis I**, homologous pairs of chromosomes (homologues) are separated from each other. **Homologues** are chromosomes that are given the same number but are of opposite parental origin.

- In **prophase I**, the same events occur as in prophase of mitosis, except that homologues come together and intertwine in a process called **synapsis**. The four chromatids are referred to as a **tetrad**, and **crossing-over** exchanges genetic material from one chromatid with material from a chromatid in the homologous chromosome. This accounts for **Mendel's second law (of independent assortment)**.
- In **metaphase I**, homologous chromosomes line up on opposite sides of the metaphase plate.
- In **anaphase I**, homologous chromosomes are segregated to opposite poles of the cell. This accounts for **Mendel's first law (of segregation)**.
- In **telophase I**, the chromosomes may or may not fully decondense, and the cell may enter **interkinesis** after cytokinesis.

In **meiosis II**, sister chromatids are separated from each other in a process that is functionally identical to mitosis. **Sister chromatids** are copies of the same DNA held together at the centromere.

The Reproductive System

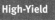

Biological sex is determined by the 23rd pair of chromosomes in humans, with XX being female and XY being male. The **X chromosome** carries a sizable amount of genetic information; mutations of X-linked genes can cause sex-linked disorders. Males are **hemizygous** with respect to the unpaired genes on the X chromosome. So they express sex-linked disorders, even if they have only one recessive, disease-carrying allele. Women with one copy of the affected recessive allele are called **carriers**.

The **Y chromosome** carries little genetic information. However, it does contain the *SRY* (**sex-determining region Y**) gene, which causes the gonads to differentiate into testes.

The male reproductive system contains both internal and external structures.

- **Sperm** develop in the **seminiferous tubules** in the **testes**. They are nourished by **Sertoli cells**.
- **Interstitial cells** (**of Leydig**) secrete **testosterone** and other male sex hormones (**androgens**).
- The testes are located in the **scrotum**, which hangs outside of the abdominal cavity and has a temperature 2°C–4°C lower than the rest of the body.
- Once formed, sperm gain motility in the **epididymis** and are stored there until ejaculation.
- During **ejaculation**, sperm travel through the **vas deferens** to the **ejaculatory duct** to the **urethra** and out through the **penis.**
- The **seminal vesicles** contribute fructose to nourish sperm and produce alkaline fluid.
- The **prostate gland** also produces alkaline fluid.
- The **bulbourethral glands** produce a clear viscous fluid that cleans out any remnants of urine and lubricates the urethra during sexual arousal.
- **Semen** is composed of sperm and **seminal fluid** from the glands above.

In **spermatogenesis**, four haploid sperm are produced from a **spermatogonium.**

- After S stage, the germ cells are called **primary spermatocytes.**
- After meiosis I, the germ cells are called **secondary spermatocytes.**
- After meiosis II, the germ cells are called **spermatids.**
- After maturation, the germ cells are called **spermatozoa.**

Sperm contain a head, midpiece, and flagellum. The **head** contains the genetic material and is covered with an acrosome—a modified Golgi apparatus that contains enzymes that help the sperm fuse to and penetrate the ovum. The **midpiece** generates ATP from fructose and contains many mitochondria. The **flagellum** promotes motility.

The female reproductive system contains only internal structures. **Ova** (eggs) are produced in **follicles** in the **ovaries**. Once each month, an egg is **ovulated** into the **peritoneal sac** and is drawn into the **fallopian tube** or **oviduct**. The fallopian tubes are connected to the **uterus**, the lower end of which is called the **cervix**. The **vaginal canal** lies below the cervix and is the site where sperm are deposited during intercourse. Birth also occurs through the vaginal canal. The external female anatomy is known as the **vulva.**

In **oogenesis**, one haploid ovum and a variable number of polar bodies are formed from an oogonium.

- At birth, all oogonia have already undergone replication and are considered **primary oocytes**. They are arrested in prophase I.
- The ovulated egg each month is a **secondary oocyte**, which is arrested in metaphase II.
- If the oocyte is fertilized, it completes meiosis II to become a true ovum.
- Cytokinesis is uneven in oogenesis. The cell receiving very little cytoplasm and organelles is called a **polar body**.
- Oocytes are surrounded by the **zona pellucida**, which is an acellular mixture of glycoproteins that protect the oocyte and contain the compounds necessary for sperm binding, and the **corona radiata**, which is a layer of cells that adheres to the oocyte during ovulation.

Gonadotropin-releasing hormone (**GnRH**) from the **hypothalamus** causes the release of **follicle-stimulating hormone** (**FSH**) and **luteinizing hormone** (**LH**), the functions of which depend on the sex of the individual. In males, FSH stimulates the Sertoli cells and triggers spermatogenesis, while LH causes the interstitial cells to produce testosterone. **Testosterone** is responsible for the maintenance and development of the male reproductive system and male secondary sex characteristics (facial and axillary hair, deepening of the voice, and changes in growth patterns). In females, FSH stimulates development of the ovarian follicles, while LH causes ovulation. These hormones also stimulate production of estrogens and progesterone.

The menstrual cycle is a periodic growth and shedding of the endometrial lining.

- In the **follicular phase**, GnRH secretion stimulates FSH and LH secretion, which promotes follicle development. Estrogen is released, stimulating vascularization and glandularization of the **decidua.**
- **Ovulation** is stimulated by a sudden surge in LH. This surge occurs because estrogen stops having negative feedback effects at a certain threshold and begins to have positive feedback effects.
- In the **luteal phase**, LH promotes the ruptured follicle to become the corpus luteum, which secretes progesterone that maintains the uterine lining. High estrogen and progesterone levels cause negative feedback on GnRH, LH, and FSH.
- **Menstruation** occurs if there is no fertilization. As the estrogen and progesterone levels drop, the endometrial lining is sloughed off and the block on GnRH production is removed.
- If fertilization does occur, the blastula produces **human chorionic gonadotropin** (**hCG**) that, as an LH analog, can maintain the corpus luteum. Near the end of the first trimester, hCG levels drop as the placenta takes over progesterone production.

Menopause occurs when the ovaries stop producing estrogen and progesterone, usually between ages 45 and 55. Menstruation stops, and FSH and LH levels rise. Physical and physiological changes accompanying menopause include flushing, hot flashes, bloating, headaches, and irritability.

EMBRYOGENESIS AND DEVELOPMENT

Early Developmental Stages

Fertilization is the joining of a sperm and an ovum. It usually occurs in the **ampulla** of the fallopian tube. The sperm uses acrosomal enzymes to penetrate the corona radiata and zona pellucida. Once it contacts the oocyte's plasma membrane, the sperm establishes the **acrosomal apparatus** and injects its pronucleus. When the first sperm penetrates, it causes a release of calcium ions, which prevent additional sperm from fertilizing the egg and increase the metabolic rate of the resulting diploid zygote. This is called the **cortical reaction.**

Fraternal (**dizygotic**) **twins** result from the fertilization of two eggs by two different sperm. **Identical** (**monozygotic**) **twins** result from the splitting of a zygote in two. Monozygotic twins can be classified by the placental structures they share (mono- vs. diamniotic, mono- vs. dichorionic).

Cleavage is defined as the early divisions of cells in the embryo. These mitotic divisions result in a larger number of smaller cells, as the overall volume does not change. The zygote becomes an embryo after the first cleavage because it is no longer unicellular. **Indeterminate cleavage** results in cells that are capable of becoming any cell in the organism, while **determinate cleavage** results in cells that are committed to differentiating into a specific cell type. (See Figure 10.4.)

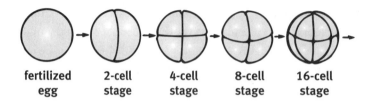

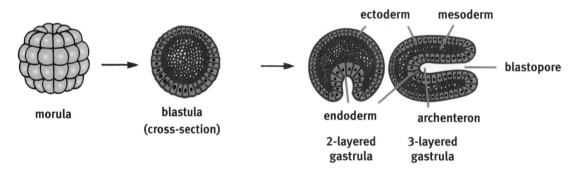

Figure 10.4. Cleavage, Morula, Blastula, and Gastrula

- The **morula** is a solid mass of cells seen in early development.
- The **blastula** (**blastocyst**) has a fluid-filled center called a **blastocoel** and has two different cell types. The **trophoblasts** become placental structures, and the **inner cell mass** becomes the developing organism.
- The blastula implants in the endometrial lining and forms the **placenta**.
- The **chorion** contains **chorionic villi**, which penetrate the endometrium and create the interface between maternal and fetal blood.
- Before the placenta is established, the embryo is supported by the **yolk sac**.
- The **allantois** is involved in early fluid exchange between the embryo and the yolk sac.
- The **amnion** lies just inside the chorion and produces amniotic fluid.
- The developing organism is connected to the placenta via the **umbilical cord**.

During **gastrulation**, the **archenteron** is formed with a **blastopore** at the end. As the archenteron grows through the blastocoel, it contacts the opposite side, establishing three primary germ layers.

- The **ectoderm** becomes epidermis, hair, and nails; the epithelia of the nose, mouth, and anal canal; the nervous system (including adrenal medulla); and the lens of the eye.
- The **mesoderm** becomes much of the musculoskeletal, circulatory, and excretory systems. Mesoderm also gives rise to the gonads, to the muscular and connective tissue layers of the digestive and respiratory systems, and to the adrenal cortex.
- The **endoderm** becomes much of the epithelial linings of the respiratory and digestive tracts and parts of the pancreas, thyroid, bladder, and distal urinary tracts.

Neurulation, or development of the nervous system, begins after the formation of the three germ layers. The **notochord** induces a group of overlying ectodermal cells to form **neural folds** surrounding a **neural groove.** The neural folds fuse to form the **neural tube**, which becomes the central nervous system. The tip of each neural fold contains **neural crest cells**, which become the peripheral nervous system (sensory ganglia, autonomic ganglia, adrenal medulla, and Schwann cells) as well as specific cell types in other tissues (calcitonin-producing cells of the thyroid, melanocytes in the skin, and others).

Teratogens are substances that interfere with development, causing defects or even death of the developing embryo. Teratogens include alcohol, certain prescription drugs, viruses, bacteria, and environmental chemicals. Maternal health can affect development, including diabetes (increased fetal size and hypoglycemia after birth) and folic acid deficiency (neural tube defects).

Mechanisms of Development

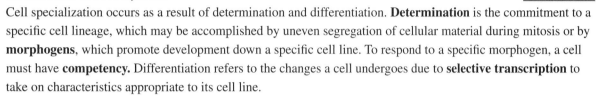

Cell specialization occurs as a result of determination and differentiation. **Determination** is the commitment to a specific cell lineage, which may be accomplished by uneven segregation of cellular material during mitosis or by **morphogens**, which promote development down a specific cell line. To respond to a specific morphogen, a cell must have **competency.** Differentiation refers to the changes a cell undergoes due to **selective transcription** to take on characteristics appropriate to its cell line.

Stem cells are cells that are capable of developing into various cell types. They can be classified by potency.

- **Totipotent cells** are able to differentiate into all cell types, including the three germ layers and placental structures.
- **Pluripotent cells** are able to differentiate into all three of the germ layers and their derivatives.
- **Multipotent cells** are able to differentiate only into a specific subset of cell types.

Cells communicate through a number of different signaling methods. An **inducer** releases factors to promote the differentiation of a competent **responder.**

- **Autocrine** signals act on the same cell that released the signal.
- **Paracrine** signals act on cells in the local area.
- **Juxtacrine** signals act through direct stimulation of the adjacent cells.
- **Endocrine** signals act on distant tissues after traveling through the bloodstream.
- Inducers are often **growth factors**, which are peptides that promote differentiation and mitosis in certain tissues.
- If two tissues both induce further differentiation in each other, this is termed **reciprocal induction.**
- Signaling often occurs via gradients.

Cells may need to migrate to arrive at their anatomically correct location. **Apoptosis** is programmed cell death via the formation of **apoptotic blebs** that can subsequently be absorbed and digested by other cells. Apoptosis can be used for sculpting certain anatomical structures, such as removing the webbing between digits. **Regenerative capacity** is the ability of an organism to regrow certain parts of the body. The liver has high regenerative capacity, while the heart has low regenerative capacity. **Senescence** is the result of multiple molecular and metabolic processes, most notably, the shortening of telomeres during cell division.

Fetal Circulation

Nutrient, gas, and waste exchange occurs at the placenta. Oxygen and carbon dioxide are passively exchanged due to concentration gradients. **Fetal hemoglobin** (**HbF**) has a higher affinity for oxygen than does adult hemoglobin (primarily HbA), which also assists in the transfer (and retention) of oxygen into the fetal circulatory system.

The placental barrier also serves as immune protection against many pathogens, and antibodies are transferred across it from mother to child. The placenta serves endocrine functions by secreting estrogen, progesterone, and human chorionic gonadotropin (hCG).

The **umbilical arteries** carry deoxygenated blood from the fetus to the placenta; the umbilical vein carries oxygenated blood from the placenta back to the fetus.

The fetal circulatory system (see Figure 10.5) differs from its adult version by having three shunts.

- The **foramen ovale** connects the right atrium to the left atrium, bypassing the lungs.
- The **ductus arteriosus** connects the pulmonary artery to the aorta, bypassing the lungs.
- The **ductus venosus** connects the umbilical vein to the inferior vena cava, bypassing the liver.

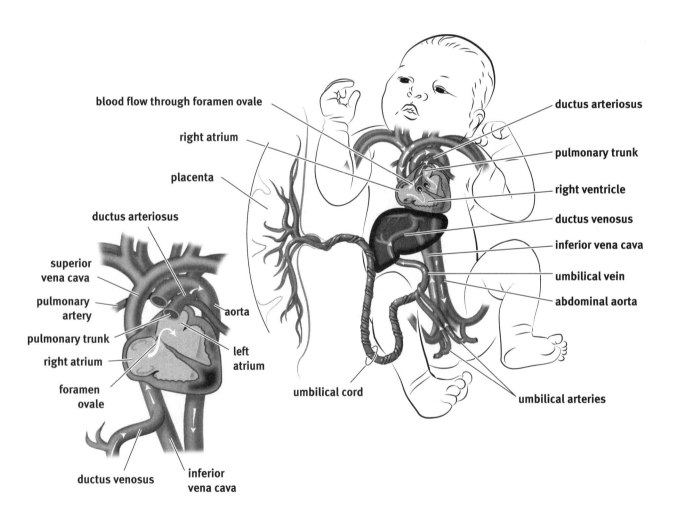

Figure 10.5. Fetal Circulatory System

Gestation and Birth

In the first trimester, organogenesis occurs (development of heart, eyes, gonads, limbs, liver, brain). In the second trimester, tremendous growth occurs, movement begins, the face becomes distinctly human, and the digits elongate. In the third trimester, rapid growth and brain development continue, and there is transfer of antibodies to the fetus. During birth, the cervix thins out and the amniotic sac ruptures. Then, uterine contractions, coordinated by prostaglandins and oxytocin, result in birth of the fetus. Finally, the placenta and umbilical cord are expelled.

THE NERVOUS SYSTEM

Cells of the Nervous System

High-Yield

Neurons are highly specialized cells responsible for the conduction of impulses. Neurons communicate using both electrical and chemical forms of communication. Electrical communication occurs via ion exchange and the generation of membrane potentials down the length of the axon. Chemical communication occurs via neurotransmitter release from the presynaptic cell and the binding of these neurotransmitters to the postsynaptic cell.

Neurons consist of many different parts, as shown in Figure 10.6.

- **Dendrites** are appendages that receive signals from other cells.
- The cell body or **soma** is the location of the nucleus as well as organelles such as the endoplasmic reticulum and ribosomes.
- The **axon hillock** is where the cell body transitions to the axon and where action potentials are initiated.
- The **axon** is a long appendage down which an action potential travels.
- The **nerve terminal** or **synaptic bouton** is the end of the axon from which neurotransmitters are released.
- **Nodes of Ranvier** are exposed areas of myelinated axons that permit saltatory conduction.
- The **synapse** consists of the nerve terminal of the presynaptic neuron, the membrane of the postsynaptic cell, and the space between the two, called the **synaptic cleft**.

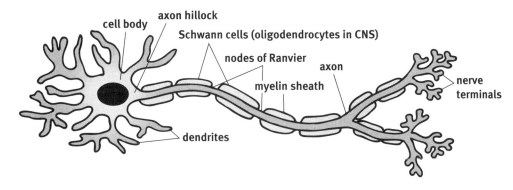

Figure 10.6. The Neuron

Many axons are coated in **myelin**, an insulating substance that prevents signal loss. Myelin prevents dissipation of the neural impulse and crossing of neural impulses from adjacent neurons.

Individual axons are bundled into **nerves** or **tracts**. A single nerve may carry multiple types of information, including sensory, motor, or both. Tracts contain only one type of information. Cell bodies of neurons of the same type within a nerve cluster form **ganglia** in the peripheral nervous system. Cell bodies of the individual neurons within a tract cluster form **nuclei** in the central nervous system.

Neuroglia or glial cells are other cells within the nervous system in addition to neurons.

- **Astrocytes** nourish neurons and form the blood-brain barrier, which controls the transmission of solutes from the bloodstream into nervous tissue.
- **Ependymal cells** line the ventricles of the brain and produce cerebrospinal fluid, which physically supports the brain and serves as a shock absorber.
- **Microglia** are phagocytic cells that ingest and break down waste products and pathogens in the central nervous system.

Transmission of Neural Impulses

`High-Yield`

All neurons exhibit a **resting membrane potential** of approximately -70 mV. Resting potential is maintained using selective permeability of ions as well as the Na^+/K^+ ATPase. The Na^+/K^+ **ATPase** pumps three sodium ions out of the cell for every two potassium ions pumped in.

Incoming signals can be either excitatory or inhibitory. Excitatory signals cause depolarization of the neuron. Inhibitory signals cause hyperpolarization of the neuron. **Temporal summation** refers to the addition of multiple signals near each other in time. **Spatial summation** refers to the addition of multiple signals near each other in space.

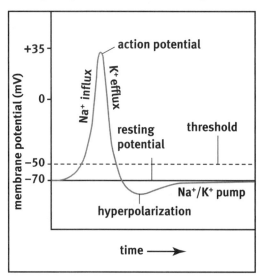

Figure 10.7. Action Potential in a Neuron

An action potential (see Figure 10.7) is used to propagate signals down the axon.

- When enough excitatory stimulation occurs, the cell is **depolarized** to the **threshold voltage** and voltage-gated sodium channels open.
- Sodium flows into the neuron due to its strong **electrochemical gradient**. This continues depolarizing the neuron.
- At the peak of the action potential (approximately +35 mV), sodium channels are inactivated and potassium channels open.
- Potassium flows out of the neuron due to its strong electrochemical gradient, **repolarizing** the cell. Potassium channels stay open long enough to overshoot the action potential, resulting in a **hyperpolarized** neuron; then the potassium channels close.
- The Na^+/K^+ ATPase brings the neuron back to the resting potential and restores the sodium and potassium gradients.
- While the axon is hyperpolarized, it is in its **refractory period**. During the **absolute refractory period**, the cell is unable to fire another action potential. During the **relative refractory period**, the cell requires a larger than normal stimulus to fire an action potential.
- The impulse propagates down the length of the axon because the influx of sodium in one segment of the axon brings the subsequent segment of the axon to threshold. The fact that the preceding segment of the axon is in its refractory period means that the action potential can travel in only one direction.

At the nerve terminal, neurotransmitters are released into the synapse. When the action potential arrives at the nerve terminal, **voltage-gated calcium channels** open. The influx of calcium causes fusion of vesicles filled with neurotransmitter with the presynaptic membrane, resulting in exocytosis of neurotransmitter into the synaptic cleft. The neurotransmitters bind to receptors on the postsynaptic cell, which may be ligand-gated ion channels or G protein-coupled receptors.

Neurotransmitters must be cleared from the postsynaptic receptors to stop the propagation of the signal. The neurotransmitter can be enzymatically broken down. The neurotransmitter can be absorbed back into the presynaptic cell by **reuptake channels.** The neurotransmitter can diffuse out of the synaptic cleft.

Organization of the Human Nervous System

There are three types of neurons in the nervous system: **motor (efferent)** neurons, **interneurons**, and **sensory (afferent) neurons. Reflex arcs** use the ability of interneurons in the spinal cord to relay information to the source of a stimulus while simultaneously routing it to the brain. In a **monosynaptic reflex arc**, the sensory (afferent, presynaptic) neuron fires directly onto the motor (efferent, postsynaptic) neuron. In a **polysynaptic reflex arc**, the sensory neuron may fire onto a motor neuron as well as interneurons that fire onto other motor neurons.

THE ENDOCRINE SYSTEM

Mechanisms of Hormone Action

High-Yield

Endocrine signaling involves the secretion of **hormones** directly into the bloodstream. The hormones travel to distant target tissues, where they bind to receptors and induce a change in gene expression or cell function (see Table 10.3).

Peptide hormones are composed of amino acids and are derived from larger precursor proteins that are cleaved during post-translational modification. Peptide hormones are polar and cannot pass through the plasma membrane. These hormones bind to extracellular receptors, where they trigger the transmission of a **second messenger.** Each step of the **signaling cascade** can demonstrate **amplification** of the signal. Peptide hormones usually have rapid onset but are short-lived. These hormones travel freely in the bloodstream and do not require a special carrier.

Steroid hormones are derived from cholesterol. Steroid hormones are minimally polar and can pass through the plasma membrane. These hormones bind to and promote a conformational change of intracellular or intranuclear receptors; the hormone-receptor complex binds to DNA, affecting the transcription of a particular gene. Steroid hormones usually have slow onset but are long-lived. These hormones cannot dissolve in the bloodstream and must be carried by specific proteins.

Amino acid–derivative hormones are modified amino acids. Their chemistry shares some features with peptide hormones and some features with steroid hormones; different amino acid–derivative hormones share different features with these other hormone classes. Common examples are epinephrine, norepinephrine, triiodothyronine, and thyroxine.

Hormones can be classified by their target tissues.

- **Direct hormones** have major effects in nonendocrine tissues.
- **Tropic hormones** have major effects in other endocrine tissues.

Endocrine Organs and Hormones

High-Yield

The **hypothalamus** is the bridge between the nervous and endocrine systems. The release of hormones from the hypothalamus is mediated by a number of factors, including projections from other parts of the brain, chemo- and baroreceptors in the blood vessels, and negative feedback from other hormones. In **negative feedback**, the final hormone (or product) of a pathway inhibits hormones (or enzymes) earlier in the pathway, maintaining **homeostasis**.

Hormone	Source	Action
Follicle-stimulating (FSH)	Anterior pituitary	Stimulates follicle maturation; spermatogenesis
Luteinizing (LH)		Stimulates ovulation; testosterone synthesis
Adrenocorticotropic (ACTH)		Stimulates adrenal cortex to make and secrete glucocorticoids
Thyroid-stimulating (TSH)		Stimulates the thyroid to produce thyroid hormones
Prolactin		Stimulates milk production and secretion
Endorphins		Inhibits the perception of pain in the brain
Growth hormone		Stimulates bone and muscle growth/lipolysis
Oxytocin	Hypothalamus; stored in posterior pituitary	Stimulates uterine contractions during labor, milk secretion during lactation
Antidiuretic (ADH, vasopressin)		Stimulates water reabsorption in kidneys
Thyroid hormones (T_3, T_4)	Thyroid	Stimulates metabolic activity
Calcitonin		Decreases (tones down) blood calcium level
Parathyroid hormone	Parathyroid	Increases blood calcium level
Glucocorticoids	Adrenal cortex	Increases blood glucose level and decreases protein synthesis; anti-inflammatory
Mineralocorticoids		Increases sodium and water reabsorption in kidneys
Epinephrine, norepinephrine	Adrenal medulla	Increases blood glucose level and heart rate
Glucagon	Pancreas	Stimulates conversion of glycogen to glucose in the lever; increases blood glucose
Insulin		Lowers blood glucose; increases glycogen stores
Somatostatin		Suppresses secretion of glucagon and insulin
Testosterone	Testes	Maintains male secondary sex characteristics
Estrogen	Ovary/placenta	Maintains female secondary sex characteristics
Progesterone		Promotes growth/maintenance of endometrium
Melatonin	Pineal	Regulates sleep-wake cycles
Atrial natriuretic peptide	Heart	Involved in osmoregulation and vasodilation
Thymosin	Thymus	Stimulates T-cell development

Table 10.3. Hormone Sources and Actions

THE RESPIRATORY SYSTEM

Anatomy and Mechanism of Breathing

Air is drawn in through the **nares** and moves through the nasal cavity and **pharynx**, where it is warmed and humidified. It is filtered by nasal hairs (**vibrissae**) and mucous membranes. It then enters the **larynx**, followed by the **trachea.** The trachea divides into two mainstem **bronchi**, which divide into **bronchioles**, which divide into continually smaller passages until reaching the alveoli.

Alveoli are small sacs that interface with the pulmonary capillaries, allowing gases to diffuse across a one-cell-thick membrane. **Surfactant** in the alveoli reduces surface tension at the liquid-gas interface, preventing collapse.

The pleurae cover the lungs and line the chest wall.

- The **visceral pleura** lies adjacent to the lung itself.
- The **parietal pleura** lines the chest wall.
- The **intrapleural space** lies between these two layers and contains a thin layer of fluid, which lubricates the two pleural surfaces.

The **diaphragm** is a thin skeletal muscle that helps to create the pressure differential required for breathing. Inhalation is an active process. The diaphragm and **external intercostal muscles** expand the thoracic cavity, increasing the volume of the intrapleural space. This decreases the intrapleural pressure. **Exhalation** may be passive or active. In passive exhalation, relaxation of the muscles of inspiration and elastic recoil of the lungs allow the chest cavity to decrease in volume, reversing the pressure differentials seen in inhalation. In active exhalation, the internal intercostal muscles and abdominal muscles can be used to decrease the volume of the thoracic cavity forcibly, pushing out air.

A **spirometer** can be used to measure lung capacities and volumes (see Figure 10.8).

- **Total lung capacity** (**TLC**) is the maximum volume of air in the lungs when one inhales completely.
- **Residual volume** (**RV**) is the minimum volume of air in the lungs when one exhales completely.
- **Vital capacity** (**VC**) is the difference between the minimum and maximum volume of air in the lungs.
- **Tidal volume** (**TV**) is the volume of air inhaled or exhaled in a normal breath.
- **Expiratory reserve volume** (**ERV**) is the volume of additional air that can be forcibly exhaled after a normal exhalation.
- **Inspiratory reserve volume** (**IRV**) is the volume of additional air that can be forcibly inhaled after a normal inhalation.

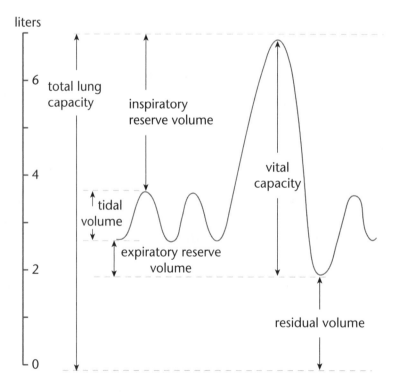

Figure 10.8. Lung Capacity and Volume

Ventilation is regulated by the **ventilation center**, a collection of neurons in the medulla oblongata. **Chemorecep-tors** respond to carbon dioxide concentrations, increasing the respiratory rate when there are high concentrations of carbon dioxide in the blood (**hypercarbia** or **hypercapnia**). The ventilation center can also respond to low oxygen concentrations in the blood (**hypoxemia**) by increasing ventilation rate. Ventilation can also be controlled consciously through the cerebrum, although the medulla oblongata will override the cerebrum during extended periods of hypo- or hyperventilation.

Functions of the Respiratory System

The lungs perform gas exchange with the blood through simple diffusion across concentration gradients. Deoxygenated blood with a high carbon dioxide concentration is brought to the lungs via the **pulmonary arteries.** Oxygenated blood with a low carbon dioxide concentration leaves the lungs via the **pulmonary veins.** The large surface area of interaction between the alveoli and capillaries allows the respiratory system to assist in thermoregu-lation through **vasodilation** and **vasoconstriction** of capillary beds.

The respiratory system must be protected from potential pathogens. Multiple mechanisms, including vibris-sae, mucous membranes, and the **mucociliary escalator**, help filter the incoming air and trap particulate matter. **Lysozyme** in the nasal cavity and saliva attacks peptidoglycan cell walls of gram-positive bacteria. **Macrophages** can engulf and digest pathogens and signal to the rest of the immune system that there is an invader. Mucosal surfaces are covered with IgA antibodies. **Mast cells** have antibodies on their surface that, when triggered, can promote the release of inflammatory chemicals. Mast cells are often involved in allergic reactions as well.

The respiratory system is involved in pH control through the bicarbonate buffer system. When blood pH decreases, the respiration rate increases to compensate by blowing off carbon dioxide. This causes a left shift in the buffer equation, reducing hydrogen ion concentration. When blood pH increases, respiration rate decreases to compensate by trapping carbon dioxide. This causes a right shift in the buffer equation, increasing hydrogen ion concentration.

THE CARDIOVASCULAR SYSTEM

Anatomy of the Cardiovascular System

`High-Yield`

The **cardiovascular system** consists of a muscular four-chambered heart, blood vessels, and blood. The **heart** is composed of **cardiac muscle** and supports two different circulations: the **pulmonary circulation** and the **systemic circulation**.

Each side of the heart (see Figure 10.9) consists of an **atrium** and a **ventricle**. The atria are separated from the ventricles by the **atrioventricular valves** (**tricuspid** on the right, **mitral** [**bicuspid**] on the left). The ventricles are separated from the vasculature by the **semilunar valves** (**pulmonary** on the right, **aortic** on the left).

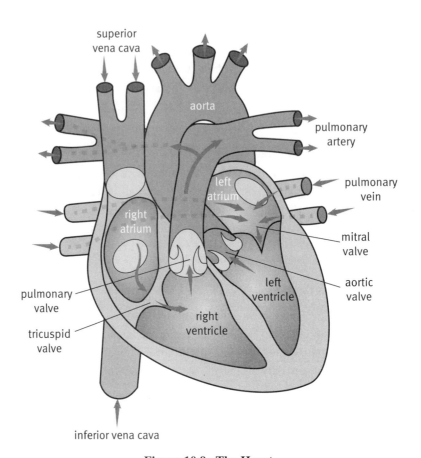

Figure 10.9. The Heart

Electrical conduction of the heart starts at the **sinoatrial** (**SA**) node and then goes to the **atrioventricular** (**AV**) node. From the AV node, electrical conduction goes to the bundle of His before traveling through the Purkinje fibers.

Systole refers to the period during ventricular contraction when the AV valves are closed. During **diastole**, the heart is relaxed and the semilunar valves are closed. The **cardiac output** is the product of **heart rate** and **stroke volume.**

The vasculature consists of arteries, veins, and capillaries.

- **Arteries** are thick, highly muscular structures with an elastic quality. This allows for recoil and helps to propel blood forward within the system. Small muscular arteries are **arterioles**, which control flow into capillary beds.
- **Capillaries** have walls that are one cell thick, making them so narrow that red blood cells must travel through them in single-file lines. Capillaries are the sites of gas and solute exchange.
- **Veins** are inelastic, thin-walled structures that transport blood to the heart. They are able to stretch in order to accommodate large volumes of blood but do not have recoil capability. Veins are compressed by surrounding skeletal muscles and have **valves** to maintain one-way flow. Small veins are called **venules.**

A portal system is one in which blood passes through two capillary beds in series. In the **hepatic portal system**, blood travels from the gut capillary beds to the liver capillary bed via the hepatic portal vein. In the **hypophyseal portal system**, blood travels from the hypothalamus to the anterior pituitary. In the **renal portal system**, blood travels from the glomerulus to the vasa recta through an efferent arteriole.

Blood

Blood is composed of cells and plasma, an aqueous mixture of nutrients, salts, respiratory gases, hormones, and blood proteins.

- **Erythrocytes** (**red blood cells**) lack mitochondria, a nucleus, and organelles in order to make room for **hemoglobin**, a protein that carries oxygen. Common measurements include hemoglobin concentration and **hematocrit**, the percentage of blood composed of erythrocytes.
- **Leukocytes** (**white blood cells**) are formed in the bone marrow. They are a crucial part of the immune system.
- Granular leukocytes, such as neutrophils, eosinophils, and basophils, play a role in nonspecific immunity.
- Agranulocytes, including lymphocytes and monocytes, also play a role in immunity, with lymphocytes playing a large role in specific immunity.
- **Thrombocytes** (**platelets**) are cell fragments from **megakaryocytes** that are required for coagulation.

Blood antigens include the surface antigens A, B, and O as well as Rh factor (D). The I^A (A) and I^B (B) alleles are codominant, while the i (O) allele is recessive. An individual has antibodies for any AB alleles he or she does not have. Positive Rh factor is dominant. An Rh-negative individual creates anti-Rh antibodies only after exposure to Rh-positive blood.

Physiology of the Cardiovascular System

Blood pressure refers to the force per unit area that is exerted on the walls of blood vessels by blood. It is divided into systolic and diastolic components. It must be high enough to overcome the resistance created by arterioles and capillaries but low enough to avoid damaging the vasculature and surrounding structures. It can be measured with a **sphygmomanometer.**

The blood pressure is maintained by baroreceptor and chemoreceptor reflexes. Low blood pressure promotes **aldosterone** and **antidiuretic hormone** (**ADH** or **vasopressin**) release. High blood osmolarity also promotes ADH release. High blood pressure promotes **atrial natriuretic peptide** (**ANP**) release.

Gas and solute exchange occurs at the level of the capillaries and relies on the existence of concentration gradients to facilitate diffusion across the capillary walls. Capillaries are also leaky, which aids in the transport of gases and solutes.

Starling forces consist of **hydrostatic pressure** and **osmotic** (**oncotic**) **pressure**. Hydrostatic pressure is the pressure of the fluid within the blood vessel, while osmotic pressure is the "sucking" pressure drawing water toward solutes. Oncotic pressure is osmotic pressure due to proteins. Hydrostatic pressure forces fluid out at the arteriolar end of a capillary bed; oncotic pressure draws the fluid back in at the venule end.

Oxygen is carried by hemoglobin, which exhibits **cooperative binding** (see Figure 10.10). In the lungs, there is a high partial pressure of oxygen, resulting in loading of oxygen onto hemoglobin. In the tissues, there is a low partial pressure of oxygen, resulting in unloading. With cooperative binding, each successive oxygen bound to hemoglobin increases the affinity of the other subunits, while each successive oxygen released decreases the affinity of the other subunits.

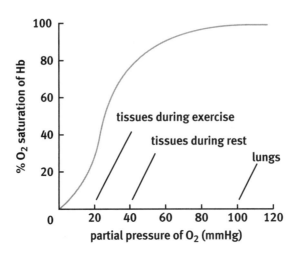

Figure 10.10. Oxygen Saturation of Hemoglobin *vs.* Partial Pressure of Oxygen

Carbon dioxide is largely carried in the blood in the form of carbonic acid, or bicarbonate and hydrogen ions. Carbon dioxide is nonpolar and not particularly soluble. In contrast, bicarbonate, hydrogen ions, and carbonic acid are polar and highly soluble.

A high $P_a\text{CO}_2$, high $[\text{H}^+]$, low pH, high temperature, and high concentration of 2,3-BPG can cause a right shift in the **oxyhemoglobin dissociation curve**, reflecting a decreased affinity for oxygen. In addition to the opposites of the causes of a right shift, a left shift can also be seen in fetal hemoglobin compared to adult hemoglobin.

Coagulation results from an activation cascade. When the endothelial lining of a blood vessel is damaged, the collagen and **tissue factor** underlying the endothelial cells are exposed. This results in a cascade of events known as the **coagulation cascade**, ultimately resulting in the formation of a clot over the damaged area. Platelets bind to the collagen and are stabilized by **fibrin**, which is activated by **thrombin**. Clots can be broken down by **plasmin.**

THE IMMUNE SYSTEM
`High-Yield`

The immune system can be divided into innate and adaptive immunity. **Innate immunity** is composed of defenses that are always active but that cannot target a specific invader and cannot maintain immunologic memory. It is also called **nonspecific immunity. Adaptive immunity** is composed of defenses that take time to activate but that target a specific invader and can maintain immunologic memory. It is also called **specific immunity.**

Immune cells come from the **bone marrow.** The **spleen** and **lymph nodes** are sites where immune responses can be mounted and in which B-cells are activated. The **thymus** is the site of T-cell maturation. Gut-associated lymphoid tissue (GALT) includes the tonsils and adenoids.

Many of the nonspecific defenses are noncellular. The skin acts as a physical barrier and secretes antimicrobial compounds, like **defensins.** Mucus on mucous membranes traps pathogens; in the respiratory system, the mucus is propelled upward by cilia and can be swallowed or expelled. Tears and saliva contain lysozyme, an antibacterial compound. The stomach produces acid, killing most pathogens. Colonization of the gut helps prevent overgrowth by pathogenic bacteria through competition. The **complement system** can punch holes into the cell walls of bacteria, making them osmotically unstable. **Interferons** are given off by virally infected cells and help prevent viral replication and dispersion to nearby cells.

Many of the nonspecific defenses are also cellular.

- **Macrophages** ingest pathogens and present them on **major histocompatibility complex** (**MHC**) molecules. They also secrete **cytokines**.
- **MHC class I** (**MHC-I**) is present in all nucleated cells and displays **endogenous antigen** (proteins from within the cell) to cytotoxic T-cells (CD8$^+$ cells).
- **MHC class II** (**MHC-II**) is present in professional antigen-presenting cells (macrophages, dendritic cells, some B-cells, and certain activated epithelial cells) and displays **exogenous antigens** (proteins from outside the cell) to helper T-cells (CD4$^+$ cells).
- **Dendritic cells** are antigen-presenting cells in the skin.
- **Natural killer cells** attack cells not presenting MHC molecules, including virally infected cells and cancer cells.
- **Granulocytes** include neutrophils, eosinophils, and basophils.
- **Neutrophils** ingest bacteria, particularly opsonized bacteria (those marked with antibodies). They can follow bacteria using **chemotaxis.**
- **Eosinophils** are used in allergic reactions and invasive parasitic infections. They release **histamine**, causing an inflammatory response.
- **Basophils** are used in allergic reactions. **Mast cells** are related cells found in the skin.

Humoral immunity is centered on antibody production by plasma cells, which are activated **B-cells. Antibodies** target a particular **antigen.** They contain two heavy chains and two light chains. They have a **constant region** and a **variable region**; the tip of the variable region is the **antigen-binding region.** When activated, the antigen-binding region undergoes **hypermutation** to improve the specificity of the antibody produced. Cells may be given signals to switch **isotypes** of antibody (IgM, IgD, IgG, IgE, IgA). Circulating antibodies can **opsonize** pathogens (mark them for destruction), cause **agglutination** (clumping) into insoluble complexes that are ingested by phagocytes, or neutralize pathogens. Cell-surface antibodies can activate immune cells or mediate allergic reactions. **Memory B-cells** lie in wait for a second exposure to a pathogen and can then mount a more rapid and vigorous immune response (**secondary response**).

Cell-mediated (cytotoxic) immunity is centered on the functions of **T-cells.** T-cells undergo maturation in the thymus through **positive selection** (only selecting for T-cells that can react to antigen presented on MHC) and **negative selection** (causing apoptosis in self-reactive T-cells). The peptide hormone **thymosin** promotes T-cell development. **Helper T-cells** (**T$_h$** or **CD4$^+$**) respond to antigen on MHC-II and coordinate the rest of the immune system, secreting **lymphokines** to activate various arms of immune defense. **T$_h$1 cells** secrete **interferon gamma**, which activates macrophages. **T$_h$2 cells** activate B-cells, primarily in parasitic infections. **Cytotoxic T-cells** (**T$_c$, CTL,** or **CD8$^+$**) respond to antigen on MHC-I and kill virally infected cells. **Suppressor** (**regulatory**) **T-cells** (**T$_{reg}$**) tone down the immune response after an infection and promote self-tolerance. **Memory T-cells** serve a similar function to memory B-cells.

In **autoimmune** conditions, a self-antigen is recognized as foreign and the immune system attacks normal cells. In **allergic** reactions, nonthreatening exposures incite an inflammatory response. Immunization is a method of inducing **active immunity** (activation of B-cells that produce antibodies to an antigen) prior to exposure to a particular pathogen. **Passive immunity** is the transfer of antibodies directly to an individual.

The **lymphatic system** is a circulatory system that consists of one-way vessels with intermittent lymph nodes. The lymphatic system connects to the cardiovascular system via the **thoracic duct** in the posterior chest. The lymphatic system equalizes fluid distribution, transports fats and fat-soluble compounds in **chylomicrons**, and provides sites for mounting immune responses.

THE DIGESTIVE SYSTEM

Intracellular digestion involves the oxidation of glucose and fatty acids to make energy. **Extracellular digestion** occurs in the lumen of the alimentary canal. **Mechanical digestion** is the physical breakdown of large food particles into smaller food particles. (See Figure 10.11.) **Chemical digestion** is the enzymatic cleavage of chemical bonds, such as the peptide bonds of proteins or the glycosidic bonds of starches.

The **enteric nervous system** is in the wall of the alimentary canal and controls peristalsis. Its activity is upregulated by the parasympathetic nervous system and downregulated by the sympathetic nervous system.

Multiple hormones regulate feeding behavior, including antidiuretic hormone (ADH or vasopressin) and aldosterone, which promote thirst; glucagon and ghrelin, which promote hunger; and leptin and cholecystokinin, which promote satiety.

- In the oral cavity, mastication starts the mechanical digestion of food, while salivary amylase and lipase start the chemical digestion of food. Food is formed into a bolus and swallowed.
- The **pharynx** connects the mouth and posterior nasal cavity to the esophagus.
- The **esophagus** propels food to the stomach using peristalsis. Food enters the stomach through the **lower esophageal (cardiac) sphincter.**
- The stomach has four parts: **fundus, body, antrum,** and **pylorus.** The stomach has a **lesser** and **greater curvature** and is thrown into folds called **rugae.** Numerous secretory cells line the stomach.
- Mucous cells produce bicarbonate-rich mucus to protect the stomach. **Chief cells** secrete **pepsinogen**, a protease activated by the acidic environment of the stomach. **Parietal cells** secrete hydrochloric acid and **intrinsic factor**, which is needed for vitamin B_{12} absorption. G-cells secrete **gastrin**, a peptide hormone that increases HCl secretion and gastric motility.

After mechanical and chemical digestion in the stomach, the food particles are now called **chyme**. Food passes into the duodenum through the **pyloric sphincter**.

The **duodenum** is the first part of the small intestine and is primarily involved in chemical digestion. Disaccharidases are brush border enzymes that break down maltose, isomaltose, lactose, and sucrose into monosaccharides. Brush border **peptidases** include aminopeptidase and dipeptidases. **Enteropeptidase** activates trypsinogen and procarboxypeptidases, initiating an activation cascade. **Secretin** stimulates the release of pancreatic juices into the digestive tract and slows motility. **Cholecystokinin** stimulates bile release from the gallbladder, release of pancreatic juices, and satiety.

Acinar cells in the pancreas produce pancreatic juices that contain bicarbonate, **pancreatic amylase**, pancreatic peptidases (**trypsinogen, chymotrypsinogen, carboxypeptidases A** and **B**), and **pancreatic lipase.** The liver synthesizes **bile**, which can be stored in the gallbladder or secreted into the duodenum directly. Bile emulsifies fats, making them soluble and increasing their surface area. The main components of bile are bile salts, pigments (especially **bilirubin** from the breakdown of hemoglobin), and cholesterol.

The liver also processes nutrients (through glycogenesis and glycogenolysis, storage and mobilization of fats, and gluconeogenesis), produces urea, detoxifies chemicals, activates or inactivates medications, produces bile, and synthesizes albumin and clotting factors.

The **jejunum** and **ileum** of the small intestine are primarily involved in absorption. The small intestine is lined with villi, which are covered with **microvilli**, increasing the surface area available for absorption. Villi contain a capillary bed and a **lacteal**, a vessel of the lymphatic system. Water-soluble compounds, such as monosaccharides, amino acids, water-soluble vitamins, small fatty acids, and water, enter the capillary bed. Fat-soluble compounds, such as fats, cholesterol, and fat-soluble vitamins, enter the lacteal.

The **large intestine** absorbs water and salts, forming semisolid feces. The **cecum** is an outpocketing that accepts fluid from the small intestine through the ileocecal valve and is the site of attachment of the appendix. The colon is divided into ascending, transverse, descending, and sigmoid portions. The **rectum** stores feces, which are then excreted through the anus. Gut bacteria produce vitamin K and biotin (vitamin B_7).

KEY CONCEPT

The gallbladder stores and concentrates bile.

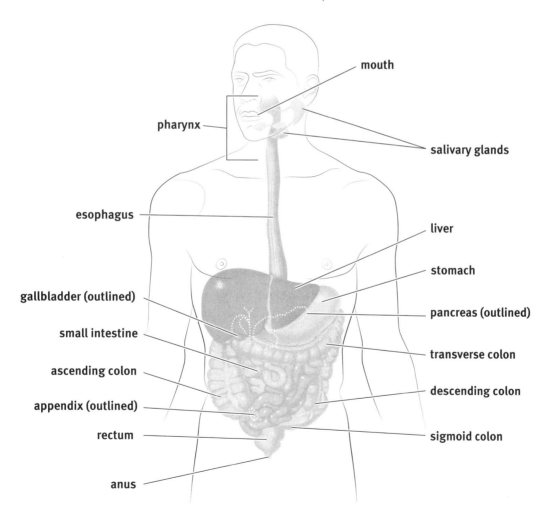

Figure 10.11. The Digestive System

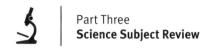

THE EXCRETORY SYSTEM

The **excretory system** serves many functions, including the regulation of blood pressure, blood osmolarity, and acid-base balance and also the removal of nitrogenous wastes. The kidney produces urine, which dumps into the **ureter** at the renal pelvis. Urine is then collected in the bladder until it is excreted through the urethra.

The kidney contains a **cortex** and a **medulla**. Each kidney has a hilum, which contains a renal artery, renal vein, and ureter. The kidney contains a portal system with two capillary beds in series. Blood from the renal artery flows into afferent arterioles, which form **glomeruli** in **Bowman's capsule** (the first capillary bed). Blood then flows through the efferent arteriole to the **vasa recta**, which surround the nephron (the second capillary bed), before leaving the kidney through the renal vein.

The **bladder** has a muscular lining known as the detrusor muscle, which is under parasympathetic control. It also has two muscular sphincters. The internal urethral sphincter consists of smooth muscle and is under involuntary (parasympathetic) control. The external urethral sphincter consists of skeletal muscle and is under voluntary control.

The kidney participates in solute movement through three processes.

- **Filtration** is the movement of solutes from blood to filtrate at Bowman's capsule. The direction and rate of filtration is determined by **Starling forces**, which account for the hydrostatic and oncotic pressure differentials between the glomerulus and Bowman's space.
- **Secretion** is the movement of solutes from blood to filtrate anywhere other than Bowman's capsule.
- **Reabsorption** is the movement of solutes from filtrate to blood.

Each segment of the nephron has a specific function.

- The **proximal convoluted tubule (PCT)** is the site of bulk reabsorption of glucose, amino acids, soluble vitamins, salt, and water. It is also the site of secretion for hydrogen ions, potassium ions, ammonia, and urea.
- The **descending limb of the loop of Henle** is permeable to water but not salt. Therefore, as the filtrate moves into the more osmotically concentrated renal medulla, water is reabsorbed from the filtrate. The vasa recta and nephron flow in opposite directions, creating a **countercurrent multiplier system** that allows maximal reabsorption of water.
- The **ascending limb of the loop of Henle** is permeable to salt but not water; therefore, salt is reabsorbed both passively and actively. The **diluting segment** is in the outer medulla. Because salt is actively reabsorbed in this site, the filtrate actually becomes hypotonic compared to the blood.
- The **distal convoluted tubule (DCT)** is responsive to aldosterone and is a site of salt reabsorption and waste product excretion, like the PCT.
- The **collecting duct** is responsive to both aldosterone and antidiuretic hormone. It has variable permeability, which allows reabsorption of the right amount of water depending on the body's needs.

The kidney is under hormonal control. When blood pressure (and volume) are low, two different hormonal systems are activated. **Aldosterone** is a steroid hormone regulated by the renin-angiotensin-aldosterone system that increases sodium reabsorption in the distal convoluted tubule and collecting duct, thereby increasing water reabsorption. This results in an increased blood volume (and pressure) but no change in blood osmolarity.

Antidiuretic hormone (ADH or vasopressin) is a peptide hormone synthesized by the hypothalamus and released by the posterior pituitary. Its release is stimulated not only by low blood volume but also by high blood osmolarity. It increases the permeability of the collecting duct to water, increasing water reabsorption. This results in an increased blood volume (and pressure) and a decreased blood osmolarity.

Skin

The skin acts as a barrier, protecting us from the elements and invasion by pathogens. The skin is composed of three major layers: the hypodermis (subcutaneous layer), dermis, and epidermis. The epidermis is composed of five layers: the **stratum basale**, **stratum spinosum**, **stratum granulosum**, **stratum lucidum**, and **stratum corneum.** The stratum basale contains stem cells that proliferate to form keratinocytes. Keratinocyte nuclei are lost in the stratum granulosum, and many thin layers form in the stratum corneum.

Melanocytes produce **melanin**, which protects the skin from DNA damage caused by ultraviolet radiation; melanin is passed to keratinocytes. **Langerhans** cells are special macrophages that serve as antigen-presenting cells in the skin.

The skin is important for thermoregulation, or the maintenance of a constant internal temperature. Cooling mechanisms include **sweating**, which absorbs heat from the body through evaporation of water from sweat, and vasodilation. Sweat glands are innervated by post-ganglionic cholinergic sympathetic neurons. Warming mechanisms include **piloerection**, in which arrector pili muscles contract and cause hairs to stand on end (trapping a layer of warmed air around the skin), vasoconstriction, shivering, and insulation provided by fat. The skin also prevents dehydration and salt loss from the body.

KEY CONCEPT

The kidney can regulate pH by selective reabsorption or secretion of bicarbonate or hydrogen ions.

KEY CONCEPT

The hypodermis contains fat and connective tissue and connects the skin to the rest of the body.

THE MUSCULAR SYSTEM

High-Yield

As shown in Table 10.4, there are three main types of muscle: skeletal muscle, smooth muscle, and cardiac muscle.

Skeletal Muscle	Cardiac Muscle	Smooth Muscle
Striated	Striated	Nonstriated
Voluntary	Involuntary	Involuntary
Somatic innervation	Autonomic innervation	Autonomic innervation
Many nuclei per cell	1–2 nuclei per cell	1 nucleus per cell
Ca^{2+} required for contraction	Ca^{2+} required for contraction	Ca^{2+} required for contraction

Table 10.4. Primary Types of Muscle

The **sarcomere**, shown in Figure 10.12, is the basic contractile unit of striated muscle. Sarcomeres are made of thick (**myosin**) and thin (**actin**) filaments. **Troponin** and **tropomyosin** are found on the thin filament and regulate actin-myosin interactions. The sarcomere can be divided into different lines, zones, and bands.

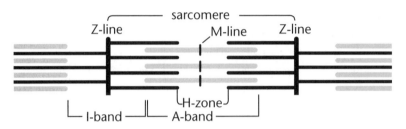

Figure 10.12. Sarcomere

Sarcomeres attach end-to-end to become **myofibrils**, and each **myocyte** (muscle cell or muscle fiber) contains many myofibrils. Myofibrils are surrounded by the sarcoplasmic reticulum, a calcium-containing modified endoplasmic reticulum. The cell membrane of a myocyte is known as the **sarcolemma.** A system of **T-tubules** is connected to the sarcolemma and oriented perpendicularly to the myofibrils, allowing the incoming signal to reach all parts of the muscle.

Muscle contraction begins at the neuromuscular junction, where the motor neuron releases acetylcholine that binds to receptors on the sarcolemma. This causes depolarization. (See Figure 10.13.)

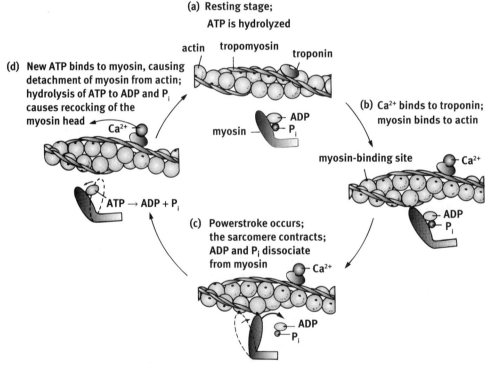

Figure 10.13. Muscle Contraction

Muscle cells exhibit an all-or-nothing response called a **simple twitch**. Addition of multiple simple twitches before the muscle has an opportunity to relax fully is called **frequency summation.** Simple twitches that occur so frequently as to not let the muscle relax at all can lead to **tetanus**, a more prolonged and stronger contraction.

Muscle cells have additional energy reserves to reduce oxygen debt (the difference between the amount of oxygen needed and the amount present) and forestall fatigue. Creatine phosphate can transfer a phosphate group to ADP, forming ATP. **Myoglobin** is a heme-containing protein that is a muscular oxygen reserve.

THE SKELETAL SYSTEM

Internal skeletons (like those in humans) are called **endoskeletons**; external skeletons (like those in arthropods) are called **exoskeletons.** The human skeletal system can be divided into **axial** and **appendicular skeletons.** The axial skeleton consists of structures in the midline such as the skull, vertebral column, ribcage, and hyoid bone. The appendicular skeleton consists of the bones of the limbs, the pectoral girdle, and the pelvis.

Bone is derived from embryonic mesoderm and includes both compact and spongy (cancellous) types.

- **Compact bone** provides strength and is dense.
- **Spongy** or **cancellous bone** has a lattice-like structure consisting of bony spicules known as **trabeculae.** The cavities are filled with bone marrow.
- Long bones contain shafts called **diaphyses** that flare to form **metaphyses** and that terminate in **epiphyses.** The epiphysis contains an **epiphyseal (growth) plate** that causes linear growth of the bone.
- Bone is surrounded by a layer of connective tissue called **periosteum.**
- Bones are attached to **muscles** by tendons and to each other by **ligaments**.

Bone matrix has both organic components, like collagen, glycoproteins, and other peptides, and inorganic components, like **hydroxyapatite.** Bone is organized into concentric rings called **lamellae** around a central **Haversian** or **Volkmann's canal.** This structural unit is called an **osteon** or **Haversian system.** Between lamellar rings are **lacunae**, where osteocytes reside. The lacunae are connected with **canaliculi** to allow for nutrient and waste transfer.

Bone remodeling is carried out by osteoblasts and osteoclasts. **Osteoblasts** build bone, while **osteoclasts** resorb bone. **Parathyroid hormone** increases resorption of bone, increasing calcium and phosphate concentrations in the blood. **Vitamin D** also increases resorption of bone, leading to increased turnover and, subsequently, the production of stronger bone. **Calcitonin** increases bone formation, decreasing calcium concentrations in the blood.

Cartilage is a firm, elastic material secreted by chondrocytes. Its matrix is called **chondrin.** Cartilage is usually found in areas that require more flexibility or cushioning. Cartilage is avascular and is not innervated.

In fetal life, bone forms from cartilage through **endochondral ossification**. Some bones, especially those of the skull, form directly from undifferentiated tissue (mesenchyme) in intramembranous ossification.

Joints may be classified as either immovable or movable. **Immovable** joints are fused together to form sutures or similar fibrous joints. **Movable** joints are usually strengthened by ligaments and contain a synovial capsule. **Synovial fluid**, secreted by the synovium, aids in motion by lubricating the joint. Each bone in the joint is coated with articular cartilage to aid in movement and provide cushioning.

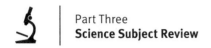

GENETICS AND EVOLUTION

Fundamental Concepts of Genetics

Chromosomes contain **genes** in a linear sequence. Alleles are alternative forms of a gene.

- A **dominant** allele requires only one copy to be expressed.
- A **recessive** allele requires two copies to be expressed.

A **genotype** is the combination of alleles an individual has at a given genetic locus.

- Having two of the same allele is termed **homozygous.**
- Having two different alleles is termed **heterozygous.**
- Having only one allele is termed **hemizygous** (such as male sex chromosomes).
- A **phenotype** is the observable manifestation of a genotype.

There are different patterns of dominance.

- **Complete dominance** has one dominant allele and one recessive allele.
- **Codominance** has more than one dominant allele.
- **Incomplete dominance** has no dominant alleles; heterozygotes have intermediate phenotypes.

Penetrance is the proportion of a population with a given genotype who express the phenotype. **Expressivity** refers to the varying phenotypic manifestations of a given genotype.

The modern interpretations of Mendel's laws help explain the inheritance of genes from parent to offspring.

- **Mendel's first law (of segregation)** states that an organism has two alleles for each gene. These alleles segregate during meiosis, resulting in gametes carrying only one allele for a trait.
- **Mendel's second law (of independent assortment)** states that the inheritance of one allele does not influence the probability of inheriting a given allele for a different trait.

Support for DNA as genetic material came through a number of experiments.

- The Griffith experiment demonstrated the transforming principle, converting nonvirulent bacteria into virulent bacteria by exposure to heat-killed virulent bacteria.
- The Avery-MacLeod-McCarty experiment demonstrated that DNA is the genetic material because degradation of DNA led to a cessation of bacterial transformation.
- The Hershey-Chase experiment confirmed that DNA is the genetic material because only radiolabeled DNA could be found in bacteriophage-infected bacteria.

Changes in the Gene Pool

All of the alleles in a given population constitute the **gene pool**. **Mutations** are changes in DNA sequence. Nucleotide mutations include **point mutations** (the substituting of one nucleotide for another) and **frameshift mutations** (moving the three-letter transcriptional reading frame). Nucleotide mutations can be classified in several ways.

- A **silent mutation** has no effect on the protein.
- A **missense mutation** results in the substitution of one amino acid for another.
- A **nonsense mutation** results in the substitution of a stop codon for an amino acid.
- **Insertions** and **deletions** result in a shift in the **reading frame**, leading to changes for all downstream amino acids.

Chromosomal mutations include much larger-scale mutations affecting whole segments of DNA.

- **Deletion mutations** occur when a large segment of DNA is lost.
- **Duplication mutations** occur when a segment of DNA is copied multiple times.
- **Inversion mutations** occur when a segment of DNA is reversed.
- **Insertion mutations** occur when a segment of DNA is moved from one chromosome to another.
- **Translocation mutations** occur when a segment of DNA is swapped with a segment of DNA from another chromosome.

Genetic **leakage** is a flow of genes between species through hybrid offspring. **Genetic drift** occurs when the composition of the gene pool changes as a result of chance. The **founder effect** results from bottlenecks that suddenly isolate a small population, leading to inbreeding and increased prevalence of certain homozygous genotypes.

Analytical Approaches in Genetics

Punnett squares visually represent the crossing of gametes from parents to show relative genotypic and phenotypic frequencies.

- The **parent generation** is represented by P; **filial** (offspring) **generations** are represented by F_1, F_2, and so on in sequence.
- A **monohybrid cross** accounts for one gene; a **dihybrid cross** accounts for two genes.
- In **sex-linked crosses**, sex chromosomes are usually used to indicate sex as well as genotype.

The **recombination frequency** (θ) is the likelihood of two alleles being separated during crossing-over in meiosis. **Genetic maps** can be made using recombination frequency as the scale in **centimorgans.** The **Hardy-Weinberg principle** states that if a population meets certain criteria (aimed at a lack of evolution), the **allele frequencies** will remain constant (**Hardy-Weinberg equilibrium**).

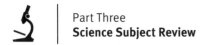

KEY CONCEPT

Punctuated equilibrium considers evolution to be a very slow process with intermittent rapid bursts of evolutionary activity.

Evolution

Natural selection states that chance variations exist among individuals and that advantageous variations—those that increase an individual's **fitness** for the environment—afford the most opportunity for reproductive success. The **modern synthesis model (neo-Darwinism)** accounts for mutation and recombination as mechanisms of variation. This model considers **differential reproduction** to be the mechanism of reproductive success. **Inclusive fitness** considers an organism's success to be based on the number of offspring, success in supporting offspring, and the ability of the offspring to then support others. Survival of offspring or relatives ensures continuation of genes in subsequent generations.

Different types of selection lead to changes in phenotypes, as shown in Figure 10.14.

- **Stabilizing selection** keeps phenotypes in a narrow range, excluding extremes.
- **Directional selection** moves the average phenotype toward one extreme.
- **Disruptive selection** moves toward two different phenotypes at the extremes and can lead to **speciation.**
- **Adaptive radiation** is the rapid emergence of multiple species from a common ancestor, each of which occupies its own ecological **niche.**

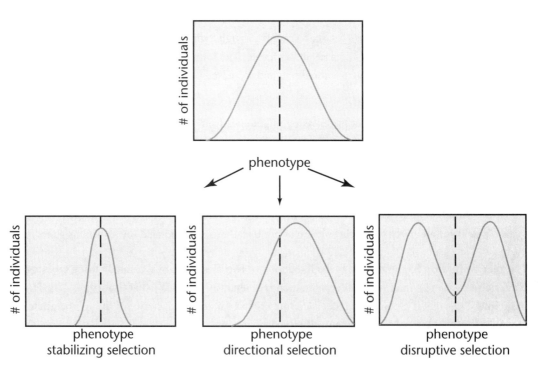

Figure 10.14. The Effects of Different Types of Selection on Phenotype

A **species** is the largest group of organisms capable of breeding to form fertile offspring. Species are reproductively isolated from each other by pre- or postzygotic mechanisms. Two species can evolve with different relationship patterns, as shown in Figure 10.15.

- **Divergent evolution** occurs when two species sharing a common ancestor become more different.
- **Parallel evolution** occurs when two species sharing a common ancestor evolve in similar ways due to analogous selection pressures.
- **Convergent evolution** occurs when two species not sharing a recent ancestor evolve to become more similar due to analogous selection pressures.

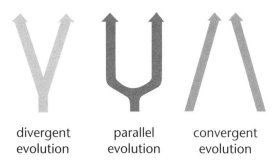

divergent evolution   parallel evolution   convergent evolution

Figure 10.15. Types of Species Evolution

According to the **molecular clock model**, the degree of difference in the genome between two species is related to the amount of time since the two species broke off from a common ancestor.

10.5 Biology Worked Examples

The following steps will walk you through the following passage using the Kaplan Passage Strategy.

PREVIEW FOR DIFFICULTY

Start by quickly glancing through the passage. Note the presence of figures demonstrating pathways for two different hypotheses. You can bet the surrounding text is going to provide insight into each of these hypotheses. A quick glance at the text reveals terms such as MS, CNS, and T-cells. Putting it all together shows that the passage appears to be about two hypotheses on multiple sclerosis.

CHOOSE YOUR APPROACH

The text is fairly dense, with details about two different hypotheses for a disease. However it does not contain experimental data. Therefore, it is an information passage and **Outlining** should be chosen.

READ AND DISTILL

P1: The purpose of this paragraph is to provide some background information on multiple sclerosis (MS). However, this content is less likely to be directly tested compared to the subsequent paragraphs on the hypotheses, so a quick skim will suffice. The last sentence indicates that the hypotheses relate to possible *causes* of MS.
Outline: Background info on MS

P2: This paragraph details the autoimmune hypothesis. Note that it involves T-cells reacting to myelin in the CNS. Move quickly through the remaining details, which should be analyzed later if they are required to answer a question.
Outline: Autoimmune hypo: T-cells attack myelin

P3: The final paragraph details the oligodendropathy hypothesis. The indicated cause of MS in this case is glial cell death leading to myelin degradation.
Outline: Oligodendropathy hypo: cell death → myelin degradation

F1/F2: The two figures summarize the two preceding paragraphs. Notice that both processes lead to inflammation. Also note the differences: the initial events, the causes of degradation, and the role of the immune system (macrophages).
Outline: Two pathways

Given that there are two hypotheses for the cause of a disease, expect that questions may give additional evidence and ask which hypothesis is supported.

PASSAGE I: THE NERVOUS SYSTEM

During development, oligodendrocyte progenitor cells are formed, which further differentiate into the glial cells responsible for creating the myelin sheaths of the nervous system. Multiple sclerosis (MS) is characterized by damage to—or destruction of—myelin sheaths in the central nervous system (CNS). This results in symptoms that vary from physical to mental manifestations. No cure currently exists for this disease, and its cause is still not completely clear.

The most widely accepted theory for the onset of MS has consistently been the classical *autoimmune hypothesis*. Recent research reports specify that nonspecific T-cells in the cervical lymph nodes, which drain the CNS, become exposed to cells with myelin-like characteristics. These T-cells then become specific against the myelinating oligodendrocytes. After entry into the CNS, an inflammatory response is induced, signaling other leukocytes and macrophages to migrate through the blood-brain barrier. The attack mounted by these cells effectively kills the oligodendrocytes and degrades the myelin sheaths. Figure 1 outlines this process.

Another theory is the *oligodendropathy hypothesis*. According to the researchers supporting this postulation, oligodendrocytes undergo apoptosis (spontaneous self-destruction) for unexplained reasons. Death of the glial cells then leads to myelin degradation. The inflammatory immune response by macrophages is simply a means to clean away the already destroyed myelin debris. Figure 2 outlines this process.

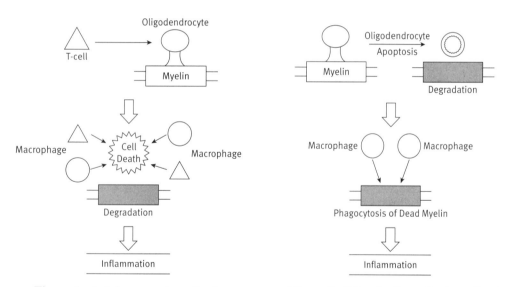

Figure 1. Autoimmune hypothesis   **Figure 2. Oligodendropathy hypothesis**

KEY CONCEPT

Myelin sheath
Action potentials

1. The propagation of action potentials in the CNS of a patient with MS compared with a control subject would be:

    A. faster, because there is less matter to inhibit its path down the axon.
    B. faster, because the lack of myelin allows ions to cross the cell membrane more easily.
    C. slower, because of the decreased number of Schwann cells.
    D. slower, because conduction is no longer saltatory.

1 Type the question

The question asks about content background regarding action potential in the context of the disease described in the passage. The answer choices have a pattern: faster or slower, with different reasons.

2 Rephrase the question stem

The task of the question requires you to understand MS from the passage and recall information about action potential. When Rephrased it asks, *Would propagation of action potential in the CNS speed up or slow down in MS and why?*

3 Investigate potential solutions

We'll need to look at the description of how MS damages the nervous system in paragraph 1 and then use our knowledge of the nervous system to find the correct answer. Paragraph 1 tells us that in MS, neurons in the CNS lose their myelin sheaths. The myelin sheath serves a number of functions, but its most notable one is to speed up the conduction of action potentials. Without the myelin sheath, conduction speed decreases dramatically. So we would predict that conduction should slow down in its absence.

Specifically, the myelin sheath speeds up conduction because conduction becomes saltatory. Ion exchange across the membrane becomes necessary only at the nodes of Ranvier, which are the periodic gaps in the myelin sheath. So a loss of myelin should result in a loss of saltatory conduction.

THINGS TO WATCH OUT FOR

Some trap answers on Test Day are designed to be so tempting that test takers will pick them and move on before ever reading the correct answer. Critical thinking will help you avoid those traps!

4 Match your prediction to an answer choice

(C) might seem tempting, but read it carefully: it refers to a decrease in Schwann cells, which are found only in the peripheral nervous system. Because MS involves the CNS, that answer is a trap. **(D)** matches both parts of our prediction and is the correct answer.

KEY CONCEPT

Nerve cell
Myelin sheath

---

2. The sequence in Figure 2 would be best supported over that of Figure 1 by which of the following?

    A. The CNS of a patient with MS was observed to have many scars and lesions.

    B. T-cells from a mouse with MS are transferred to a normal mouse that, over time, begins to display symptoms of multiple sclerosis.

    C. A study was conducted that showed large numbers of immune cells were first observed to enter the CNS only after signs of myelin degradation had been noted.

    D. Unusually high numbers of macrophages are found in the CNS of patients with MS.

---

① Type the question

This question asks us for a new finding that would support the oligodendropathy theory depicted in Figure 2 over the autoimmune hypothesis in Figure 1. Integrating new information can be tough. Together with the lack of patterns in the answer choices, this question might be a good candidate for answering after the other questions in this passage set.

② Rephrase the question stem

The task of the question requires us to examine the two figures to find the key differences. We'll then need to find an answer choice that illustrates one of those differences. When Rephrased it asks, *Which answer choice supports the oligodendropathy theory?*

③ Investigate potential solutions

Look at the two figures; the key difference is how the cells die. In the autoimmune hypothesis (Figure 1), the T-cells kill the oligodendrocytes. In the oligodendropathy hypothesis (Figure 2), the cells undergo apoptosis first (for unknown reasons) and then the T-cells attack. Our correct answer should illustrate the latter theory only.

④ Match your prediction to an answer choice

For **(A)**, the presence of scars and lesions in the CNS could fit with either hypothesis. Their presence is simply an effect of demyelination in general, no matter how the scars and lesions occurred. **(A)** is incorrect.

Next, look at **(B)**. Here, a previously normal mouse develops MS after it is exposed to T-cells from an affected mouse. This suggests that the T-cells caused the onset of MS. Figure 1 shows this is the first step of the autoimmune hypothesis, so **(B)** should be eliminated.

(**C**) describes a scenario in which demyelination has already occurred before the immune cells arrive. This matches what Figure 2 shows us and contradicts Figure 1. (**C**) must be the correct answer.

(**D**) is too general. Both figures show macrophages in the CNS, so this cannot be the answer.

KEY CONCEPT

Nervous system structure and function

---

3. In Guillain-Barré syndrome, demyelination occurs in the peripheral nervous system only. A patient with this condition would be LEAST likely to exhibit a decrease in:

  A. motor coordination.
  B. autonomic function.
  C. efferent motor responses.
  D. afferent sensory responses.

---

1 Type the question

Based on the patterns in the answer choices, this question is testing the functions of the peripheral and central nervous systems. Note that because this is a LEAST question, we're looking for the one answer that doesn't fit. Also note that this is a pseudodiscrete question; we don't need any information from the passage.

2 Rephrase the question stem

The additional information about the syndrome tells us that it's specific to the peripheral nervous system. Since it's a LEAST question, when Rephrased it asks, *What is one function that is not part of the peripheral nervous system?*

3 Investigate potential solutions

The CNS includes the brain and the spinal cord, whereas the peripheral nervous system contains the sensory and motor systems. So we're looking for an answer involving the brain and/or the spinal cord. We can eliminate any answers that involve the sensory and motor systems.

4 Match your prediction to an answer choice

Autonomic function is controlled by both the CNS and the peripheral nervous system, so (**B**) is wrong. Efferent motor responses and afferent sensory responses are both relayed by the peripheral nervous system (and processed in the CNS). So we can eliminate (**C**) and (**D**).

THINGS TO WATCH OUT FOR

Read questions carefully to catch keywords, such as NOT or EXCEPT.

Motor coordination takes place in the cerebellum of the brain, which is part of the CNS. Thus (**A**) is correct.

> **4.** Researchers develop a drug that slows the progression of multiple sclerosis by stimulating production of myelin in the CNS. This treatment addresses the primary cause of the condition described by:
>
> **A.** the autoimmune hypothesis only.
> **B.** the oligodendropathy hypothesis only.
> **C.** both hypotheses.
> **D.** neither hypothesis.

❶ Type the question

This question asks us to determine whether the phenomenon described in the question stem supports the theories described in the passage, which is the focus of the answer choices.

❷ Rephrase the question stem

The question describes a new drug. We're given the results and asked to consider which theory is supported by the outcome. When Rephrased it asks, *Which theory aligns with increased myelin production to address MS?*

❸ Investigate potential solutions

To answer this question, we'll need to see if stimulating CNS production of myelin supports the autoimmune hypothesis (by checking paragraph 2) and/or the oligodendropathy hypothesis (by checking paragraph 3). Paragraph 2 tells us that according to the autoimmune hypothesis, MS is triggered by T-cells attacking myelin-producing oligodendrocytes. Would creating more myelin prevent this attack? No. So the drug does not treat the cause, according to this theory.

Paragraph 3 describes the oligodendropathy hypothesis, which argues that MS is triggered by apoptosis, or spontaneous self-destruction, of oligodendrocytes. Would creating more myelin prevent this from happening? No, myelin does not play a role in apoptosis. So the new drug wouldn't treat the cause in this theory either.

❹ Match your prediction to an answer choice

Once we know that the drug's action doesn't treat the cause according to the autoimmune hypothesis, we can eliminate (**A**) and (**C**). Knowing that it doesn't treat the cause in the oligodendropathy hypothesis means we can also eliminate (**B**), leaving (**D**) as the correct answer.

TAKEAWAYS

Whenever a passage discusses multiple processes or theories, be sure to understand the key features of each as well as their key similarities and differences.

5. The following diagram depicts a somatic reflex arc.

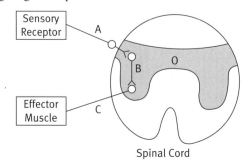

In a patient with MS, the reflex arc would most likely:

- **A.** remain unchanged.
- **B.** exhibit a delay at neuron A.
- **C.** exhibit a delay at interneuron B.
- **D.** exhibit a delay at neuron C.

❶ Type the question

This question introduces a diagram of a reflex arc and then asks us how MS would affect the diagram. The answer choices range from having no effect to describing a delay at specific parts of the diagram.

❷ Rephrase the question stem

This question requires you to understand the components of reflex arcs from content background and to consider the passage information with MS. When Rephrased the question asks, *What effect will MS have on reflex arcs?*

❸ Investigate potential solutions

We'll need the description of MS in paragraph 1 as well as our knowledge of reflex arcs to answer this question. MS affects only the CNS—that is, the brain and the spinal cord—according to paragraph 1. That means it does not affect the peripheral nervous system, with its motor and sensory components. As a result, we can predict that MS would affect a neuron that is part of the CNS, if there is one. If there isn't such a neuron, then there should be no change.

❹ Match your prediction to an answer choice

In the diagram, neuron A is a sensory neuron and neuron C is a motor neuron. Both of these are part of the peripheral nervous system. So we can eliminate (**B**) and (**D**). Neuron B, however, is an interneuron, which is part of the CNS. Therefore, we would expect it to be involved. So (**C**) is the correct answer.

This chapter continues on the next page. ▶ ▶ ▶

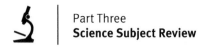

BIOLOGY PASSAGE II: THE ENDOCRINE SYSTEM

Aldosterone release from the adrenal cortex plays a key role in controlling blood pressure. This important hormone is regulated as shown in Figure 1.

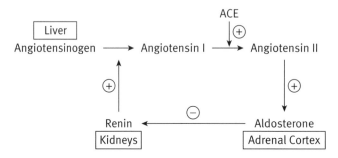

Figure 1. The renin-angiotensin feedback system

Low blood volume through the kidneys triggers juxtaglomerular cells to secrete renin into circulation. Angiotensinogen released from the liver is converted by this enzyme into the peptide angiotensin I. Angiotensin-converting enzyme (ACE) then converts angiotensin I into angiotensin II, which stimulates the adrenal cortex to release aldosterone. The ultimate increase in blood volume caused by aldosterone shuts off the secretion of renin from the juxtaglomerular cells. Angiotensin II also increases arteriolar vasoconstriction, sympathetic nervous activity, and reabsorption of sodium and chloride. Aldosterone, in addition to its effects on sodium, also increases potassium excretion.

Researchers at a pharmaceutical company are investigating the use of compounds thought to inhibit steps in the renin-angiotensin-aldosterone (RAA) pathway as a means of treating hypertension. A clinical trial has been approved to test the effects of four such drugs. Eighty subjects, each exhibiting chronic hypertension with systolic pressures greater than 160 mm Hg and diastolic pressures greater than 100 mmHg, were recruited; the subjects were divided into four groups of 20 patients each. Each group received a 10 mg daily dose of one of the four drugs. Blood pressure, urine volume, and concentration of urine potassium were measured every day for each patient in each group. At the end of the trial, the average results of these measurements over the last week of the trial were calculated; the results are shown in Table 1.

	Average Systolic/Diastolic Blood Pressure (mmHg)	Average Daily Urine Volume (L)	Average Daily Urine Potassium Concentration (mEq/L)
Drug A	118/75	2.5	175
Drug B	145/95	2.2	50
Drug C	116/80	2.5	40
Drug D	122/78	1.1	135
Normal ranges	–	0.8–2.0	25–125

Table 1. Results of a Clinical Trial of Four Drugs to Treat Hypertension

1. Based on the results in Table 1, which of the following conclusions about Drug A and Drug C is most reasonable?

   A. Drug A inhibits renin release, and Drug C inhibits ADH release.

   B. Drug A inhibits ADH release, and Drug C inhibits ACE release.

   C. Drug A inhibits ACE release, and Drug C inhibits renin release.

   D. Drug A inhibits aldosterone release, and Drug C inhibits ADH release.

2. Suppose that a certain substance is capable of preventing the binding of all hormones to receptors on the cell membrane. Such a drug would directly influence the function of:

   A. ADH but not aldosterone.

   B. aldosterone but not ADH.

   C. both ADH and aldosterone.

   D. neither ADH nor aldosterone.

3. A successful inhibitor of the RAA system could reasonably be expected to cause all of the following EXCEPT:

   A. increased dilation of arterioles.

   B. decreased urine sodium concentration.

   C. decreased pupil dilation.

   D. increased urine volume.

4. Although Drug B was the least successful for treating hypertension, the results obtained suggest it would be most useful in treating:

   A. hypotension.

   B. dehydration.

   C. edema.

   D. hyperkalemia (high plasma K^+ levels).

5. A researcher believes she knows the mechanism by which Drug D lowers blood pressure. To confirm her hypothesis, she should perform an experiment, with appropriate controls, to measure:

   A. angiotensinogen release from the liver.

   B. renin release from the kidneys.

   C. arteriolar pressure increases caused by angiotensin II.

   D. the concentration of ACE in the plasma

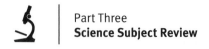

USING THE KAPLAN METHOD

Preview the passage: At a glance, this is an endocrine passage involving the RAA pathway in the first paragraph and figure. The second paragraph sets up an experiment, with a table at the end containing results. As such, this is an experimental passage.

Choose your approach: Interrogate

Read and Distill:

P1: Keep the author's intent in mind while you interrogate this passage, as many details are mentioned for a reason. This introductory statement about the role aldosterone plays with controlling blood pressure probably isn't new. However, it should give you a hint that the testable principles in the passage may be about feedback, regulatory mechanisms, and the circulatory system.

F1: We see a diagram that should be fairly familiar describing the RAA system, but keep that anticipation sharp! Think about how you can get disruptions in the pathway and be able to predict the effect.

P2: Notice how the description of the RAA system here is particularly centered around its effect on blood pressure, including vasoconstriction, blood volume, and solute concentration. Interrogate by asking, *Why would the author include these details?* We can probably anticipate that the experiment coming up will deal with hypertension. Make sure to refer back to this paragraph to help understand the context!

P3: Here we see the setup of the experiment, including the purpose, which was to use a variety of drugs to inhibit steps in RAA and thereby look to treat hypertension. Notice how the ion concentration, blood pressure, and urine volume are all measured, which is a link to P2.

T1: Interrogation of the table should focus on identifying the key trends in the data. Begin with the variables. The independent variables are the four drugs. The dependent variables are the measurements: average BP, urine volume, urine [K^+]. Make sure to assess each measurement. Drug B has higher BP compared to the other three drugs, though all four are lower than the average chronic hypertension pressures listed in P3. Drug D had normal range urine volume. Drugs B and C had normal ranges for urine [K^+]. Link this back to the passage. Since each of the drugs had differing effects on the dependent variables, the drugs are likely targeting different enzymes in the RAA pathway described in P1. Be prepared for questions that ask you to make that kind of connection.

TAKEAWAYS

When a passage presents an experiment, expect questions testing your ability to interpret the results, especially if the passage doesn't draw any conclusions for you.

> 1. Based on the results in Table 1, which of the following conclusions about Drug A and Drug C is most reasonable?
>
>   A. Drug A inhibits renin release, and Drug C inhibits ADH release.
>   B. Drug A inhibits ADH release, and Drug C inhibits ACE release.
>   C. Drug A inhibits ACE release, and Drug C inhibits renin release.
>   D. Drug A inhibits aldosterone release, and Drug C inhibits ADH release.

KEY CONCEPT

Osmoregulation
Secretion and reabsorption of solutes

① Type the question

The question refers to the data in Table 1, and all of the answer choices deal with inhibiting the release of hormones in response to Drugs A and C.

② Rephrase the question stem

Based on the data, which hormones do Drugs A and C inhibit?

③ Investigate potential solutions

To answer this question, we'll need to examine the differences in Table 1 between Drugs A and C. We will also need to use Figure 1, which shows how the various hormones are regulated, and paragraph 3, which gives us the normal urine output and potassium content. We may also need paragraph 2, which describes the functions of some of these hormones. Look at Table 1; the average blood pressure for patients taking Drugs A and C is approximately the same. The average urine output is the same for both drugs and is elevated in both cases. The only difference in the table is the urine concentration of K^+ ions. The urine of Drug A patients has an elevated potassium level, whereas the urine of Drug C patients has a potassium level at the low end of the average range. Our correct answer thus needs to explain how Drug A causes K^+ excretion to rise whereas Drug C does not.

The key to answering this question is tucked into the end of paragraph 2: increased K^+ excretion is caused by aldosterone. Therefore, Drug A's effects should not include inhibiting aldosterone.

④ Match your prediction to an answer choice

We can immediately eliminate (**D**) because we've established that Drug A should not inhibit aldosterone. Renin (**A**) and ACE (**C**) are both needed to stimulate aldosterone release. Inhibiting either of them should result in reduced aldosterone activity, which would make it unlikely that Drug A would cause elevated urine potassium levels. Eliminating those answers leaves (**B**) as the correct answer.

Note that we didn't even need to consider Drug C here. However, if it was inhibiting ACE, we'd expect to see decreased aldosterone activity, which doesn't contradict the information in the table.

THINGS TO WATCH OUT FOR

Watch out when an experimental passage presents results for multiple variables. Odds are there will be at least one question that requires a conclusion to be drawn from a comparison of those results.

2. Suppose that a certain substance is capable of preventing the binding of all hormones to receptors on the cell membrane. Such a drug would directly influence the function of:

   A. ADH but not aldosterone.
   B. aldosterone but not ADH.
   C. both ADH and aldosterone.
   D. neither ADH nor aldosterone.

❶ Type the question

The question stem introduces new information about a substance, which we know from the word "suppose." The answer choices ask whether this substance would affect ADH, aldosterone, both, or neither. This is actually a pseudodiscrete question; we don't need any information directly from the passage.

❷ Rephrase the question stem

How would ADH and/or aldosterone function be affected by a substance that prevents binding of hormones to cell surface receptors?

❸ Investigate potential solutions

We need only two pieces of information: (1) an understanding of what hormones bind to cell membrane receptors and (2) the hormone classes to which ADH and aldosterone belong. Then we can apply that information to the new scenario in the question stem. There are two major classes of hormones: steroid hormones and peptide (amino acid) hormones. Steroid hormones have intracellular receptors because steroids are permeable and cross the cell membrane. Peptide hormones, however, have membrane-bound receptors; amino acids are too polar to cross the cell membrane.

So if our hypothetical compound can block all hormone binding at the cell membrane, it would affect peptide hormones but not steroid hormones. Aldosterone, like all adrenal cortex hormones, is a steroid; ADH, like all hormones produced in the hypothalamus, is a peptide. Keeping this in mind, we would expect the drug to impact only ADH and not aldosterone.

❹ Match your prediction to an answer choice

(A) matches our prediction exactly, choose it and move on.

> **3.** A successful inhibitor of the RAA system could reasonably be expected to cause all of the following EXCEPT:
>
>   **A.** increased dilation of arterioles.
>   **B.** decreased urine sodium concentration.
>   **C.** decreased pupil dilation.
>   **D.** increased urine volume.

① Type the question

Take note of the word "EXCEPT" in the question stem. The answer choices are all physiological responses, possibly drawing from paragraph 2. Note that EXCEPT questions can be excellent candidates to save for later in the passage set.

② Rephrase the question stem

Given that this an EXCEPT question, Rephrase it as, *Which of the following physiological responses would occur if RAA is inhibited?* Then eliminate the true statements.

③ Execute the plan

Figure 1 shows the various steps of the RAA system, whereas paragraph 2 describes the effects of the hormones. Because we're looking for something that blocking the system will not cause, the wrong answers are things that inhibiting the pathway will cause. The correct answer is therefore either a normal effect of the RAA system or something that is not affected by it at all.

④ Answer by matching, eliminating, or guessing

Paragraph 2 tells us that angiotensin II increases arteriole vasoconstriction. So inhibiting RAA would mean a lack of constriction—in other words, we expect vasodilation. That means **(A)** would happen and is therefore incorrect.

The end effect of the RAA system is the release of aldosterone, which increases sodium reabsorption in the kidney. Inhibiting the system would mean decreased sodium reabsorption and, therefore, higher excretion. **(B)** says we'd expect lower sodium excretion. This is the normal RAA effect we predicted that we'd see as the correct answer.

Paragraph 2 tells us that angiotensin II increases sympathetic nervous activity. Pupil dilation is a sympathetic effect. So inhibiting RAA would decrease dilation, which rules out **(C)**.

Because aldosterone increases sodium reabsorption, it also indirectly increases water reabsorption. We would thus expect the RAA pathway to decrease urine volume. **(D)** also is incorrect.

(B) is the correct answer.

Osmoregulation
Mechanisms of hormone action
Feedback control regulation

4. Although Drug B was the least successful for treating hypertension, the results obtained suggest it would be most useful in treating:

   A. hypotension.

   B. dehydration.

   C. edema.

   D. hyperkalemia (high plasma K^+ levels).

1 Type the question

The question asks about the results in Table 1 regarding Drug B, and the answer choices are all abnormal conditions.

2 Rephrase the question stem

Which of these conditions would Drug B be best at treating?

3 Investigate potential solutions

To answer this question, we'll need to look at the results for Drug B in Table 1 and then use our knowledge of the conditions in the answer choices. Look at Table 1; patients taking Drug B had slightly elevated urine output but normal urine potassium levels. So the correct answer is a condition that can be treated solely by increasing urine output.

4 Match your prediction to an answer choice

Look at the answer choices. The only one that can be treated solely by increasing urine output is edema, which is an accumulation of fluid in interstitial spaces. The correct answer is (**C**).

(**A**) might sound tempting; if Drug B doesn't reduce blood pressure, maybe it can be used to raise blood pressure. However, the passage told us that the patients involved in the trial have blood pressures greater than 160/100. So Drug B still managed to reduce blood pressure, meaning it cannot be the answer. To treat dehydration, (**B**), we would want a drug that increases water retention in the body. Drug B resulted in high urine volume, so it would not increase water retention.

In hyperkalemia, plasma potassium levels are elevated. Drug B did not elevate urine potassium levels, so it is unlikely that it would be effective in ridding the body of excess potassium. Thus, (**D**) is eliminated.

If you're not familiar with a concept in an answer choice, don't reflexively select or reject that answer.

KEY CONCEPT

Mechanisms of hormone action
Feedback control regulation

> 5. A researcher believes she knows the mechanism by which Drug D lowers blood
>   pressure. To confirm her hypothesis, she should perform an experiment, with
>   appropriate controls, to measure:
>
>   **A.** angiotensinogen release from the liver.
>   **B.** renin release from the kidneys.
>   **C.** arteriolar pressure increases caused by angiotensin II.
>   **D.** the concentration of ACE in the plasma.

1 Type the question

This is an experimental design question involving the data in Table 1. All of the answer
choices involve hormones shown in Figure 1.

2 Rephrase the question stem

How does the Drug D data link to one of the RAA system hormones?

3 Investigate potential solutions

To answer this question, we need to know how Drug D works. That information isn't explicitly given to us in the passage, so we'll need to use the data in Table 1 to help us figure out
how Drug D works. Then we can use our knowledge of the hormones in the answer choices
to determine the correct answer. In Table 1, patients on Drug D had significantly reduced
blood pressure. However, they also had high urine potassium levels and normal urine volume. We're therefore looking for an answer that doesn't involve excess urine excretion.

4 Match your prediction to an answer choice

Look at the answer choices. The most promising answer is **(C)**, which doesn't directly
involve the kidneys at all. Angiotensin II, according to paragraph 2, causes vasoconstriction;
inhibiting angiotensin II could directly result in vasodilation.

Changes in angiotensinogen release **(A)** and renin release **(B)** should both alter aldosterone
levels. So it would not be likely that these would produce a decrease in blood pressure without increasing urine volume. Finally, although **(D)** sounds tempting, the actual concentration
of ACE is irrelevant; what matters is its activity. It is possible that there are large amounts of
ACE in the blood, but the vast majority of it could be inhibited. **(C)** is the correct response.

10.6 **Biology on Your Own**

BIOLOGY PASSAGE III (QUESTIONS 1–6)

Yeasts, which are unicellular fungi, can reproduce by budding or by performing mitosis and meiosis. *Saccharomyces cerevisiae*, for example, will undergo mitosis when resources are plentiful but can undergo meiosis to form haploid spores when the primary fuel sources support fermentation rather than aerobic respiration.

Both mitosis and meiosis depend on formation of a complex, Cdk1-Clb, between the proteins Cdk1 and cyclin B to activate spindle formation. In mitosis, Cdk1-Clb is activated within minutes, but in meiosis, it typically takes at least three hours. The human analog of Cdk1, Cdc2, can substitute for Cdk1 in yeast.

The entry of yeast into meiosis I depends on the expression of Ndt80, a transcription factor expressed only during meiosis, which triggers the formation of the meiotic spindle and disassembly of synaptonemal complexes. It is regulated in part by positive feedback: Ndt80 acts as an activator for its own gene. Another required protein is Ama1, which activates the anaphase-promoting complex (APC/C), which is required for the cell to enter anaphase I. During prophase I, APC/C suppresses the signals that cause yeast cells to undergo mitosis; it also helps inhibit entry into S phase.

In an experiment, a researcher cultured *S. cerevisiae* cells in glucose-rich medium. One population was mutated to lack the gene for Ndt80; the other lacked genes for both Ndt80 and Ama1. Two hundred cells from each sample were then transferred to media designed to induce meiosis. The researcher then counted the number of cells in each sample that exhibited the presence of a meiotic spindle; the results are shown in Figure 1.

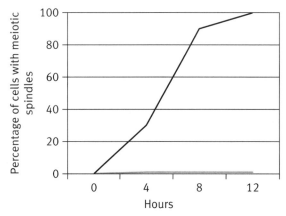

Figure 1. Development of the meiotic spindle in
–Ndt80 /–Ama1 (——) and –Ndt80 (——) cells

1. Suppose researchers discover a compound that prevents binding of Cdk1 to cyclin B. Although they use the drug in their research, they do not pursue using it as a treatment for fungal infections. Which of the following would be the most likely reason for that decision?

    A. The drug might not quantitatively kill fungal cells.

    B. The drug might be too expensive to mass produce.

    C. The drug might pose too great a risk to subjects.

    D. The drug might cause dangerous genetic mutations in the yeast cells.

2. Based on information in the passage, which of the following is most likely to be true of meiotic cells lacking Ndt80 and Ama1?

    A. Cells lacking only Ndt80 will arrest in prophase I; cells lacking both proteins will arrest in anaphase I.

    B. Cells lacking only Ndt80 will arrest in anaphase I; cells lacking both proteins will arrest in metaphase I.

    C. Cells lacking only Ndt80 will arrest in prophase I; cells lacking both proteins will arrest in metaphase I.

    D. Cells lacking only Ndt80 will arrest in metaphase I; cells lacking both proteins will arrest in anaphase I.

3. Which of the following, if true, would be the best explanation for how Ama1 is regulated prior to entry into anaphase?

    A. The cell can detect chromosomes not attached to spindle fibers and produces a signal that inhibits Ama1 when it does.

    B. The cell can detect chromosomes not attached to spindle fibers and produces a signal that activates Ama1 when it does.

    C. The cell can detect the attachment of chromosomes to spindle fibers and produces a signal that activates Ama1 when it does.

    D. The cell can detect the attachment of chromosomes to spindle fibers and produces a signal that inhibits Ama1 when it does.

4. A sample of *S. cerevisiae* grown in a medium containing only acetate and no glucose would most likely exhibit:

    A. formation of Cdk1-Clb in less than an hour.

    B. activation of APC/C in prophase I.

    C. exclusively mitosis.

    D. decreased expression of Ndt80.

5. A certain yeast cell is unable to proceed to metaphase I of meiosis and is unable to proceed to metaphase I of mitosis. It most likely contains a mutation in the gene for:

    A. Ama1.

    B. Ndt80.

    C. tubulin.

    D. Cdc2.

6. Based on information in the passage, is it reasonable to conclude that after telophase I:

    I. APC/C remains active into meiosis II.

    II. Ndt80 remains active into meiosis II.

    III. Additional Ama1 must be synthesized.

    A. II only

    B. I and II only

    C. I and III only

    D. I, II, and III

Biology Practice Passage Explanations

1. (C)

One of the keys to antimicrobial therapy, in general, is that it must be relatively safe for the host and attack a mechanism that the infected organism's cells do not use. For example, the bacterial ribosome is not identical to the human ribosome, so drugs that target the bacterial ribosome generally pose little threat to humans. Here, however, paragraph 2 tells us that the human analog of Cdk1, Cdc2, can work like Cdk1 in yeast cells. That implies there is a high degree of homology between the yeast pathway and the mitotic pathway in humans and other mammals. As a result, such a drug would likely affect both yeast cells and human cells; it could cause damage to organs that require frequent cell divisions (such as the stomach). **(C)** is the best answer.

(A) might be true. However, even if it could kill the yeast cells (and perhaps especially if it could kill the yeast cells!), it would still pose a risk to the subjects. Even if **(B)** were true, it would not be the best reason to avoid testing the drug. The formation of the mitotic spindle is independent of DNA synthesis, and no information in the passage suggests the drug would be capable of causing mutations in the yeast cells **(D)**.

2. (C)

First, note that all of the answers state that the cells will arrest at some stage of meiosis. To answer this question, we need to know the key events of prophase I and metaphase I. To exit prophase I, chromosomes must condense, the nuclear envelope needs to disintegrate, and the spindle bodies need to form. According to Figure 1, in cells lacking only Ndt80, the spindle never forms; in cells lacking both Ndt80 and Ama1, though, it does form. Therefore, we can conclude that Ndt80 cells should arrest in prophase I. According to paragraph 3, Ama1 activates APC/C, which is needed for entry into anaphase I. Therefore, it is most reasonable to conclude that in the absence of Ama1, the cells will arrest in metaphase I. This matches **(C)**.

Ndt80 cells will arrest in prophase I. However, the lack of Ama1 prevents activation of APC/C, which is needed for entry into anaphase I. So **(A)** is incorrect. Without Ndt80, the spindle never forms, so cells cannot leave prophase I. This means **(B)** is impossible. Without Ndt80, the spindle never forms, so cells cannot leave prophase I. Moreover, without Ama1, cells cannot enter anaphase I. Thus, **(D)** is incorrect.

3. (A)

During anaphase, the cell needs to avoid nondisjunction, the incorrect separation of chromosomes during cell division. To do this, the cell needs to make sure that every chromosome is attached to a spindle fiber. Because the number of chromosomes in cells varies widely, the easiest way to do this would be to depend on a signal that disappears when all chromosomes have been attached, rather than a signal that appears when chromosomes are attached. As a result, we can eliminate **(C)** and **(D)**. Because paragraph 3 tells us that Ama1 activates APC/C, which initiates anaphase, we would expect that the signal should be an inhibitory one. Once all of the chromosomes have attached, the inhibitory signal disappears; Ama1 will become active. This matches **(A)**.

4. (B)

Paragraph 1 states that when fermentable fuel sources predominate, yeast cells are more likely to undergo sporulation. Acetate would be an example of such a fuel source, especially in the absence of glucose. Thus, we would expect the yeast to undergo meiosis. The only answer choice that corresponds to the induction of meiosis is **(B)**.

According to paragraph 2, Cdk1-Clb forms within minutes in mitosis, not meiosis, thus eliminating **(A)**. We would expect to see exclusively meiosis, not mitosis, which means **(C)** is incorrect. Ndt80 is required for meiosis. So this would be a signal for mitosis, thus nullifying **(D)**.

5. (C)

According to the information in Figure 1, neither Ama1 nor Ndt80 is necessary for the formation of the meiotic spindle. That rules out both **(A)** and **(B)**. A close reading of paragraph 2 shows that Cdc2 is a gene found in humans, not in yeast, which eliminates **(D)**. That leaves **(C)** as the correct answer; tubulin is the protein required for actual formation of the spindle fibers.

6. (B)

This question tests your understanding of meiosis II. In particular, to answer this question correctly, you need to know that there is no S phase preceding meiosis II as there is preceding meiosis I. Therefore, we would expect that APC/C (item I) would remain active to prevent the cell from undergoing S phase. That eliminates **(A)**. We also would expect that Ndt80 (item II) would be active; because a second meiotic spindle is needed for meiosis II, we can eliminate **(C)**. On the other hand, we have no reason to conclude that additional Ama1 is needed to activate the APC/C (item III). It is possible that Ama1 activation of APC/C during prophase I lasts throughout meiosis I and meiosis II. **(B)** is the best answer.

CHAPTER 11

General Chemistry

One of the main characteristics of the MCAT is that many of the questions, even in the physical sciences, are related to living systems. Thus, passages presenting an inorganic chemical reaction with stoichiometry questions are far less likely to appear. Most questions related to general chemistry also involve biochemistry or biology. In addition, general chemistry questions appear in both the Chemical and Physical Foundations of Biological Systems and the Biological and Biochemical Foundations of Living Systems sections. Approximately 5 percent of the questions in the Biological and Biochemical Foundations of Living Systems section are strictly general chemistry, and approximately 30 percent of the questions in the Chemical and Physical Foundations of Biological Systems section are general chemistry. However, it is important to remember that knowledge of general chemistry concepts is essential for success in organic chemistry and biochemistry. As such, fewer questions in general chemistry does not necessarily mean that less knowledge is required. It simply means that the test maker is likely to be more creative in testing general chemistry concepts in the context of organic chemistry or biochemistry.

11.1 Reading the Passage

One of the most difficult aspects of the MCAT is reading the passages. Test takers tend to waste a lot of time reading passages in the same way that one would read a textbook or a newspaper, by attempting to understand completely every argument made and every detail given. However, the goal of the MCAT is not reading the passages; it is answering questions by using the passage as a piece of reference material. MCAT science passages are full of information that will always be there if required to answer questions. When you read a passage, take a broad look at what is happening and think about the basic science concepts that are being applied to situations presented within the passage. For information passages, aim to Read and Distill the passage quickly!

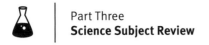

PASSAGE TYPES

As in the other sciences, general chemistry concepts can appear in both information and experiment passages on the MCAT. With that said, the MCAT presents general chemistry in the context of living systems. This means that most passages require the test taker to have the knowledge and the ability to apply the fundamental concepts of biology and biochemistry within the context of general chemistry. Because only 5 percent of the questions in the Biological and Biochemical Foundations of Living Systems section are related to general chemistry, it is unlikely that any single passage in that section is strictly general chemistry. Passages that are strictly general chemistry are more likely to be found in the Physical and Chemical Foundations of Biological Systems section. (See Table 11.1.)

Information Passages

- Read like a textbook or journal article.
- Usually explain the general chemistry behind a natural phenomenon.
- May be associated with one or more figures, such as a reaction, equation, table, chart, graph, or diagram. The text of the passage usually describes these figures.

Experiment Passages

- Consists of brief background information, frequently linking the chemical process presented in the experiment with a biological process.
- The procedure is described, and the results are presented.
- The hypothesis of the experiment is usually stated fairly early in the passage.
- Numerical results may be presented in a table or a graph.

	Biology and Biochemical Foundations of Living Systems	Chemical and Physical Foundations of Biological Systems
Percentage of questions in general chemistry	5%	30%
Passages	Possibly one; unlikely to see a passage that is strictly general chemistry.	More than one; general chemistry topics are also likely to be mixed with biochemistry and physics topics.
Questions	Very few questions that require only general chemistry knowledge. Many more questions may require you to integrate general chemistry concepts with other sciences.	Some questions require only general chemistry knowledge, but many discuss living systems. Expect to integrate general chemistry with biochemistry and organic chemistry.

Table 11.1. General Chemistry in the Biology and Biochemical Foundations of Living Systems Section and the Chemical and Physical Foundations of Biological Systems Section

READING AND DISTILLING THE PASSAGE

Regardless of how the passages in this section differ from those found in the other sections, the same Kaplan Method should be applied across all sciences. Read the passage quickly and efficiently; apply the Distill approach best suited to the kind of information being conveyed.

- **Preview** for difficulty
  - Note the structure of the passage, the location of the paragraphs, and any figures such as charts, graphs, tables, or diagrams.
  - Determine whether the passage is an *experiment* or an *information* passage.
  - Determine the topic and the degree of difficulty.
  - Identify whether this passage will require a large time investment.
  - Decide whether this passage is one to do now or later.

- **Choose** your approach
  - Using information from the Preview step, Choose an appropriate Distill approach for the passage (Interrogate, Outline, or Highlight).
  - **Interrogation** should be chosen for experiment passages.
  - **Outlining** should be chosen for information passages that are dense or detail heavy.
  - **Highlighting** should be chosen for information passages that are light on details.

- **Read and Distill** key themes
  - While reading the passage, your aim is to distill the major takeaway of each paragraph and identify testable information using one of the following approaches.
  - **Interrogate**: Thoroughly examine the experiment passage by identifying the key components of experimental design and interrogating *why* specific procedures were done and *how* they connect to the overall purpose of the experiment.
  - **Outline**: Create a brief label for each paragraph that summarizes the contents of the paragraph, allowing you to return quickly to the passage when demanded by a question.
  - **Highlight**: Highlight one to three terms per paragraph that can pull your attention back to testable information when demanded by a question.

MCAT EXPERTISE

Passages containing general chemistry concepts often include diagrams or figures that relate to the text. To approach the passage efficiently while maximizing your Read and Distill steps, do the following:

- Identify each chart, graph, table, or diagram, and determine what is represented in each one.
- Identify any relationships between the text and the image. For example, an entire paragraph may be devoted to explaining variables or the results of an experiment. These same ideas may also be represented visually, meaning that the same information is presented in two different formats.
- If information is presented in two different formats, this is a cue that you may skim the information in the paragraph, as it can may be better explained visually in a graph or figure.

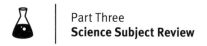
11.2 **Answering the Questions**

Similar to the other sciences, general chemistry questions fall into one of four categories.

- **Discrete questions**
  - ○ Questions not associated with a descriptive passage.
  - ○ Are preceded by a warning such as, "Questions 12–15 do not refer to a passage and are independent of each other."
  - ○ Likely to ask for you to recall a specific piece of information or apply your knowledge to a new situation.
  - ○ Not likely to require analysis of an experiment.

- **Questions that stand alone from the passage**
  - ○ Questions associated with a passage, but the passage is not required to answer the question.
  - ○ Often thematically related to the passage but often designed to test an additional aspect of the topic that is not mentioned in the passage.

- **Questions that require data from the passage**
  - ○ Often require data analysis or conceptual understanding of ideas presented in the passage.
  - ○ You are required to apply your knowledge to information within the passage.
  - ○ Do not require the goal of the passage.

- **Questions that require the goal of the passage**
  - ○ Require a deeper understanding of the passage as a whole, especially the overall goal of the passage.
  - ○ Usually the most time-consuming of the question types in general chemistry.

ATTACKING THE QUESTIONS

Each question is designed to test a specific skill and information set. The MCAT is designed to test your ability to apply your knowledge in a logical manner to answer questions. The Kaplan Method provides you with a logical method for applying your knowledge to maximize your points on Test Day.

- **Type** the question
  - Read the question; peek at the answer choices for patterns, but don't analyze closely.
  - Assess the topic and the degree of difficulty.
  - Identify the level of time involvement: is this question likely to take a tremendous amount of time to identify the answer? If so, skip it and come back after you do the other questions in the passage set.
  - Good questions to do now in general chemistry are those that stand alone from the passage because these are generally quick and easy points.

- **Rephrase** the question stem
  - Rephrase the question, focusing on the task(s) to be accomplished.
  - Simplify the phrasing of the original question stem.
  - Translate the question into a specific set of tasks to be accomplished using the passage and your background knowledge.

- **Investigate** potential solutions
  - Complete the task(s) identified in your Rephrase step.
  - Analyze the data; evaluate the experimental design; locate the information required; and connect the information, data, and experimental design with the information you already know.
  - Predict what you can about the answer.
  - Be flexible if your initial approach fails.

- **Match** your prediction to an answer choice
  - Search the answer choices for a response that is synonymous with your prediction or eliminate answers that are not correct.
  - Select an answer and move on.
  - If you cannot find a match to your prediction, eliminate wrong answers, select a response from the remaining choices, and move on.

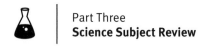
11.3 Getting the Edge in General Chemistry

Over the years, the amount of general chemistry on the MCAT has declined and shifted in scope. Currently, the majority of general chemistry tested on the MCAT has a direct application to the life sciences. Thus, performing calculations using the Henderson-Hasselbalch equation are still important, but they are typically applied to topics such as determining how changes in the concentration of bicarbonate and carbonic acid affect the pH of blood. Therefore, the type of learning required to succeed on general chemistry passages is different.

General chemistry passages often feature multiple images, and you are required to interpret these images. However, interpretation is necessary only if a question requires it. Note the image, what it summarizes, and move on; there is no need to interpret the image when reading the passage. The only figures that should require additional time spent are figures with experimental data as identifying the key trends will allow you to understand the passage better while reading.

KEY CONCEPT

Topic-specific passage practice is vital for developing mastery on any topic, and therefore it's vital for Test Day success. Be sure to include both discrete and passage-based questions in your study resources.

Mastering general chemistry on the MCAT means being able to use critical reasoning skills and to apply the principles of general chemistry to living systems. This requires practice. Top-scoring test takers often refine their skills by reading passages and answering questions about the topic at hand. Reading a textbook or review book is helpful. However, the MCAT requires you to apply knowledge, not to memorize it.

11.4 Preparing for the MCAT: General Chemistry

The following presents the general chemistry content you are likely to see on Test Day. The High-Yield badges point out the topics that are tested most frequently.

ATOMIC STRUCTURE

A **proton** has a positive charge and a mass of around 1 amu; a **neutron** has no charge and a mass of around 1 amu; an **electron** has a negative charge and negligible mass. The **nucleus** contains the protons and neutrons, while the electrons move around the nucleus. The **atomic number** is the number of protons in a given element, while the **mass number** is the sum of an element's protons and neutrons.

Atomic mass is essentially equal to the mass number, which is the sum of an element's protons and neutrons. Atomic mass varies due to isotopes. **Isotopes** are atoms of a given element (elements with the same atomic number) that have different mass numbers. They differ in the number of neutrons. Most isotopes are identified by the element followed by the mass number (such as carbon-12, carbon-13, and carbon-14). **Atomic weight** is the weighted average of the naturally occurring isotopes of an element. The periodic table lists atomic weights, not atomic masses.

In the **Bohr model of the atom**, a dense, positively charged nucleus is surrounded by electrons revolving around the nucleus in orbits with distinct energy levels. The energy difference between energy levels is called a **quantum**, first described by Planck.

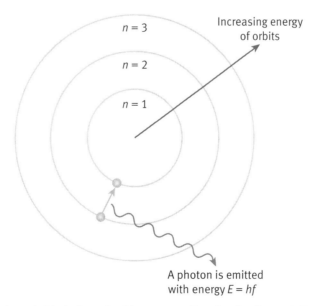

Figure 11.1. Atomic Emission of a Photon as a Result of a Ground-State Transition

Quantization means that there is not an infinite range of energy levels available to an electron; electrons can exist only at certain energy levels. The energy of an electron increases the farther it is from the nucleus. The **atomic absorption spectrum** of an element is unique. For an electron to jump from a lower energy level to a higher one, it must absorb an amount of energy precisely equal to the energy difference between the two levels. When electrons

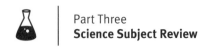
return from the excited state to the ground state, they emit an amount of energy that is exactly equal to the energy difference between the two levels. Every element has a characteristic **atomic emission spectrum** (see Figure 11.1). Sometimes the electromagnetic energy emitted corresponds to a frequency in the visible light range.

The **quantum mechanical model** posits that electrons are localized in orbitals and do not travel in definite orbits; an **orbital** is a region of space around the nucleus defined by the probability of finding an electron in that region of space. The **Heisenberg uncertainty principle** says it is impossible to know both an electron's position and its momentum exactly at the same time. The **principal quantum number**, *n*, is one of four quantum numbers. It describes the average energy of a **shell**; as *n* increases, the average distance between the electron and the nucleus increases as does the potential energy of the electron.

Electrons fill from lower- to higher-energy subshells, according to the **Aufbau principle**. Each subshell fills completely before electrons begin to enter the next one. Electrons fill orbitals according to **Hund's rule**: subshells with multiple orbitals fill electrons so that every orbital in a subshell gets one electron before any orbital gets a second.

Valence electrons are those in the outermost shell available for interaction (bonding) with other atoms. Many atoms form bonds that complete an octet in the valence shell.

THE PERIODIC TABLE

The **periodic table of the elements** organizes the elements according to their atomic numbers. It reveals a pattern of similar chemical and physical properties among elements. Rows are called **periods** and are based on the same principal energy level, *n*, while columns are called **groups**. Elements in the same group have the same valence shell electron configuration.

The elements on the periodic table (see Figure 11.2) belong to one of three types.

- **Metals** are shiny (lustrous), conduct electricity well, and both malleable and ductile. Metals are found on the left side and the middle of the periodic table.
- **Nonmetals** are dull, poor conductors of electricity, and brittle. Nonmetals are found on right side of the periodic table.
- **Metalloids** possess characteristics of both metals and nonmetals. They are found in a stair-step pattern starting with boron (B).

Atomic radius is the distance between the center of the nucleus and the outermost electron. **Ionic radius** is the size of a charged species. Cations (positive charge) are generally smaller than their corresponding neutral atom; anions (negative charge) are generally larger than their corresponding neutral atom. **Ionization energy** is the amount of energy necessary to remove an electron from the valence shell of a gaseous species. **Electron affinity** is the amount of energy released when a gaseous species gains an electron in its valence shell. **Electronegativity** is a measure of the attractive force of the nucleus for electrons within a bond. (See Figure 11.2.)

KEY CONCEPT

Effective nuclear charge (Z_{eff}) is the net positive charge experienced by electrons in the valence shell; it forms the foundation for all periodic trends. Z_{eff} increases from left to right across a period, with little change in value from top to bottom in a group. Valence electrons become increasingly separated from the nucleus as the principal energy level, *n*, increases from top to bottom in a group.

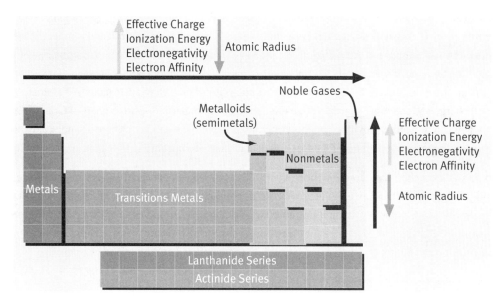

Figure 11.2. The Periodic Table of the Elements

Alkali metals typically take on an oxidation state of $+1$ and prefer to lose an electron to achieve a noble gas configuration (an octet). Both alkali metals and the alkaline earth metals are the most reactive of all metals. **Alkaline earth metals** take on an oxidation state of $+2$ and can lose two electrons to achieve noble gas configurations. **Transition metals** are unique because they take on multiple oxidation states.

Chalcogens take on oxidation states of -2 or $+6$ (depending on whether they are nonmetals or metals, respectively) in order to achieve a noble gas configuration. **Halogens** take on an oxidation state of -1 and prefer to gain an electron to achieve noble gas configurations; these nonmetals have the highest electronegativities. **Noble gases** have a fully filled valence shell in their standard state and prefer not to give up or take on additional electrons. Noble gases have very high ionization energies and virtually nonexistent electronegativities and electron affinities.

BONDING AND CHEMICAL INTERACTIONS

`High-Yield`

Elements form bonds to attain a noble gas electron configuration (an octet), and these bonds are either ionic or covalent. The **octet rule** states that elements are most stable with eight valence electrons. There are, however, a few exceptions. Some elements with an incomplete octet are stable (H, He, Li, Be, and B). Elements with an expanded octet are stable with more than eight electrons (all elements in Period 3 or greater). Compounds with an odd number of electrons cannot have eight electrons on each element.

An **ionic bond** is formed via the transfer of one or more electrons from an element with a relatively low ionization energy to an element with a relatively high electron affinity—usually between metals and nonmetals. The resulting electrostatic attraction between the ions causes them to remain in close proximity, forming the ionic bond and often **crystalline lattices**—large, organized arrays of ions. Ionic compounds have unique physical and chemical properties such as high melting points and the tendency to dissociate in polar solvents.

A **covalent bond** is formed via the sharing of electrons between two elements of similar electronegativities. **Bond order** refers to whether a covalent bond is a single bond, double bond, or triple bond. As bond order increases, **bond strength** increases, **bond energy** increases, and **bond length** decreases.

Covalent bonds can be categorized as either nonpolar or polar based on the nature of the elements involved. **Nonpolar bonds** result in molecules in which both atoms have exactly the same electronegativity. Some bonds are considered nonpolar when there is a very small difference in electronegativity between the atoms, even though they are technically slightly polar. **Polar bonds** form when there is a significant difference in electronegativities but not enough to transfer electrons and form an ionic bond. In a polar bond, the more electronegative element takes on a partial negative charge and the less electronegative element takes on a partial positive charge. **Coordinate covalent bonds** result when a single atom provides both bonding electrons while the other atom does not contribute any; coordinate covalent bonds are most often found in Lewis acid-base chemistry.

Lewis dot symbols are a chemical representation of an atom's valence electrons; they require a balance of valence, bonding, and nonbonding electrons in a molecule or ion. **Formal charges** exist when an atom is surrounded by either more or fewer valence electrons than it has in its neutral state (assuming equal sharing of electrons in a bond). For any molecule with a π (pi) system of electrons, **resonance structures** exist. These represent all of the possible configurations of electrons—stable and unstable—that contribute to the overall structure.

The **valence shell electron pair repulsion (VSEPR) theory** predicts the three-dimensional molecular geometry of covalently bonded molecules. In this theory, electrons—whether bonding or nonbonding—arrange themselves to be as far apart as possible from each other in three-dimensional space, leading to characteristic geometries. Nonbonding electrons exert more repulsion than bonding electrons because nonbonding electrons reside closer to the nucleus. **Electronic geometry** refers to the position of all electrons in a molecule, whether bonding or nonbonding. **Molecular geometry** refers to the position of only the bonding pairs of electrons in a molecule.

The **polarity of molecules** depends on the dipole moment of each bond and the sum of the dipole moments in a molecular structure. All polar molecules contain polar bonds. However, nonpolar molecules may contain nonpolar bonds or may contain polar bonds with dipole moments that cancel each other. σ and π bonds describe the patterns of overlap observed when molecular bonds are formed. **Sigma (σ) bonds** are the result of head-to-head overlap, while **pi (π) bonds** are the result of the overlap of two parallel electron cloud densities.

Intermolecular forces are electrostatic attractions between molecules. They are significantly weaker than covalent bonds (which are weaker than ionic bonds). **London dispersion forces** are the weakest interactions but are present in all atoms and molecules. As the size of the atom or structure increases, so does the corresponding London dispersion force. **Dipole–dipole interactions**, which occur between the oppositely charged ends of polar molecules, are stronger than London dispersion forces. These interactions are evident in the solid and liquid phases but negligible in the gas phase due to the distance between particles. **Hydrogen bonds** are a specialized subset of dipole–dipole interactions involved in intra- and intermolecular attraction. Hydrogen bonding occurs when H is bonded to one of three very electronegative atoms—F, O, or N.

COMPOUNDS AND STOICHIOMETRY

Compounds are substances composed of two or more elements in a fixed proportion. **Molecular weight** is the mass (in amu) of the constituent atoms in a compound as indicated by the molecular formula. **Molar mass** is the mass of 1 mole (**Avogadro's number** or 6.022×10^{23} particles) of a compound, usually measured in grams per mole.

Gram equivalent weight is a measure of the mass of a substance that can donate one equivalent of the species of interest. **Normality** is the ratio of equivalents per liter; normality is molarity multiplied by the number of equivalents present per mole of compound. **Equivalents** are moles of the species of interest, most often seen in acid-base chemistry (hydrogen ions or hydroxide ions) and oxidation-reduction reactions (moles of electrons).

The **law of constant composition** states that any pure sample of a compound contains the same elements in the same mass ratio. The **empirical formula** is the smallest whole-number ratio of the elements in a compound. The **molecular formula** is either the same as or a multiple of the empirical formula; it gives the exact number of atoms of each element in a compound. To calculate **percent composition** by mass, determine the mass of the individual element and divide by the molar mass of the compound.

Combination reactions occur when two or more reactants combine to form one product. **Decomposition reactions** occur when one reactant is chemically broken down into two or more products. **Combustion reactions** occur when a fuel and an oxidant (typically oxygen) react, forming the products water and carbon dioxide (if the fuel is a hydrocarbon). **Neutralization reactions** are those in which an acid reacts with a base to form a salt and, usually, water.

Displacement reactions occur when one or more atoms or ions of one compound are replaced with one or more atoms or ions of another compound. **Single-displacement reactions** occur when an ion of one compound is replaced with another element. **Double-displacement reactions** occur when elements from two different compounds trade places with each other to form two new compounds.

Chemical equations must be balanced to perform stoichiometric calculations. **Balanced equations** are determined using the following steps in order:

1. Balance the least common atoms.
2. Balance the more common atoms.
3. Balance the charge, if necessary.

Balanced equations can be used to determine the **limiting reagent**, which is the reactant that is consumed first in a chemical reaction. The other reactants present are termed **excess reagents**. The **theoretical yield** is the amount of product generated if all of the limiting reactant is consumed with no side reactions. However, the **actual yield** is typically lower than theoretical yield. **Percent yield** is the actual yield divided by the theoretical yield, which is then converted to a percentage.

Ionic charges are predictable by group number and type of element (metal or nonmetal) for representative elements. However, they are generally unpredictable for nonrepresentative elements. Metals form positively charged cations based on group number, while nonmetals form negatively charged anions based on the number of electrons needed to achieve an octet. **Electrolytes** contain equivalents of ions from molecules that dissociate in solution. The strength of an electrolyte depends on its degree of dissociation or **solvation.**

CHEMICAL KINETICS

High-Yield

Chemical mechanisms propose a series of steps that make up the overall reaction. **Intermediates** are molecules that exist within the course of a reaction but are neither reactants nor products overall. The slowest step, also known as the **rate-determining step**, limits the maximum rate at which the reaction can proceed.

The **collision theory** states that a reaction rate is proportional to the number of effective collisions between the reacting molecules. For a collision to be effective, molecules must be in the proper orientation and have sufficient kinetic energy to exceed the **activation energy.** The **Arrhenius equation** is a mathematical way of representing collision theory.

KEY CONCEPT

Reaction rates can be affected by a number of factors. Increasing the concentration of reactant increases the reaction rate (except for zero-order reactions) because there are more effective collisions per time. Increasing the temperature increases the reaction rate because the particles' kinetic energy is increased. Changing the medium can increase or decrease reaction rate, depending on how the reactants interact with the medium. Adding a catalyst increases the reaction rate because it lowers the activation energy (see Figure 11.3).

The **transition state theory** states that molecules form a **transition state** or an **activated complex** during a reaction in which the old bonds are partially dissociated and the new bonds are partially formed. From the transition state, the reaction can proceed toward products or revert back to reactants. The transition state is the highest point on a free-energy reaction diagram.

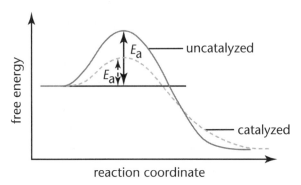

Figure 11.3. Reaction Diagram for a Catalyzed and an Uncatalyzed Reaction

Reaction rates are measured in terms of the rate of reactant disappearance or product appearance. **Rate laws** take the form of rate $= k[A]^x[B]^y$ and must be determined from experimental data. The **rate orders** usually do not match the stoichiometric coefficients. The rate order of a reaction is the sum of all individual rate orders in the rate law. **Zero-order reactions** have a constant rate that does not depend on the concentration of reactant; their rates can be affected only by changing the temperature or by adding a catalyst. A concentration $vs.$ time curve of a zero-order reaction is a straight line; the slope of such a line is equal to $-k$.

First-order reactions have a nonconstant rate that depends on the concentration of reactant. A concentration $vs.$ time curve of a first-order reaction is nonlinear, and the slope of a ln [A] $vs.$ time plot is $-k$ for a first-order reaction. **Second-order reactions** have a nonconstant rate that depends on the concentration of reactant. A concentration $vs.$ time curve of a second-order reaction is nonlinear, and the slope of a $\dfrac{1}{[A]}$ $vs.$ time plot is k for a second-order reaction.

EQUILIBRIUM

Reversible reactions eventually reach a state in which energy is minimized and entropy is maximized. Chemical equilibria are **dynamic**—the reactions are still occurring, just at a constant rate. In equilibrium, the concentrations of reactants and products remain constant because the rate of the forward reaction equals the rate of the reverse reaction.

The **law of mass action** gives the expression for the equilibrium constant, K_{eq}. The reaction quotient, Q, has the same form but can be calculated at any concentrations of reactants and products. Q is a calculated value that relates the reactant and product concentrations at any given time during a reaction. In contrast, K_{eq} is the ratio of products to reactants at equilibrium, with each species raised to its stoichiometric coefficient. Pure solids and liquids do not appear in the law of mass action; only gases and aqueous species do.

Comparison of Q to K_{eq} provides information about where the reaction is with respect to its equilibrium state. If $Q < K_{eq}$, $\Delta G < 0$ and the reaction proceeds in the forward direction. If $Q = K_{eq}$, $\Delta G = 0$ and the reaction is in dynamic equilibrium. If $Q > K_{eq}$, $\Delta G > 0$ and the reaction proceeds in the reverse direction.

Equilibrium calculations are broadly applicable to many areas of chemistry but are often formulaic in their application. The magnitude of K_{eq} determines the balance of a reaction and whether the amount that has reacted can be treated as negligible when compared to other concentrations. If $K_{eq} > 1$, the products are present in greater concentration at equilibrium. If $K_{eq} < 1$, the reactants are present in greater concentration at equilibrium.

Le Châtelier's Principle states that when a chemical system experiences a stress, it will react so as to restore equilibrium. Three main types of stresses can be applied to a system: changes in concentration, changes in pressure and volume, and changes in temperature. Increasing the concentration of reactants or decreasing the concentration of products will shift the reaction to the right. By the same logic, decreasing the concentration of reactants or increasing the concentration of products will shift the reaction to the left. Increasing pressure on a gaseous system (decreasing its volume) will shift the reaction toward the side with fewer moles of gas and vice versa. Increasing the temperature of an endothermic reaction or decreasing the temperature of an exothermic reaction will shift the reaction to the right and vice versa.

Reactions may have both kinetic and thermodynamic products that can be regulated by temperature and the presence of a catalyst. **Kinetic products** are higher in free energy than thermodynamic products and can form at lower temperatures. Kinetic products are sometimes termed "fast" products because they can form more quickly under such conditions. **Thermodynamic products** are more stable and lower in free energy than kinetic products. Despite proceeding more slowly than the kinetic pathway, the thermodynamic pathway is more spontaneous (more negative ΔG). (See Figure 11.4.)

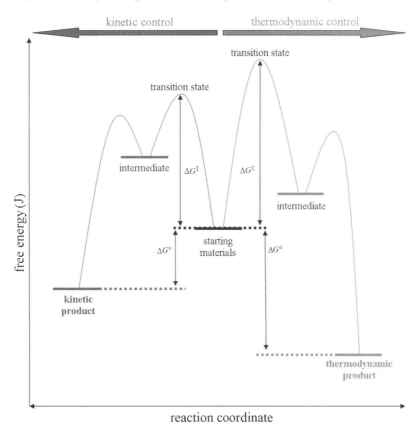

Figure 11.4. Kinetic and Thermodynamic Control of a Reaction

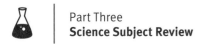

THERMOCHEMISTRY

Systems are classified based on what is or is not exchanged with the surroundings. **Isolated systems** exchange neither matter nor energy with the environment. **Closed systems** can exchange energy but not matter with the environment. **Open systems** can exchange both energy and matter with the environment.

Processes can be characterized based on a single constant property. **Isothermal** processes occur at constant temperature. **Adiabatic** processes exchange no heat with the environment. **Isobaric** processes occur at constant pressure. **Isovolumetric** processes occur at constant volume.

State functions describe the physical properties of an equilibrium state. They are pathway independent and include pressure, density, temperature, volume, enthalpy, internal energy, Gibbs free energy, and entropy. **Standard conditions** are defined as 298 K, 1 atm, and 1 M concentrations. The **standard state** of an element is its most prevalent form under standard conditions; **standard enthalpy**, **standard entropy**, and **standard free energy** are all calculated under standard conditions.

Phase changes exist at characteristic temperatures and pressures. **Fusion** (**melting**) and freezing (**crystallization** or **solidification**) occur at the boundary between the solid and the liquid phases. **Vaporization** (**evaporation** or **boiling**) and **condensation** occur at the boundary between the liquid and the gas phases. **Sublimation** and **deposition** occur at the boundary between the solid and gas phases. At temperatures above the **critical point**, liquid and gas phases are no longer distinguishable. At the **triple point**, all three phases of matter exist in equilibrium. **Phase diagrams** (see Figure 11.5) graph the phases and phase equilibria as a function of temperature and pressure.

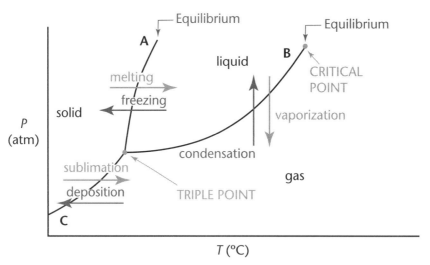

Figure 11.5. Phase Diagram for a Single Compound

Temperature is a scaled measure of the average kinetic energy of a substance. **Heat** is the transfer of energy that results from temperature differences between two substances. The total heat of a system undergoing heating, cooling, or phase changes is the sum of all energy changes.

Enthalpy (**ΔH**) is a measure of the potential energy of a system found in intermolecular attractions and chemical bonds. **Hess's law** states that the total change in potential energy of a system is equal to the changes of potential energies of the individual steps of the process. Enthalpy can also be calculated using heats of formation, heats of combustion, or bond dissociation energies. **Entropy (ΔS)**, which is often thought of as disorder, is actually a measure of the degree to which energy has been spread throughout a system or between a system and its surroundings. Entropy is a ratio of heat transferred per mole per unit kelvin. Entropy is maximized at equilibrium.

Gibbs free energy (*G*) is derived from both enthalpy and entropy values for a system. The change in Gibbs free energy determines whether a process is or is not spontaneous (see Table 11.2). At $\Delta G < 0$, a reaction proceeds in the forward direction (is spontaneous). At $\Delta G = 0$, a reaction is in dynamic equilibrium. At $\Delta G > 0$, a reaction proceeds in the reverse direction (is nonspontaneous). ΔG depends on temperature. Temperature-dependent processes change between spontaneous and nonspontaneous depending on the temperature. ΔG determines whether or not a reaction is spontaneous.

Enthalpy (ΔH)	Entropy (ΔS)	Outcome
+	+	Spontaneous at high temperatures
+	−	Nonspontaneous at all temperatures
−	+	Spontaneous at all temperatures
−	−	Spontaneous at low temperatures

Table 11.2. The Effects of Enthalpy, Entropy, and Temperature on the Spontaneity of Reactions

THE GAS PHASE

Gases are the least dense phase of matter. They are fluids and therefore conform to the shapes of their containers. However, gases are easily compressible. Gas systems are described by the variables **temperature (*T*)**, **pressure (*P*)**, **volume (*V*)**, and **number of moles (*n*)**. Important pressure equivalencies include 1 atm = 760 mmHg ≡ 760 torr = 101.325 kPa.

Standard temperature and pressure (STP) is 273 K (0°C) and 1 atm. Equations for ideal gases assume negligible mass and volume of gas molecules. Regardless of the identity of the gas, equimolar amounts of two gases occupy the same volume at the same temperature and pressure. At STP, 1 mole of an ideal gas occupies 22.4 L.

The **ideal gas law** describes the relationship between the four variables of the gas state for an ideal gas ($PV = nRT$).

- **Avogadro's principle** is a special case of the ideal gas law for which the pressure and temperature are held constant; it shows a direct relationship between the number of moles of gas and volume.
- **Boyle's law** is a special case of the ideal gas law for which temperature and number of moles are held constant; it shows an inverse relationship between pressure and volume ($P_1V_1 = P_2V_2$).
- **Charles's law** is a special case of the ideal gas law for which pressure and number of moles are held constant; it shows a direct relationship between temperature and volume $\left(\frac{V_1}{T_1} = \frac{V_2}{T_2}\right)$.
- **Gay-Lussac's law** is a special case of the ideal gas law for which volume and number of moles are held constant; it shows a direct relationship between temperature and pressure $\left(\frac{P_1}{T_1} = \frac{P_2}{T_2}\right)$.

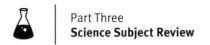

- **Dalton's law of partial pressures** states that individual gas components of a mixture of gases exert individual pressures in proportion to their **mole fractions**. The total pressure of a mixture of gases is equal to the sum of the partial pressures of the component gases.
- **Henry's law** states that the amount of gas dissolved in solution is directly proportional to the partial pressure of that gas at the surface of a solution.
- **Graham's law** describes the behavior of gas diffusion or effusion, stating that gases with lower molar masses diffuse or effuse faster than gases with higher molar masses at the same temperature.

Diffusion is the spreading out of particles from high to low concentration. **Effusion** is the movement of gas from one compartment to another through a small opening under pressure.

The **kinetic molecular theory** attempts to explain the behavior of gas particles. It makes a number of assumptions about the gas particles: gas particles have negligible volume, gas particles do not have intermolecular attractions or repulsions, gas particles undergo random collisions with each other and the walls of the container, collisions between gas particles (and with the walls of the container) are elastic, and the average kinetic energy of the gas particles is directly proportional to temperature.

Real gases deviate from ideal behavior under high pressure (low volume) and low temperature conditions. At moderately high pressures, low volumes, or low temperatures, real gases occupy less volume than predicted by the ideal gas law because the particles have intermolecular attractions. At extremely high pressures, low volumes, or low temperatures, real gases occupy more volume than predicted by the ideal gas law because the particles occupy physical space. The **van der Waals equation of state** is used to correct the ideal gas law for intermolecular attractions (*a*) and molecular volume (*b*).

SOLUTIONS

`High-Yield`

Solutions are homogeneous **mixtures** composed of two or more substances. They combine to form a single phase, generally the liquid phase. **Solvent** particles surround **solute** particles via electrostatic interactions in a process called **solvation** or **dissolution.** Most dissolutions are endothermic, although the dissolution of gas into liquid is exothermic. **Solubility** is the maximum amount of a solute that can be dissolved in a given solvent at a given temperature; it is often expressed as **molar solubility**—the molarity of the solute at saturation.

Complex ions are composed of metallic ions bonded to various neutral compounds and anions, referred to as **ligands.** Formation of **complex ions** increases the solubility of otherwise insoluble ions (the opposite of the common ion effect). The process of forming a complex ion involves electron pair donors and electron pair acceptors such as in **coordinate covalent bonding.**

Concentration can be expressed in many ways. **Percent composition by mass** (mass of solute per mass of solution times 100%) is used for aqueous solutions and solid-in-solid solutions. The **mole fraction** (moles of solute per total moles) is used for calculating vapor pressure depression and partial pressures of gases in a system. **Molarity** (moles of solute per liters of solution) is the most common unit for concentration and is used for rate laws, the law of mass action, osmotic pressure, pH and pOH, and the Nernst equation. **Molality** (moles of solute per kilograms of solvent) is used for boiling point elevation and freezing point depression. **Normality** (number of equivalents per liters of solution) is the molarity of the species of interest and is used for acid-base and oxidation-reduction reactions.

Saturated solutions are in equilibrium at that particular temperature. The **solubility product constant (K_{sp})** is simply the equilibrium constant for a dissociation reaction. Comparison of the **ion product (IP)** to K_{sp} determines the level of saturation and behavior of the solution. When $IP < K_{sp}$, the solution is unsaturated; if more solute is added, that solute will dissolve. When $IP = K_{sp}$, the solution is saturated (at equilibrium); if more solute is added, that solute will not dissolve unless another change occurs to the system (change in temperature or amount of solvent, for instance). When $IP > K_{sp}$, the solution is supersaturated, and disruptions of the solution will lead to precipitation.

Formation of a complex ion in solution greatly increases solubility. The **formation or stability constant (K_f)** is the equilibrium constant for complex formation. Its value is usually much greater than K_{sp}. The formation of a complex increases the solubility of other salts containing the same ions because the complex uses up the products of those dissolution reactions, shifting the equilibrium to the right (the opposite of the common ion effect). The **common ion effect** decreases the solubility of a compound in a solution that already contains one of the ions in the compound. The presence of that ion in solution shifts the dissolution reaction to the left, decreasing dissociation.

Colligative properties are physical properties of solutions that depend on the concentration of dissolved particles but not on their chemical identity. **Vapor pressure depression** follows **Raoult's law** (see Figure 11.6). The presence of other solutes decreases the evaporation rate of a solvent without affecting its condensation rate, thus decreasing its vapor pressure. Vapor pressure depression also explains boiling point elevation—as the vapor pressure decreases, the temperature (energy) required to boil the liquid must be raised.

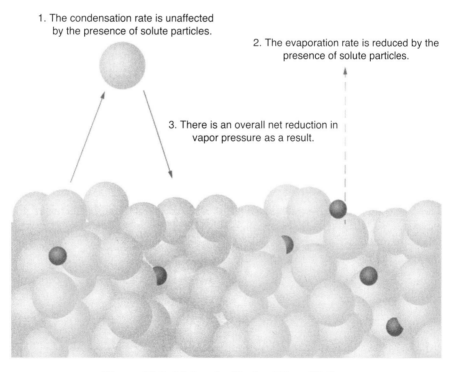

1. The condensation rate is unaffected by the presence of solute particles.

2. The evaporation rate is reduced by the presence of solute particles.

3. There is an overall net reduction in vapor pressure as a result.

Figure 11.6. Molecular Basis of Raoult's Law

Freezing point depression and **boiling point elevation** are shifts in the phase equilibria dependent on the molality of the solution. **Osmotic pressure** is primarily dependent on the molarity of the solution. For solutes that dissociate, the **van't Hoff factor (i)** is used in freezing point depression, boiling point elevation, and osmotic pressure calculations.

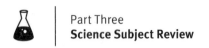
ACIDS AND BASES

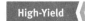

Arrhenius acids dissociate to produce excess of hydrogen ions in solution. **Arrhenius bases** dissociate to produce an excess of hydroxide ions in solution. **Brønsted-Lowry acids** are species that can donate hydrogen ions. **Brønsted-Lowry bases** are species that can accept hydrogen ions. **Lewis acids** are electron-pair acceptors. **Lewis bases** are electron-pair donors. All Arrhenius acids and bases are Brønsted-Lowry acids and bases, respectively; all Brønsted-Lowry acids and bases are Lewis acids and bases, respectively. However, the converse of these statements is not necessarily true.

Amphoteric species are those that can behave as either an acid or a base. **Amphiprotic** species are amphoteric species that specifically behave as a Brønsted-Lowry acid or base. Water is a classic example of an amphoteric, amphiprotic species—it can accept a hydrogen ion to become a hydronium ion, or it can donate a hydrogen ion to become a hydroxide ion. Conjugate species of polyvalent acids and bases can also behave as amphoteric and amphiprotic species.

The **water dissociation constant**, K_w, is 10^{-14} at 298 K. Like other equilibrium constants, K_w is affected only by changes in temperature. **pH** and **pOH** can be calculated using the concentrations of H_3O^+ and OH^- ions, respectively. In aqueous solutions, pH + pOH = 14 at 298 K. Strong acids and bases completely dissociate in solution. **Weak acids and bases** do not completely dissociate in solution and have corresponding **dissociation constants** (K_a and K_b, respectively).

In the Brønsted-Lowry definition, acids have conjugate bases that are formed when the acid is deprotonated. Bases have conjugate acids that are formed when the base is protonated. Strong acids and bases have very weak (inert) conjugates, and weak acids and bases have weak conjugates. **Neutralization reactions** form salts and (sometimes) water.

An **equivalent** is defined as 1 mole of the species of interest. In acid-base chemistry, **normality** is the concentration of acid or base equivalents in solution. **Polyvalent** acids and bases are those that can donate or accept multiple electrons.

Titrations are used to determine the concentration of a known reactant in a solution. The **titrant** has a known concentration and is added slowly to the titrand to reach the equivalence point. The **titrand** has an unknown concentration but a known volume. The **half-equivalence point** is the midpoint of the **buffering region**, in which half of the titrant has been protonated (or deprotonated); thus, [HA] = [A⁻] and a buffer is formed.

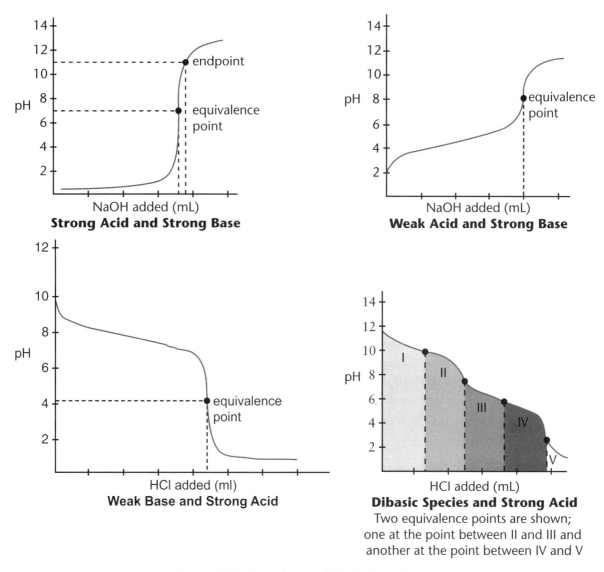

Figure 11.7. Titrations and Equivalence Points

The **equivalence point** is indicated by the steepest slope in a titration curve (see Figure 11.7). It is reached when the number of acid equivalents in the original solution equals the number of base equivalents added, or vice versa. Strong acid and strong base titrations have equivalence points at pH = 7. Weak acid and strong base titrations have equivalence points at pH > 7. Weak base and strong acid titrations have equivalence points at pH < 7. Weak acid and weak base titrations can have equivalence points above or below 7, depending on the relative strength of the acid and base.

Indicators are weak acids or bases that display different colors in protonated and deprotonated forms. The indicator chosen for a titration should have a pK_a close to the pH of the expected equivalence point. The **endpoint** of a titration is when the indicator reaches its final color. Multiple buffering regions and equivalence points are observed in polyvalent titrations (see Figure 11.7).

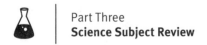

Buffer solutions consist of a mixture of a weak acid and its conjugate salt or a weak base and its conjugate salt; they resist large fluctuations in pH. **Buffering capacity** refers to the ability of a buffer to resist changes in pH; maximal buffering capacity is seen within 1 pH point of the pK_a of the acid in the buffer solution. The **Henderson-Hasselbalch equation** quantifies the relationship between pH and pK_a for weak acids and between pOH and pK_b for weak bases. When a solution is optimally buffered, $pH = pK_a$ and $pOH = pK_b$.

OXIDATION-REDUCTION REACTIONS

Oxidation is a loss of electrons, and **reduction** is a gain of electrons; the two are paired together in what is known as an **oxidation-reduction (redox)** reaction. An **oxidizing agent** facilitates the oxidation of another compound and is reduced itself in the process; a **reducing agent** facilitates the reduction of another compound and is itself oxidized in the process. Common oxidizing agents almost all contain oxygen or a similarly electronegative element. Common reducing agents often contain metal ions or hydrides (H^-).

To assign oxidation numbers, one must know the common oxidation states of the representative elements. Any free element or diatomic species has an oxidation number of zero. The oxidation number of a monatomic ion is equal to the charge of the ion.

When in compounds, Group IA metals have an oxidation number of $+1$; Group IIA metals have an oxidation number of $+2$. When in compounds, Group VIIA elements have an oxidation number of -1 (unless combined with an element with higher electronegativity). The oxidation state of hydrogen is $+1$ unless it is paired with a less electronegative element, in which case the oxidation state of hydrogen is -1. The oxidation state of oxygen is usually -2, except in peroxides (when its charge is -1) or in compounds with more electronegative elements. The sum of the oxidation numbers of all the atoms present in a compound is equal to the overall charge of that compound.

A **complete ionic equation** accounts for all of the ions present in a reaction. To write a complete ionic reaction, split all aqueous compounds into their relevant ions, but keep all solid salts intact. **Net ionic equations** ignore spectator ions to focus on only the species that actually participate in the reaction. To obtain a net ionic reaction, subtract the ions appearing on both sides of the reaction, which are called **spectator ions.** For reactions that contain no aqueous salts, the net ionic equation is generally the same as the overall balanced reaction. For double-displacement (metathesis) reactions that do not form a solid salt, there is no net ionic reaction because all ions remain in solution and do not change oxidation number.

Disproportionation (dismutation) reactions are a type of redox reaction in which one element is both oxidized and reduced, forming at least two molecules containing the element with different oxidation states. **Oxidation-reduction titrations** are similar in methodology to acid-base titrations. These titrations follow the transfer of charge. Indicators used in such titrations change color when certain voltages of solutions are achieved. **Potentiometric titration** is a form of redox titration in which a voltmeter or an external cell measures the electromotive force (emf) of a solution. No indicator is used, and the equivalence point is determined by a sharp voltage change.

ELECTROCHEMISTRY

An **electrochemical cell** describes any cell in which oxidation-reduction reactions take place. Certain characteristics are shared among all types of electrochemical cells. **Electrodes** are strips of metal or other conductive materials placed into an **electrolyte** solution. The **anode**, which attracts anions, is always the site of oxidation. The **cathode**, which attracts cations, is always the site of reduction. Electrons flow from the anode to the cathode, while current flows from the cathode to the anode.

Cell diagrams are shorthand notation that represent the reactions taking place in an electrochemical cell. They are written from anode to cathode with electrolytes (the solution) in between. A vertical line represents a phase boundary, and a double vertical line represents a salt bridge or other physical boundary.

Galvanic (voltaic) cells house spontaneous reactions ($\Delta G < 0$) with a positive electromotive force. **Electrolytic cells** house nonspontaneous reactions ($\Delta G > 0$) with a negative electromotive force. These nonspontaneous cells can be used to create useful products through electrolysis. **Concentration cells** are a specialized form of a galvanic cell in which both electrodes are made of the same material. Rather than a potential difference causing the movement of charge, the concentration gradient between the two solutions causes the movement of charge.

The charge on an electrode depends on the type of electrochemical cell one is studying. For galvanic cells, the anode is negatively charged and the cathode is positively charged. For electrolytic cells, the anode is positively charged and the cathode is negatively charged.

Rechargeable batteries are electrochemical cells that can experience both **charging** (electrolytic) and **discharging** (galvanic) states (see Figure 11.8). Rechargeable batteries are often ranked by **energy density**—the amount of energy a cell can produce relative to the mass of battery material.

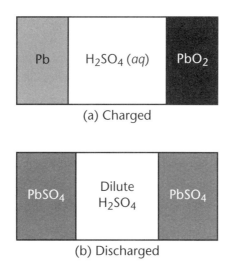

Figure 11.8. Lead-Acid Battery

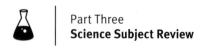
A **reduction potential** quantifies the tendency for a species to gain electrons and be reduced. The higher the reduction potential, the more a given species wants to be reduced. **Standard reduction potentials ($E°_{red}$)** are calculated by comparison to the **standard hydrogen electrode (SHE)** under the standard conditions of 298 K, 1 atm pressure, and 1 M concentrations. The standard hydrogen electrode has a standard reduction potential of 0 V.

Standard electromotive force ($E°_{cell}$) is the difference in standard reduction potential between the two half-cells. For galvanic cells, the difference of the reduction potentials of the two half-reactions is positive; for electrolytic cells, the difference of the reduction potentials of the two half-reactions is negative.

Electromotive force and change in free energy always have opposite signs.

- When $E°_{cell}$ is positive, $\Delta G°$ is negative. This is the case in galvanic cells.
- When $E°_{cell}$ is negative, $\Delta G°$ is positive. This is the case in electrolytic cells.
- When $E°_{cell}$ is 0, $\Delta G°$ is 0. This is the case in concentration cells.

The **Nernst equation** describes the relationship between the concentration of species in a solution under nonstandard conditions and the electromotive force. The equilibrium constant (K_{eq}) is the ratio of the products' concentrations at equilibrium over the reactants' concentrations, raised to their stoichiometric coefficients. There exists a relationship between the equilibrium constant (K_{eq}) and $E°_{cell}$.

- When K_{eq} is greater than 1, $E°_{cell}$ is positive.
- When K_{eq} is less than 1, $E°_{cell}$ is negative.
- When K_{eq} is equal to 1, $E°_{cell}$ is 0.

This chapter continues on the next page. ▶ ▶ ▶

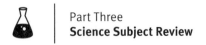

11.5   General Chemistry Worked Examples

The following steps will walk you through the following passage using the Kaplan Passage Strategy.

PREVIEW FOR DIFFICULTY

At a glance, the reaction at the beginning of the passage provides a clue as to the content of this passage: chemistry. Reading a bit more we see "equilibrium," "acidosis," and "alkalosis." So we should be thinking acid-base chemistry. In addition, this passage appears to be purely informational, with many short paragraphs each containing numerical values.

CHOOSE YOUR APPROACH

Highlighting would be ideal for this passage as it is an information passage and has many short paragraphs. In addition, since each paragraph contains numerical values, it is likely that many questions require pulling out this information. **Highlighting** is ideal for this!

READ AND DISTILL

P1: The first paragraph is essentially filler. You should be aware of the role of carbon dioxide in metabolism and the bicarb buffering system (Reaction 1). Keep reading, a little more quickly now, looking for new information.
Highlight: Nothing

R1: This simply shows the bicarb buffering system. No need to waste time analyzing it.
 Highlight: Nothing

P2: The next paragraph gives an apparent equilibrium constant and quantitative relationship between carbon dioxide and carbonic acid based on solubility. Reference values are also given, which are important to note as they may be needed for calculations. Specifically, note the contrast between CO_2 in arterial and venous blood.
Highlight: "Carbonic acid is proportional to," "Henry's law constant," "arterial blood," and "venous blood"

P3: The third paragraph discusses bicarb transport and provides values for serum levels of bicarb and chloride as well as pH.
Highlight: "Bicarbonate ions are exchanged for chloride ions," "respectively," and "arterial pH stabilized at 7.40"

P4: The fourth paragraph discusses acidosis, specifically respiratory and metabolic.
Highlight: "Respiratory acidosis, and "metabolic acidosis"

P5: The last paragraph discusses alkalosis, once again with a comparison of respiratory and metabolic.
 Highlight: "Respiratory alkalosis" and "metabolic alkalosis"

Given the formula and values, it's likely that calculations will be required—make sure you're using the correct reference values. Further, the comparisons between respiratory and metabolic disturbances are a likely target for questions.

PASSAGE I: ACIDS AND BASES

Carbon dioxide gas is a by-product of metabolism in the human body. After diffusing out of metabolically active tissue, the majority of carbon dioxide enters red blood cells, where it is rapidly hydrated by the enzyme carbonic anhydrase, as shown in Reaction 1.

$$H_2O \ (aq) + CO_2 \ (g) \rightleftharpoons H_2CO_3 \ (aq) \rightleftharpoons HCO_3^- \ (aq) + H^+ \ (aq)$$

Reaction 1

The apparent equilibrium constant for the dissociation of carbonic acid is $K_a = 7.9 \times 10^{-7}$, and the concentration of carbonic acid is proportional to the amount of carbon dioxide:

$$[H_2CO_3] = k_{H \ CO_2} \times pCO_2$$

where k_H is the Henry's law constant for carbon dioxide solubility, which is approximately $0.03 \ \dfrac{mmol}{L \cdot mm \ Hg}$, and pCO_2 is the partial pressure of CO_2 in the blood. The latter varies with location in the circulatory system but typically measures between 35 and 44 mmHg for arterial blood and between 39 and 52 mmHg for venous blood.

Bicarbonate ions are transported out of red blood cells, where they help maintain a constant serum pH. During transport, bicarbonate ions are exchanged for chloride ions. Equilibrium keeps bicarbonate and chloride ion serum levels at approximately 25 mM and 100 mM, respectively. This buffer system, along with the body's compensatory mechanisms, results in a normal arterial pH stabilized at 7.40.

Acidosis is a condition in which the body's arterial pH drops below 7.35. Respiratory acidosis is a specific condition that occurs when pCO_2 is too great. Metabolic acidosis is a similar condition in which an acid is being either overproduced by the body or insufficiently excreted by it.

Conversely, *alkalosis* is a condition in which the body's pH rises above 7.45. Respiratory alkalosis is a specific condition that can develop when carbon dioxide is removed too quickly from the body, such as hyperventilation during periods of significant stress, which commonly exacerbates this condition. Metabolic alkalosis also has many causative agents, including bicarbonate ion and chloride ion imbalances. In general, metabolic imbalances can be compensatory mechanisms for respiratory abnormalities.

1. Which of the following provides the best approximation for the pH of venous blood in a physiologically normal individual?

    A. $\text{pH} = -\log\left(7.9 \times 10^{-7}\right) + \log\left(\dfrac{25}{0.03 \times 35}\right)$

    B. $\text{pH} = -\log\left(7.9 \times 10^{-7}\right) + \log\left(\dfrac{0.03 \times 35}{25}\right)$

    C. $\text{pH} = -\log\left(7.9 \times 10^{-7}\right) + \log\left(\dfrac{25}{0.03 \times 44}\right)$

    D. $\text{pH} = -\log\left(7.9 \times 10^{-7}\right) + \log\left(\dfrac{0.03 \times 44}{25}\right)$

❶ Type the question

At a glance, this is an acid-base problem with the answer choices resembling the Henderson-Hasselbalch equation. Although it might be possible to make a quick guess at physiological pH (slightly less than 7.4), that is insufficient because our logarithmic calculations will not be accurate enough to differentiate among the answers. Notice the similarities within the answers: they all contain $-\log\left(7.9 \times 10^{-7}\right)$.

❷ Rephrase the question stem

After assessing the similarities and differences among the answer choices, it can be seen that each answer choice is a Henderson-Hasselbalch equation differing in the acid and conjugate base concentrations. When combined with the *venous* reference in the question stem, we can Rephrase this question as, *What is the acid and conjugate base concentration in venous blood?*

❸ Investigate potential solutions

All of the answers include the same term; that term is the pK_a for carbonic acid. The equation includes pH, pK_a for an acid, and the log of a ratio. This information and the context of the passage (buffering) leads one to the Henderson-Hasselbalch equation. The equation becomes $\text{pH} = pK_a + \log\left(\dfrac{[\text{HCO}_3^-]}{[\text{H}_2\text{CO}_3]}\right)$. The passage gives the bicarbonate concentration as 25 mM, but the carbonic acid concentration is more elusive. To solve for the carbonic acid concentration, it is necessary to combine $[\text{H}_2\text{CO}_3] = k_{\text{H CO}_2} \times p\text{CO}_2$ and the given values for $p\text{CO}_2$.

❹ Match your prediction to an answer choice

Armed with our prediction of the conjugate base being 25 mM, eliminate choices (B) and (D) because they have the concentration of bicarbonate in the denominator. The difference between (A) and (C) is the $p\text{CO}_2$, which can be deduced from the passage; it is either 39 mmHg or 44 mmHg. Use the reference values; 35 mmHg is too low for venous blood. So the correct answer is (C).

> **2.** Why is the chloride ion required by the cell for Reaction 1 to continue?
>
> **A.** Chloride ions act as catalysts for the system.
> **B.** Anion exchange prevents the accumulation of products.
> **C.** Chloride ions relieve the excessive charge buildup.
> **D.** The chloride ion is a base, which helps neutralize acidic products.

❶ Type the question

The question asks about reasoning. The correct answer must match the role of the chloride ion and must make sense. Glance at the answer choices; the reasoning should be based on a fundamental chemical understanding.

❷ Rephrase the question stem

The question stems asks us for the function of the chloride ion in Reaction 1. This goes beyond the scope of discrete MCAT content, so this must be a passage-based question. Rephrasing the question stem itself is fairly redundant, *What do chloride ions do?* However, it does give us an actionable step: find the chloride ion reference in the passage!

❸ Investigate potential solutions

Locate the chloride passage reference and how it relates to Reaction 1. Paragraph 3 explicitly states that an exchange of chloride ions occurs during transport of the bicarbonate ion out of the cell. This can serve as our prediction. The correct answer will reasonably explain why the removal of bicarbonate and/or the addition of chloride ions is necessary for the reaction to continue.

❹ Match your prediction to an answer choice

Starting with (**A**), chloride ion as a catalyst is not implausible; however, there is not enough information to confirm this. Because of that and the statement that chloride is exchanged, this an unlikely answer.

For (**B**), because bicarbonate is a product of Reaction 1 and the chloride ion does help remove it, this answer is plausible based on Le Châtelier's Principle.

(**C**) can be eliminated because there is no difference electrically. Although loss of bicarbonate without chloride exchange may lead to an electrical imbalance, this answer choice indicates that there is a preexisting *excessive* charge difference.

Finally, in (**D**), the chloride ion is the conjugate base of a strong acid (HCl), which makes it a very weak base—to the point that it is inert. So this is not correct.

Although our prediction did not immediately lead to a Match, it allowed us to eliminate (**A**), (**C**), and (**D**), indicating that (**B**) is correct.

3. Which of the following is the approximate arterial partial pressure of carbon
   dioxide in blood?
   A. 0.0052 kPa
   B. 0.052 kPa
   C. 5.3 kPa
   D. 40 kPa

① Type the question

This question asks for pCO_2, the partial pressure of CO_2 in the blood. The answers are numbers that differ in order of magnitude. So we should pay more attention to that than the exact value. Also, the answers are in kilopascals, not mmHg as in the passage.

② Rephrase the question stem

Reading the question stem carefully indicates that we need to limit our consideration to arterial partial pressure when considering CO_2. A Rephrase of this question could be: *Calculate the pCO_2 in kPa for arterial blood.*

③ Investigate potential solutions

Paragraph 2 states that pCO_2 is between 35 and 44 mmHg. Given the spacing between answer choices, we can just pick a number that is within the range and easy to use; 40 mmHg will do.

The conversion needed is 760 mmHg = 101.5 kPa. This should be known content because 1 atm = 760 Torr = 760 mmHg = 101.5 kPa. Setting up a proportion gives:

$$\frac{101.5 \text{ kPa}}{760 \text{ mmHg}} = \frac{x \text{ kPa}}{40 \text{ mmHg}}$$

Solving this for x gives:

$$x = \frac{(40)(100)}{760} = \frac{1(100)}{19} \approx \frac{100}{20} = 5 \text{ kPa}$$

④ Match your prediction to an answer choice

The only answer close to 5 kPa is (**C**). Note that (**D**) assumes that 1 kPa = 1 mmHg, which is incorrect. (**A**) and (**B**) are both based on using incorrect proportions for mmHg and kPa.

> **4.** During the last century, carbon dioxide emissions have noticeably increased the carbon dioxide concentration in the atmosphere. What effect has this had on the oceans?
>
> **A.** Marine life dependent on CO_3^{2-} have proliferated.
>
> **B.** The oceans have become more basic.
>
> **C.** There has been an increase in bicarbonate levels.
>
> **D.** The rise in atmospheric CO_2 has been exacerbated by global warming.

① Type the question

This question relies on your ability to relate passage information of carbon dioxide concentrations to the world. At first glance, this may seem like a discrete question. However, climate change is beyond the scope of the MCAT. Therefore this must be a passage-based question.

② Rephrase the question stem

Glance back at the passage; pCO_2 was explicitly mentioned in Henry's law, which states that the partial pressures of a gas above a liquid is proportional to the concentration of the gas within the liquid. This question can be Rephrased as, *What would happen if a greater amount of CO_2 was dissolved in the oceans?*

③ Investigate potential solutions

If the atmospheric concentration of CO_2 increases, the amount of CO_2 dissolved in the oceans would also increase. If the amount of dissolved CO_2 increases, according to Reaction 1 so does the amount of H_2CO_3 and, ultimately, both HCO_3^- and acidity. If the acidity of the oceans increases, the pH decreases. This can serve as your prediction.

④ Match your prediction to an answer choice

Using your prediction, Match to **(C)**.

(A) can be eliminated after further consideration because an increase in the acidity of the oceans would promote the formation of HCO_3^- from CO_3^{2-} and H^+, rendering less of the carbonate ion available for marine life.

(B) can be eliminated because it is opposite of the prediction.

(D) relates solubility to temperature. Although the two are related, if there was an increase in global temperatures, that would reduce the solubility of CO_2 and raise atmospheric concentrations. However, this does not address the effect on the oceans, so it cannot be the correct answer.

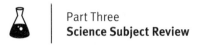
> **5.** Given a typical plasma volume of 5 L, a typical adult has an amount of bicarbonate with a buffering capability equivalent to how many 500 mg calcium carbonate antacid tablets?
>
> **A.** 12.5
>
> **B.** 25
>
> **C.** 125
>
> **D.** 6×10^3

❶ Type the question

The question is asking about the limit of a buffer system. The answer choices and the context of the passage indicate you'll need to do a stoichiometry calculation to solve this problem. In addition, the unit of 500 mg/tablet implies unit analysis must be done. At a quick glance, this question (and questions like it) should be triaged for later.

❷ Rephrase the question stem

To answer a unit analysis (also known as dimensional analysis) question, map out how to relate the provided values to your needed values. This can serve as the Rephrase: *How many $CaCO_3$ tablets are needed to match the equivalents of HCO_3^- found in 5 L of plasma?*

❸ Investigate potential solutions

Relating liters of bicarbonate to milligrams of calcium carbonate requires some important steps in between. Naturally, we can begin by evaluating each of these compounds. HCO_3^- has the buffering capability of 1 equivalent as it can gain only a single proton. In contrast, CO_3^{2-} from calcium carbonate has the buffering capability of 2 equivalents. After seeing how these two buffers can be related through equivalents, a natural next step would be to calculate the equivalents of HCO_3^- and CO_3^{2-} in the 5 L of plasma and 500 mg antacid tablet, respectively.

First let's determine how much bicarbonate would be found in a typical adult (5 L of plasma). This will require some information from the passage plus a conversion from volume and concentration to amount. Paragraph 3 indicates that the typical level of bicarbonate is 25 mM, and the question provides an average volume of 5 L. Combining these gives 25 mmoles/L × 5 L = 125 mmoles of bicarbonate. Because bicarbonate's formula is HCO_3^-, 1 mole can neutralize 1 mole of acid, and 1 mmol = 1 mEq. Therefore, we have 125 mEq of base.

Next, use stoichiometry to determine the equivalent amount of antacid. To calculate the number of calcium carbonate tablets needed, we need to know that carbonate is CO_3^{2-}, so 1 mmol = 2 mEq. In addition, the molecular mass of CO_3^{2-} is 100 g/mol (or 100 mg/mmol). Now we can do a stoichiometry calculation:

$$125 \text{ mEq} \times \frac{1 \text{ mmol CaCO}_3}{2 \text{ mEq}} \times \frac{100 \text{ mg CaCO}_3}{1 \text{ mmol CaCO}_3} \times \frac{1 \text{ tablet}}{500 \text{ mg}} = 12.5 \text{ tablets}$$

④ Match your prediction to an answer choice

Our prediction of 12.5 tablets matches (**A**). Notice common errors that may lead you to pick a wrong answer. (**B**) incorrectly assumes that 1 mole of calcium carbonate neutralizes 1 equivalent of acid. (**C**) is the number of milliequivalents of bicarbonate in blood. (**D**) is the milligrams of calcium carbonate required, not the number of 500 mg tablets.

---

6. Metabolic acidosis is characterized by a:

A. high plasma $[HCO_3^-]$, a low plasma $[H^+]$, and increased breathing rate.

B. high plasma $[HCO_3^-]$, a high plasma $[H^+]$, and decreased breathing rate.

C. low plasma $[HCO_3^-]$, high plasma $[H^+]$, and increased breathing rate.

D. low plasma $[HCO_3^-]$, high plasma $[H^+]$, and decreased breathing rate.

---

① Type the question

Although the question stem is extremely general, only indicating metabolic acidosis, the answer choices show important patterns. Each answer choice mentions $[HCO_3^-]$, $[H^+]$, and breathing, indicating that this question tests the bicarbonate buffering system as well the impact of breathing on blood pH.

② Rephrase the question stem

Utilizing the question and answer choice patterns above, we can Rephrase this question as: *According to Reaction 1 (bicarbonate buffering system), how does metabolic acidosis affect $[HCO_3^-]$, $[H^+]$, and breathing?*

③ Investigate potential solutions

The term *acidosis* is enough to predict a decrease in pH and an increase in $[H^+]$. The passage states that "metabolic acidosis is a similar condition in which an acid is being either overproduced by the body or insufficiently excreted by it." Use the equilibrium in Reaction 1 to determine the effect of increased acid production on bicarbonate concentrations. According to Le Châtelier's Principle, an increase in $[H^+]$ would shift the equilibrium back toward H_2O and CO_2, so $[HCO_3^-]$ would decrease. Finally, an increase of blood CO_2 would result in increased ventilation to remove the excess CO_2.

④ Match your prediction to an answer choice

Using the prediction from our Investigate step, Match to (**C**).

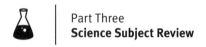

GENERAL CHEMISTRY PASSAGE II: SOLUBILITY

Adequate solubility of ions and macromolecules, along with their ability to permeate epithelial layers in various sections of the digestive and excretory systems, helps prevent malnutrition and other dangerous conditions.

The human body needs to absorb regular doses of certain vitamins and minerals. *Vitamins* are organic molecules that an organism cannot sufficiently synthesize; they are not broken down for energy but are needed for normal cellular operation. Some vitamins have hormone-like functionality (vitamin D, for example), whereas others act as antioxidants (vitamin C) or as precursors to enzyme cofactors (vitamin B_{12}).

Dietary minerals are elements (other than C, H, N, and O) required for living; *trace minerals* are dietary minerals essential only in minute quantities. Most of them must be taken as parts of compounds because many free elements can react with substances in the digestive tract to form by-products, some of which are toxic. Approximately 30 elements are known to be—or are suspected to be—essential to normal biological function. Most minerals are naturally occurring in the diet, although foods may be fortified.

The chemical and physical nature of required nutrients affects their solubility and ability to permeate membranes. It can also alter their *bioavailability*, the fraction of the ingested dose that reaches systemic circulation unaltered. Any process that alters the compound or hinders its absorption will reduce bioavailability. Certain food additives can alter bioavailability; for example, the fat substitute Olestra (molecular formula: $C_{13}H_{14}O_{11}$) reduces vitamin K absorption. Each gram of Olestra in food can reduce absorption of vitamin K by 3.3 μg. Table 1 displays some of the nutritional and chemical characteristics of important vitamins and minerals. (Note: The average adult has a blood volume of approximately 5 L.)

Nutrient Source	Oral Bioavailability	Recommended Daily Intake (RDI)	Molecular Mass (g/mol)
Vitamin A acetate	0.99	900 μg	328.49
Vitamin B_6	0.85	1.7 mg	123.11
Vitamin C	0.99	90.0 mg	176.12
Vitamins D_2 and D_3	0.99	10.0 μg	396.65
Vitamin E	0.67	15.0 mg	430.71
Vitamin K	0.90	120 μg	444.65
Potassium chloride	0.90	4700 mg	74.55
Sodium chloride	0.99	1500 mg	58.44
Calcium carbonate	0.35	1300 mg	100.09
Zinc sulfate	0.37	5.0 mg	161.47

Table 1. Nutritional and Chemical Values of Selected Vitamins and Minerals

1. Vitamin C formulations are administered in a variety of ways, including pure ascorbic acid administered orally and ascorbyl palmitate (vitamin C ester) administered topically. How does the addition of the palmitate group affect the oral and topical bioavailability of vitamin C?

Palmitic Acid

A. The palmitate group decreases oral bioavailability by reducing solubility in the digestive tract but increases topical bioavailability by minimizing free radicals in the epidermis.

B. The palmitate group increases oral bioavailability by increasing absorption in the digestive tract and increases topical bioavailability by increasing vitamin C stability in topical solutions.

C. The palmitate group decreases oral bioavailability by decreasing absorption in the digestive tract and has little effect on topical bioavailability because ascorbyl palmitate penetrates the skin as effectively as pure vitamin C.

D. The palmitate group has little effect on oral bioavailability because the palmitate group is removed by hydrolysis in the digestive tract and increases topical bioavailability by increasing the stability of vitamin C in topical solutions.

2. Normal serum levels of vitamin E range from 12–46 μmol/L. Vitamin E toxicity can lead to muscle weakness, fatigue, nausea, diarrhea, and excess bleeding, while vitamin E deficiency can cause neurological damage, muscle weakness, and retinal changes. The upper limit of recommended vitamin E supplementation is 1,000 mg/day. Will this lead to toxicity in an individual with severe vitamin E deficiency?

A. Yes, because any amount above the normal serum level will be toxic.

B. No, because the serum level from the supplement must be above normal to make up for the deficiency.

C. Yes, because these individuals are more at risk for vitamin E toxicity.

D. No, because this individual is likely to have lower bioavailability for vitamin E than a healthy individual.

3. Which of the following would best explain the relatively low bioavailability of zinc sulfate?

A. Zinc sulfate is insoluble in aqueous solution, and thus, its ions cannot be digested and absorbed.

B. Other substances interact with the ions in the oral route, inhibiting absorption.

C. Zn^{2+} ions do not have enough valence electrons to interact sufficiently with intestinal ion channels.

D. Zn^{2+} ions are immediately deposited in bone and other tissue, thus lowering the bioavailability.

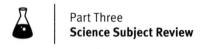

4. Hyperoxaluria causes calcium oxalate (CaC_2O_4) to deposit in urine. A 0.75 L urine sample free of oxalate was collected. The Ca^{2+} concentration of the urine was determined to be 1 mM, and then oxalate was added until crystals formed. If 0.15 mg was added, what is the K_{sp} of CaC_2O_4?

   A. $K_{sp} = 2.9 \times 10^{-7}$
   B. $K_{sp} = 2.4 \times 10^{-9}$
   C. $K_{sp} = 2.9 \times 10^{-9}$
   D. $K_{sp} = 2.4 \times 10^{-11}$

5. Olestra, once a popular food additive, has been found to reduce the absorption of certain nutrients. For example, each mole of Olestra effectively removes 2.5 μmol of vitamin K from the digestive tract. How much vitamin K must be ingested to achieve the RDI if 34 g of Olestra is taken concurrently?

   A. 0.01 mg
   B. 0.1 mg
   C. 0.25 mg
   D. 3.5 g

USING THE KAPLAN METHOD

Preview the passage: At a glance, the paragraphs are information dense and seem to discuss nutritional science. The associated Table 1 includes data, but it is information that you'd expect to find in a textbook. This is an information passage.

Choose your approach: Outlining

Read and Distill:

P1: Solubility = excretory/digestive tract section dependence

P2: Vitamins = organic; various functions; examples

P3: Minerals ≠ C, H, O, N; description

P4: Chemical composition dictates bioavailability

T1: Values for minerals and vitamins

1. Vitamin C formulations are administered in a variety of ways, including pure ascorbic acid administered orally and ascorbyl palmitate (vitamin C ester) administered topically. How does the addition of the palmitate group affect the oral and topical bioavailability of vitamin C?

Palmitic Acid

   A. The palmitate group decreases oral bioavailability by reducing solubility in the digestive tract but increases topical bioavailability by minimizing free radicals in the epidermis.
   B. The palmitate group increases oral bioavailability by increasing absorption in the digestive tract and increases topical bioavailability by increasing vitamin C stability in topical solutions.
   C. The palmitate group decreases oral bioavailability by decreasing absorption in the digestive tract and has little effect on topical bioavailability because ascorbyl palmitate penetrates the skin as effectively as pure vitamin C.
   D. The palmitate group has little effect on oral bioavailability because the palmitate group is removed by hydrolysis in the digestive tract and increases topical bioavailability by increasing the stability of vitamin C in topical solutions.

❶ Type the question

This question has long answer choices that deal with changes in oral and topical bioavailability. Notice, though, that each answer choice has a total of four parts (change in oral bioavailability, explanation, change in topical bioavailability, explanation). In answering this question, we'll probably want to start with just one part rather than try to predict everything at once.

❷ Rephrase the question stem

The question stem states that vitamin C in the form of ascorbic acid is orally administered and vitamin C in the form of ascorbyl palmitate is topically administered. Despite the additional information on ascorbic acid, the question asks only about the addition of the palmitate group or, more specifically, ascorbyl palmitate (vitamin C ester). Thus, we can Rephrase the question as, *How does the ester in ascorbyl palmitate affect oral and topical bioavailability?*

❸ Investigate potential solutions

Begin by considering the oral and topical administration routes and how the palmitate group would affect the bioavailability.

Starting with the oral route, what will happen when the ester reaches the stomach? It's in an aqueous solution that contains significant amounts of acid. That's the perfect recipe for hydrolysis of the ester, which results in vitamin C and palmitic acid. As a result, vitamin C should be available in the stomach in its pure form, so its bioavailability should remain approximately the same.

Next, consider the palmitate's effect on topical availability. The question states that ascorbyl palmitate is administered topically. Thus we can infer that the vitamin C can be absorbed in this manner. Perhaps a prediction could be that the additional carbon chain makes ascorbyl palmitate more fat soluble, allowing it to better be absorbed via the skin.

TAKEAWAYS

For predictions about absorption and solubility, use the chemical structures. Be mindful of chemical reactions that could alter the physical properties.

❹ Match your prediction to an answer choice

Only (**D**) matches the prediction. Moreover, the second half of the statement is correct as well: the palmitate group should increase the stability of vitamin C in topical solutions.

Let's quickly look at the wrong answers. (**B**) would be unlikely on general principle. The oral bioavailability is already 99 percent. So it's unlikely that palmitate—or anything else for that matter—could significantly increase that percentage. On the other hand, (**A**) and (**C**) both claim a significant decrease. (**A**) claims this occurs because the ester is less soluble in water. As stated previously, esters undergo hydrolysis in water, so this is incorrect. (**C**), on the other hand, claims that it is because of decreased absorption of the ester. In fact, the reverse is true. If anything, the vitamin C ester, because of its large hydrophobic group, should be better absorbed.

> **2.** Normal serum levels of vitamin E range from 12–46 µmol/L. Vitamin E toxicity can lead to muscle weakness, fatigue, nausea, diarrhea, and excess bleeding, while vitamin E deficiency can cause neurological damage, muscle weakness, and retinal changes. The upper limit of recommended vitamin E supplementation is 1,000 mg/day. Will this lead to toxicity in an individual with severe vitamin E deficiency?
>
> **A.** Yes, because any amount above the normal serum level will be toxic.
> **B.** No, because the serum level from the supplement must be above normal to make up for the deficiency.
> **C.** Yes, because these individuals are more at risk for vitamin E toxicity.
> **D.** No, because this individual is likely to have lower bioavailability for vitamin E than a normal individual.

1 Type the question

This is a Yes/No question, which at first glance appears to have patterns that can be exploited to eliminate answers. However, Yes/No questions are actually critical-reasoning questions based on the second part of the answer. Given their challenging nature, these question types can be ideal to save for later in the passage set.

2 Rephrase the question stem

Much of the information in the question stem is unneeded and can be ignored. Based on two of the answer choices, the serum level of vitamin E might be an issue. However, if reasoning can be used instead, it is a better and faster approach to the question than doing any calculations. As such, we can Rephrase this question as, *Would consuming 1,000 mg/day of vitamin E lead to toxicity for a patient with severe vitamin E deficiency?*

3 Investigate potential solutions

Although forming a focused prediction is possible through consideration of the cause of severe vitamin E deficiency in the individual, it is more efficient to eliminate unreasonable answer choices. Look for opportunities to eliminate answer choices as unreasonable and for answer choices that fit with the premise of the question.

4 Match your prediction to an answer choice

(**A**) makes an extreme statement that any amount above the normal serum level will lead to toxicity. This is unlikely to be true as a small increase above normal should not lead to a severe problem. Eliminate (**A**).

TAKEAWAYS

Look at the answer choices and the information given. Always ensure that your calculations include units to ensure that you have achieved the answer as desired.

(**B**) sounds appealing, especially because a quick calculation shows that the serum level would be above normal based on the bioavailability shown in Table 1:

$$\frac{1{,}000\ \text{mg}}{5\ \text{L}} \times \frac{1\ \text{mmole}}{430\ \text{mg}} \times 0.67 \approx \frac{0.3\ \text{mmole}}{\text{L}} = 300\ \mu\text{mole/L}$$

THINGS TO WATCH OUT FOR

Scientific notation makes math much simpler. Using dimensional analysis in these situations is critical. Always assess carefully to determine whether math is actually necessary before performing a calculation.

This is significantly above the normal serum level for vitamin E. Even without calculations, this answer choice can be eliminated as the goal is to reach standard serum levels of vitamin E rather than to exceed them. Eliminate (**B**).

(**C**) is again appealing at first glance as the individual in question has problems with vitamin E. However, this choice is opposite the correct answer. The individual is deficient in vitamin E, which does not make him or her more likely to be affected by toxicity.

(**D**) is the only remaining option and thus must be the correct answer. It is a reasonable inference that an individual with severe vitamin E deficiency would have lower bioavailability than normal due to an inability to absorb vitamin E. (**D**) is correct.

KEY CONCEPT

Stoichiometry and dimensional analysis are skills used in various topics.

3. Which of the following would best explain the relatively low bioavailability of zinc sulfate?

   A. Zinc sulfate is insoluble in aqueous solution, and thus, its ions cannot be digested and absorbed.
   B. Other substances interact with the ions in the oral route, inhibiting absorption.
   C. Zn^{2+} ions do not have enough valence electrons to interact sufficiently with intestinal ion channels.
   D. Zn^{2+} ions are immediately deposited in bone and other tissue, thus lowering the bioavailability.

① Type the question

This question asks us why zinc sulfate has low bioavailability. The answers are reasons, which means we need an answer that is both scientifically plausible and relevant to the question at hand.

② Rephrase the question stem

Bioavailability is defined in paragraph 4. Zinc sulfate is considered a mineral, which is discussed in the third paragraph. Table 1 confirms that it does, in fact, have low bioavailability. The MCAT does not expect us to have specific knowledge on zinc bioavailability but, rather, the chemical category zinc belongs to. Thus, we can Rephrase this question as, *Why do positive ions (Zn^{2+}) have lower bioavailability?*

③ Investigate potential solutions

Paragraph 4 states that processes that hinder absorption or alter a substance reduce bio-availability. Paragraph 3 notes that elements can react with molecules in the digestive tract, sometimes forming toxic by-products. It's reasonable to believe that the same might happen with ions as well as free elements. Therefore, we can predict that the correct answer should indicate either a reaction involving Zn^{2+} ions or some factor that hinders absorption.

④ Match your prediction to an answer choice

Consider the answer choices one at a time. (**A**) is false. Sulfates are generally soluble. (**B**) matches our prediction; it gives us a reason why Zn^{2+} would be poorly absorbed. (**C**) is incorrect. Cations are moved by electrostatic forces as a result of their positive charges, not their electrons. Finally, (**D**) also is incorrect. Bone does not act as a storage pool for zinc.

---

4. Hyperoxaluria causes calcium oxalate (CaC_2O_4) to deposit in urine. A 0.75 L urine sample free of oxalate was collected. The Ca^{2+} concentration of the urine was determined to be 1 mM, and then oxalate was added until crystals formed. If 0.15 mg was added, what is the K_{sp} of CaC_2O_4?

    A. $K_{sp} = 2.9 \times 10^{-7}$
    B. $K_{sp} = 2.4 \times 10^{-9}$
    C. $K_{sp} = 2.9 \times 10^{-9}$
    D. $K_{sp} = 2.4 \times 10^{-11}$

---

① Type the question

This is a calculation question. In addition, the answer choices are relatively close together, meaning that precision is needed during the calculation (limit rounding). To solve for the K_{sp}, it is necessary to determine the ion product at the time of precipitation. This involves calculating the concentrations of both ions present. The question provides the calcium concentration, and the concentration of oxalate can be calculated from the information in the question stem. Given the math involved, save this question for late in the passage set.

② Rephrase the question stem

It is necessary to have the K_{sp} expression for CaC_2O_4 (which can be derived from the balanced reaction) and the concentrations of each ion in the equation. The calcium concentration is given. The concentration of oxalate can be calculated from the molar mass of oxalate along with the mass and volume of the oxalate sample. This calculation question can be Rephrased to the task, *Find the Ca^{2+} and oxalate concentrations to calculate K_{sp}.*

TAKEAWAYS

When left with four confusing choices, eliminate the ones that are certainly wrong.

THINGS TO WATCH OUT FOR

Solubility rules are often—but not always—necessary to solve solution problems. When in doubt, start with what you are most confident with and work from there.

KEY CONCEPT

Questions that task you with explaining discrepancies require critical thinking and a firm understanding of the passage. If unsure how to approach these, mark them for review and return to them when you have more time.

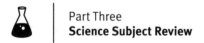

3 Investigate potential solutions

$$CaC_2O_4 \rightleftharpoons Ca^{2+} + C_2O_4^{2-}$$

$$K_{sp} = \left[Ca^{2+}\right]\left[C_2O_4^{2-}\right]$$

$$\left[C_2O_4^{2-}\right] = \frac{0.15 \text{ mg } C_2O_4^{2-}}{0.75 \text{ L}} \times \frac{1 \text{ mol}}{88 \text{ g}} \times \frac{1 \text{ g}}{10^3 \text{ mg}}$$

$$\approx \frac{1}{5} \times \frac{1}{90} \times 10^{-3} = 0.2 \times 0.011 \times 10^{-3} = 2.2 \times 10^{-6} \text{ M}$$

From the question stem, $[Ca^{2+}] = 1 \times 10^{-3}$ M. Determine the K_{sp}:

$$K_{sp} = \left[Ca^{2+}\right]\left[C_2O_4^{2-}\right] = \left(1 \times 10^{-3}\right)\left(2.2 \times 10^{-6}\right) = 2.2 \times 10^{-9}$$

4 Match your prediction to an answer choice

Executing the plan leads to a prediction of 2.2×10^{-9}. There is no exact match to this answer. However, answer (**B**) is a reasonable choice given the estimation and rounding done in this problem.

---

5. Olestra, once a popular food additive, has been found to reduce the absorption of certain nutrients. For example, each mole of Olestra effectively removes 2.5 μmol of vitamin K from the digestive tract. How much vitamin K must be ingested to achieve the RDI if 34 g of Olestra is taken concurrently?

    A. 0.01 mg
    B. 0.1 mg
    C. 0.25 mg
    D. 3.5 mg

---

1 Type the question

The question stem provides a mole ratio between Olestra and vitamin K removed. The question stem also mentions RDI and provides the mass of Olestra in grams. In addition, the answer choices are all in milligrams. Therefore this is a stoichiometry problem and a convoluted one at that. Triage this question for later.

2 Rephrase the question stem

TAKEAWAYS

Conversion factors may sometimes be given in a passage or question stem. Be sure to use them appropriately (using labels whenever necessary).

Based on the information provided in the passage and question stem, as well as the small range of answer choices, this is a stoichiometry question that can be Rephrased as, *Find the mass of vitamin K needed to achieve 120 µmol (vitamin K RDI) while taking 34 g of Olestra.*

3 Investigate potential solutions

Olestra removes vitamin K in a ratio given in the passage using grams, so the information given in the question stem is extraneous. In other words, there is no need to calculate moles. Instead, use the ratio to determine how much vitamin K will be removed by Olestra. Then look at the RDI and bioavailability of vitamin K to determine how much more must be consumed.

Start with the ratio given in the passage, and set up a proportion to determine the amount of vitamin K needed:

$$\frac{1 \text{ g Olestra}}{3.3 \text{ } \mu\text{g vit K}} = \frac{34 \text{ g Olestra}}{x \text{ } \mu\text{g vit K}}$$
$$x = 34 \times 3.3 \approx 110 \text{ } \mu\text{g vit K}$$

THINGS TO WATCH OUT FOR

Rounding error will need to be taken into account at times. It's best to keep notes (mental or on your noteboard) about the approximations that you have made so that you can make adjustments quickly and accurately.

110 µg is the mass of vitamin K that 34 g of Olestra will remove. Therefore, 110 µg of additional vitamin K must be ingested to reach RDI. The RDI for vitamin K from Table 1 is 120 µg. Thus the total vitamin K ingested is the sum of these two values, 110 µg + 120 µg = 230 µg.

Finally, convert 230 µg to mg, which is 0.230 mg. Let this be your prediction.

4 Match your prediction to an answer choice

Match your prediction to (**C**).

(**A**) and (**B**) are incorrect because they are well below the estimated calculation for the amount required, while (**D**) is too large.

THINGS TO WATCH OUT FOR

Don't rush through stoichiometry calculations. Make sure that you're using the correct ratios and that the proper units cancel out in each step.

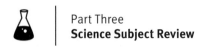

11.6 General Chemistry on Your Own

GENERAL CHEMISTRY PASSAGE III (QUESTIONS 1–6)

The conversion of reactants to products can be mediated by various factors. In a reaction that has a high free energy of activation for the conversion of reactants to transition state, the observed reaction rate is based on the concentration of the transition state in solution. Take the following example:

$$\text{Reactants} \rightleftharpoons \text{Transition State} \rightarrow \text{Products}$$

where there is an equilibrium constant, K^I, for the equilibrium between the reactants and the transition state. The rate of the overall reaction, V, is dictated as follows:

$$V = v[A]$$

where v is the rate constant and $[A]$ is the concentration of the transition state. The activation energy required to complete this reaction is the difference between the free energy of the reactants and that of the transition state. Depending on the reaction, this free energy of activation may be very large. A large free energy of activation implies that relatively few of the reactants will have sufficient energy to overcome the barrier and (ultimately) become products. The free activation energy and the equilibrium constant (for the reactants and the intermediate) are related as follows:

$$\Delta G^I = -RT \ln K^I$$

This equation, combined with the equation for the overall reaction rate, shows that the rate can be affected by changing the activation energy of the system; the lower the activation energy, the quicker the reaction will proceed.

In biological systems, enzymes work to lower activation energies and therefore allow reactions to reach equilibrium more quickly. Reaction rates and enzyme activity alike depend on the temperature of the system. For reaction rates, the temperature affects K_{eq}, thereby establishing a new equilibrium. For optimal enzyme activity, only a certain range of temperatures is suitable. As the enzyme is heated, the enzyme denatures and the conformation of the active site is compromised.

1. Which of the following equations relates the rate of the reaction to the activation energy?

    A. $v[I]RT\ln K_{eq}$

    B. $v[I]e^{-(\Delta G^{\ddagger}/RT)}$

    C. $v[R]e^{(\Delta G^{\ddagger}/RT)}$

    D. $v[R]10^{-(\Delta G^{\ddagger}/2.3RT)}$

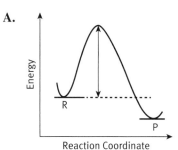

2. A scientist studying the kinetics of a two-substrate reaction observes rates for three trials in the ratio 4:1:16. In the second trial, the only change was a reduction in the concentration of A (by a factor of four) relative to the first trial. For the third trial, the concentration of A was unchanged from the second trial and the concentration of B was quadrupled. Which of the following best represents the rate law for this reaction?

    A. $k[A][B]$

    B. $k[A]^2[B]$

    C. $k[A][B]^2$

    D. $k[A]^2[B]^2$

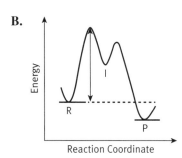

3. All of the following quantities do NOT change after the addition of the appropriate enzyme, EXCEPT:

    A. K_{eq}.

    B. $\Delta G^{\ddagger}$.

    C. V.

    D. ΔG°.

4. The interactions between an enzyme and the substrate typically involve multiple weak and reversible interactions. Which factor is the LEAST abundant between the substrate and enzyme?

    A. Van der Waals forces

    B. Hydrophobic effects

    C. Covalent bonding

    D. Hydrogen bonding

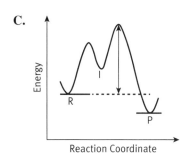

5. If the example reaction described in the passage is a multi-step exothermic process with a rate-limiting first step, which of the following could represent the energy profile for the reaction?

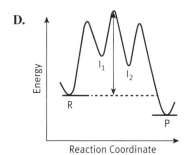

6. Suppose an enzyme is active only when a given carboxylic acid residue is in the carboxylate form. If the K_a of the acid is 4×10^{-5}, which of the following correctly matches the pH of the solution with the ratio of active to inactive enzymes?

    A. pH 5.0 and 1:1

    B. pH 4.4 and 10:1

    C. pH 4.0 and 1:1

    D. pH 3.4 and 1:10

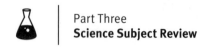

General Chemistry Practice Passage Explanations

1. (D)

The reaction velocity, or rate, is given as $V = v[A]$, which is the jumping-off point for this question. The passage gives K^I as the equilibrium constant for the transition between $[R]$ and $[A]$. By looking at the second equation in the passage, it can be seen that K^I and ΔG^I, the activation energy, are related. To get K^I and, subsequently, ΔG^I into the equation, solve for $[A]$ in terms of K^I. Because K^I is the equilibrium constant, its expression is governed by $K^I = \dfrac{[A]}{[R]}$, which can be rearranged to $[A] = [R]K^I$. Solving for K^I in terms of ΔG^I requires the rearrangement of $\Delta G^I = -RT\ln K^I$ to $\ln K^I = \dfrac{-\Delta G^I}{RT}$. Solving to get rid of the natural log gives $K^I = e^{-(\Delta G^I/RT)}$. Combining that equation with the earlier expression for the rate gives $ve^{-(\Delta G^I/RT)}$. However, this doesn't match any answers. One more step is then required to solve this. When solving for $\ln K^I = \dfrac{-\Delta G^I}{RT}$, one can multiply by a factor of 2.3 to change from natural log to log base 10, giving $2.3 \log K^I = \dfrac{-\Delta G^I}{RT}$, which yields (D), or $v[R]10^{-(\Delta G^I/RT)}$. Alternatively, use the process of elimination. (A) does

not relate the rate of the reaction to the activation energy. (B) implies $e^{-(\Delta G^I/RT)} = 1$ (to satisfy $v[A]e^{-(\Delta G^I/RT)} = v[A]$), which means the activation energy is always zero. So it cannot be correct. Finally, the passage states that the "lower the activation energy, the quicker the reaction." So (C) is eliminated because it shows a direct relationship between the two.

2. (C)

To determine the rate law of a reaction, each reactant's concentration is varied and the change in the rate of reaction is determined. From the first to the second trial, the concentration of A is decreased by a factor of 4 and the rate likewise decreases by a factor of 4. This indicates that the rate law is first order with respect to A. At this point, (B) and (D) can be eliminated as both show reactions that are second order with respect to A. In the third trial, the concentration of B is increased by a factor of 4; at the same time, the rate increases by a factor of 16. This indicates that the rate law is second order with respect to B. This matches (C) and eliminates (A).

3. (C)

Eliminate those answer choices that are not increased. (A) can be eliminated because enzymes do not alter the equilibrium constant; they just allow the reaction to reach equilibrium more quickly. From the passage, it can be seen that ΔG^I is lowered, so eliminate (B). Also, enzymes do not change the difference in free energy between the reactants and products, $\Delta G°$, just the free energy of activation—so (D) is eliminated. Enzymes increase the reaction rate, so V increases, meaning it's the exception to those that do not increase, which matches (C).

4. (C)

Stabilizing transition states in biological systems involves making sure unstable parts of the molecules, that is, atoms or regions that have charges that they don't want, have something to interact with to stabilize them. Although covalent bonds are made and broken as the reaction proceeds, holding the substrate in place in the active site and stabilizing it is the job of noncovalent forces. This means weak interactions are more abundant than those that actually bond. There are many more instances of the noncovalent forces because these are usually present in numerous places in an enzyme's active site to help stabilize. Covalent bonding (C) is the least prevalent.

5. (B)

The question stem states that this is a multi-step reaction but does not specify the exact number of steps. This eliminates **(A)** because it has too few steps. The next thing to consider is the question stem. It indicates that the first step of the reaction, the conversion of reactant to intermediate, is the rate-limiting step. This means that it is the slowest step and thus has the largest activation energy, which means that **(B)** is correct.

6. (D)

The pK_a is a function of the K_a, which describes the ratio of concentration of conjugate base to acid at equilibrium. Given the K_a, the pK_a can be estimated to be between 4 and 5, or approximately 4.5. At a certain pH, the actual ratio of conjugate base to acid is described by the Henderson-Hasselbalch equation. The equation

$$pH = pK_a + \log\left(\frac{[\text{conj. base}]}{[\text{acid}]}\right)$$ can be rearranged to yield

$\dfrac{[\text{conj. base}]}{[\text{acid}]} = 10^{pH-pK_a}$. So at a pH = pK_a (4.5), the

ratio of active to inactive is 1:1. This means we can

eliminate **(A)**, **(B)**, and **(C)**. According to the Henderson-Hasselbalch equation, at a pH one point below the pK_a (approximately 3.5), the ratio of active to inactive is 1:10, which matches **(D)**.

CHAPTER 12

Organic Chemistry

Organic chemistry has long been regarded as a significant hurdle to medical school, full of long hours in the lab and challenging synthesis pathways. Over the years, the AAMC has been placing less significance on organic chemistry and more emphasis on molecular biology, biochemistry, and genetics. On the MCAT, 5 percent of the questions in the Biological and Biochemical Foundations of Living Systems section and 15 percent of the questions in the Chemical and Physical Foundations of Biological Systems section are related to organic chemistry. Regardless of these changes, organic chemistry is still important to achieving a high score. Organic chemistry knowledge is required to evaluate chemical structures and predict the behavior of molecules within a biological system. You can expect the MCAT to test organic chemistry that is necessary for an understanding of biochemistry and reactions essential for an medical testing and pharmacology.

12.1 Reading the Passage

Passages related to organic chemistry may come in the form of a passage that is exclusively related to organic chemistry or a passage that covers multiple subject areas, especially biochemistry. There is a clear relationship between these two sciences; an understanding of organic chemistry structures and reactions is essential to understanding the behavior of biochemical systems. Therefore, success in organic chemistry on the MCAT depends on your ability to apply your knowledge of organic chemistry to biochemical systems.

PASSAGE TYPES

Organic chemistry passages are either information passages or experiment passages. (See Table 12.1.)

Information Passages
- Often short and accompanied by diagrams illustrating reactions or mechanisms.
- May be integrated with other subject areas, such as biochemistry or biology.
- May present a new reaction or a series of related reactions, or may describe a compound or an experimental technique.

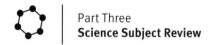

Experiment Passages

- Presentation of one or more experiments.
- Experimental data may be in the form of percentage yield from a synthesis, a written summary of the reaction, or a description of the appearance or the spectroscopic properties of a product.
- The product of a synthesis may then be used in a biochemistry experiment, meaning that the synthesis reaction and the biochemistry experiment go hand in hand.

	Information Passages	**Experiment Passages**
Content	Read like a textbook; may integrate concepts of organic chemistry and biochemistry.	Read like a lab report or a journal article that summarizes an experimental procedure. The product of an organic chemistry reaction may be the substrate for a biochemistry experiment.
Questions	Many questions do not require information from the passage. Those that do are likely to be more theoretical.	Often focus on the hypothesis, procedure, and outcome. If multiple experiments are described, questions are likely to focus on the relationships among the experiments.

Table 12.1. Organic Chemistry Passage Types

READING AND DISTILLING THE PASSAGE

Organic chemistry passages often feature synthesis pathways or molecular structures. In addition, the passage may be a mixture of organic chemistry and biochemistry rather than a pure organic chemistry passage. When approaching a passage, be sure to think about how the organic chemistry science applies to a living system, and look for the connections between the sciences presented in the passage.

- **Preview** for difficulty
  - Note the structure of the passage, the location of the paragraphs, and any figures such as charts, graphs, tables, or diagrams.
  - Determine whether the passage is an *experiment* or an *information* passage.
  - Determine the topic and the degree of difficulty.
  - Identify whether this passage requires a large time investment.
  - Decide whether this passage is one to do now or later.

- **Choose** your approach
  - Using information from the Preview step, Choose an appropriate Distill approach for the passage (Interrogate, Outline, or Highlight).
  - **Interrogation** should be chosen for experiment passages.
  - **Outlining** should be chosen for information passages that are dense or detail heavy.
  - **Highlighting** should be chosen for information passages that are light on details.

- **Read and Distill** key themes
  - While reading the passage, your aim is to distill the major takeaway of each paragraph and identify testable information using one of the following approaches.
  - **Interrogate**: Thoroughly examine the experimental passage by identifying the key components of experimental design and interrogating *why* specific procedures were done and *how* they connect to the overall purpose of the experiment.
  - **Outline**: Create a brief label for each paragraph that summarizes the contents of the paragraph, allowing you to return quickly to the passage when demanded by a question.
  - **Highlight**: Highlight one to three terms per paragraph that can pull your attention back to testable information when demanded by a question.

12.2 Answering the Questions

Questions that are exclusively related to organic chemistry are often very straightforward. However, questions that require integration of organic chemistry with another topic may be more difficult. Once again, the same question types seen in the other sciences apply.

- **Discrete questions**
  - Questions not associated with a descriptive passage.
  - Are preceded with a warning such as, "Questions 12–15 do not refer to a passage and are independent of each other."
  - Likely to test basic principles of organic chemistry, such as structures and reactions.

- **Questions that stand alone from the passage**
  - One of the most common organic chemistry questions types.
  - Often requires analysis of structures.
  - When evaluating structures, many of the wrong answer choices contain structures that are simply not possible given the basic concepts of organic chemistry.

- **Questions that require data from the passage**
  - Often require analysis of data or an experimental design.
  - Often require evaluation of a synthesis process with a different substrate, thus requiring the application of information from the passage to a new situation.

- **Questions that require the goal of the passage**
  - The nature of these questions depends on what else is in the passage.
  - If the passage is exclusively organic chemistry, the goal of the passage is likely to be the outcome of an experiment or a synthetic pathway.
  - If the passage contains organic chemistry integrated with biology or biochemistry, the goal of the passage depends on the content of the passage as a whole and the context in which organic chemistry is discussed.

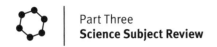
ATTACKING THE QUESTIONS

MCAT organic chemistry questions may be related only to organic chemistry or may be organic chemistry in the context of another subject area. In addition, language is often used to disguise simple organic chemistry questions as more difficult ones. Pay special attention to the task of the question to ensure that questions like these are discovered and answered correctly.

- **Type** the question
  - ○ Read the question; peek at the answer choices for patterns, but don't analyze closely.
  - ○ Assess the topic and the degree of difficulty.
  - ○ Identify the level of time involvement: is this question likely to take a tremendous amount of time to identify the answer? If so, skip it and come back after you do the other questions in the passage set.
  - ○ Good questions to do now in organic chemistry are those that stand alone from the passage because these are generally quick and easy points.

- **Rephrase** the question stem
  - ○ Rephrase the question, focusing on the task(s) to be accomplished.
  - ○ Simplify the phrasing of the original question stem.
  - ○ Translate the question into a specific set of tasks to be accomplished using the passage and your background knowledge.

- **Investigate** potential solutions
  - ○ Complete the task(s) identified in your Rephrase step.
  - ○ Analyze the data; evaluate the experimental design; locate the information required; and connect the information, data, and experimental design with the information you already know.
  - ○ Predict what you can about the answer.
  - ○ Be flexible if your initial approach fails.

- **Match** your prediction to an answer choice
  - ○ Search the answer choices for a response that is synonymous with your prediction, or eliminate answers that are not correct.
  - ○ Select an answer and move on.
  - ○ If you cannot find a match to your prediction, eliminate wrong answers, select a response from the remaining choices, and move on.

12.3   Getting the Edge in Organic Chemistry

With the addition of biochemistry to the MCAT, many organic chemistry questions require integration with concepts of biochemistry and biology. In this context, expect questions that assess your understanding of the implications of organic chemistry in biochemistry and biology. Simpler organic chemistry questions are likely to be disguised as more complicated ones. Using the task of the question, paraphrase these questions in a simpler form. Doing so will help you identify these questions and determine the correct answer. Many test takers become overwhelmed by these questions, whereas a critical thinker who rephrases questions sees the simpler question and answers it correctly.

Organic chemistry questions often contain structures as answer choices. Many wrong answer choices among these questions are structures that are not possible given the basic fundamentals of organic chemistry. Applying the basic fundamentals of organic chemistry to these answer choices can allow for quick elimination of wrong answer choices.

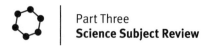
12.4 Preparing for the MCAT: Organic Chemistry

The following presents the organic chemistry content you are likely to see on Test Day. Organic chemistry is the least commonly tested topic on the MCAT. The High-Yield badges will direct you to the specific organic chemistry topics that are tested most frequently.

NOMENCLATURE

The **International Union of Pure and Applied Chemistry (IUPAC)** has designated five steps for naming chemical compounds. First, find the longest carbon chain in the compound that contains the highest-priority functional group (see Figure 12.1). This is called the **parent chain**.

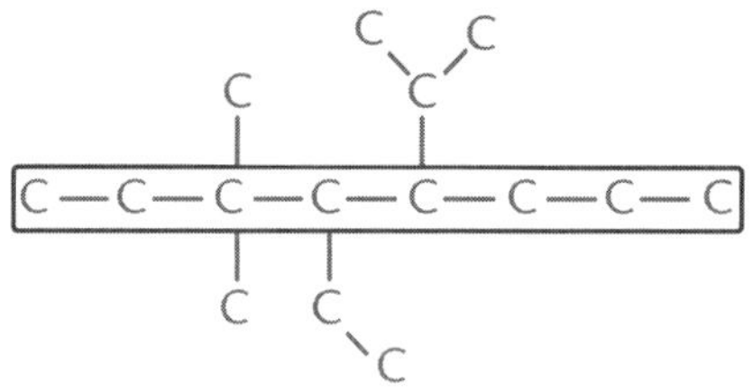

Figure 12.1. Finding the Longest Carbon Chain

Second, number the chain in such a way that the highest-priority functional group receives the lowest possible number (see Figure 12.2). This group determines the **suffix** of the molecule.

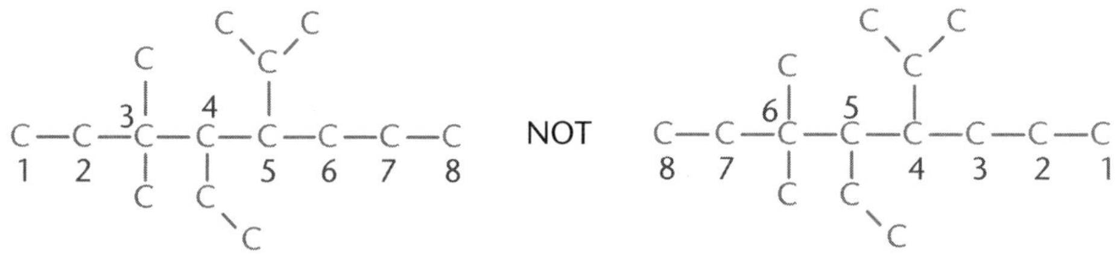

Figure 12.2. Numbering the Longest Carbon Chain

Third, name the **substituents** with a **prefix** (see Figure 12.3). Multiple substituents of a single type receive another prefix denoting how many are present (*di–*, *tri–*, *tetra–*, and so on).

$$CH_3- \qquad CH_3CH_2- \qquad CH_3CH_2CH_2-$$
$$\text{methyl} \qquad \text{ethyl} \qquad \textit{n}\text{-propyl}$$

Figure 12.3. Common Alkyl Substituents

Fourth, assign a number to each of the substituents depending on the carbon to which it is bonded. Finally, complete the name by alphabetizing the substituents and separating numbers from each other by commas and from words by hyphens.

Alkanes are **hydrocarbons** without any double or triple bonds. They have the general formula $C_nH_{(2n+2)}$ and are named according to the number of carbons present followed by the suffix *–ane*. The first four alkanes are methane (CH_4), ethane (C_2H_6), propane (C_3H_8), and butane (C_4H_{10}). Larger alkanes use the Greek root for the number (pentane, hexane, heptane, octane, and so on).

Alkenes and **alkynes** contain double and triple bonds, respectively. Alkenes are named by substituting *–ene* for the suffix and numbering the double bond by its lowest-numbered carbon. Alkynes substitute *–yne* with the same numbering.

Alcohols contain a hydroxyl (–OH) group, which substitutes for one or more of the hydrogens in the hydrocarbon chain. Alcohols are named by substituting the suffix *–ol* or by using the prefix *hydroxy–* if a higher-priority group is present. Alcohols have higher priority than double or triple bonds and alkanes. **Diols** contain two hydroxyl groups.

Aldehydes and ketones contain a **carbonyl group**—which is a carbon double bonded to an oxygen. **Aldehydes** have the carbonyl group on a terminal carbon that is also attached to a hydrogen atom. They are named with the suffix *–al* or by using the prefix *oxo–* if a higher-priority group is present. **Ketones** have the carbonyl group on a nonterminal carbon and are named with the suffix *–one* and share the prefix *oxo–* if a higher-priority group is present. Ketones can also be indicated by the prefix *keto–*. Acetone is significant as the smallest ketone. Its IUPAC name is propanone. Carbonyl-containing compounds (aldehydes, ketones, carboxylic acids, and derivatives) also create a lettering scheme for carbons. The carbon adjacent to the carbonyl carbon is the α-**carbon**.

Carboxylic acids are the highest-priority functional group because they contain three bonds to oxygen: one from a hydroxyl group and two from a carbonyl group. Carboxylic acids are always terminal, although their **derivatives** may occur within a molecule. They are named with the suffix *–oic acid* and are very rarely named with a prefix.

Esters are carboxylic acid derivatives where –OH is replaced with –OR, which is an **alkoxy group**. Esters use the suffix *–oate* or the prefix *alkoxycarbonyl–*. **Amides** replace the hydroxyl group of a carboxylic acid with an amino group that may or may not be substituted. Amides use the suffix *–amide* or the prefix *carbamoyl–* or *amido–*. Substituents attached to the amide nitrogen are designated with a capital *N–*.

Anhydrides are formed from two carboxylic acids by dehydration. They may be symmetric (two of the same acid), asymmetric (two different acids), or cyclic (intramolecular reaction of a dicarboxylic acid). Anhydrides are named using the suffix *anhydride* in place of *acid*. If the anhydride is formed from more than one carboxylic acid, both are named in alphabetical order in the name before the word *anhydride*.

Table 12.2 lists the functional groups that you will need to know for the MCAT in order of priority, with prefixes and suffixes. Carboxylic acids are the highest-priority functional group on the MCAT. In nomenclature, use the suffix if the functional group is the highest-priority group in the molecule; otherwise, name the group as a substituent using its prefix.

Functional Group	Prefix	Suffix
Carboxylic acid	*carboxy–*	*–oic acid*
Anhydride	*alkanoyloxycarbonyl–*	*anhydride*
Ester	*alkoxycarbonyl–*	*–oate*
Amide	*carbamoyl–* or *amido–*	*–amide*
Aldehyde	*oxo–*	*–al*
Ketone	*oxo–* or *keto–*	*–one*
Alcohol	*hydroxy–*	*–ol*
Alkene*	*alkenyl–*	*–ene*
Alkyne*	*alkynyl–*	*–yne*
Alkane	*alkyl–*	*–ane*
* Note: Alkenes and alkynes are considered to be tied for priority except in cyclic compounds, where alkenes have higher priority.		

Table 12.2. Functional Groups Listed in Order of Priority

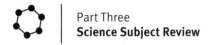
ISOMERS

High-Yield

Structural isomers share a molecular formula but have different physical and chemical properties.

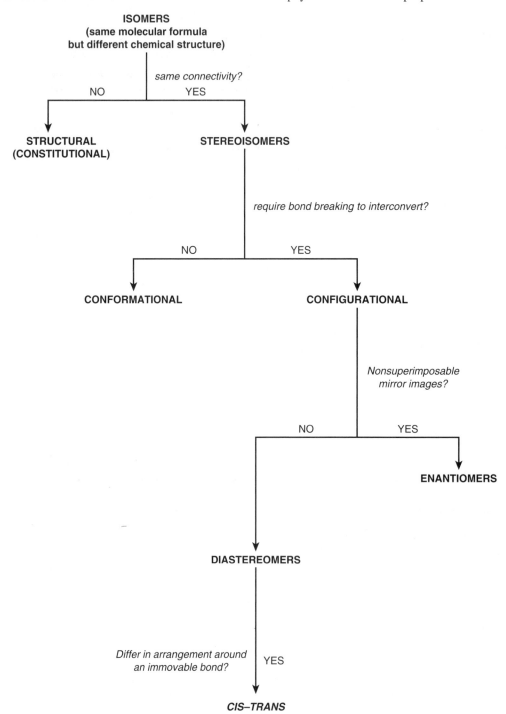

Figure 12.4. Flowchart of Isomer Relationships

Conformational isomers differ by rotation around a single (σ) bond (see Figure 12.5). **Staggered conformations** have groups 60° apart, as seen in a **Newman projection**. In *anti* **staggered** molecules, the two largest groups are 180° apart and strain is minimized. In *gauche* **staggered** molecules, the two largest groups are 60° apart. **Eclipsed conformations** have groups directly in front of each other as seen in a Newman projection. In **totally eclipsed conformations**, the two largest groups are directly in front of each other and strain is maximized.

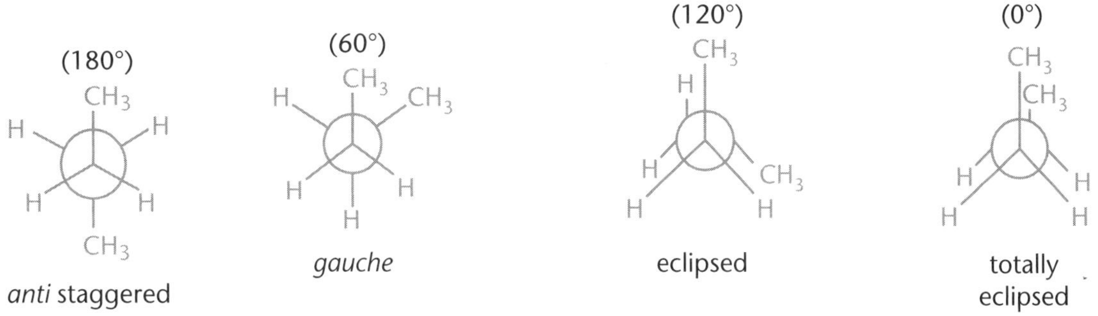

Figure 12.5. Conformational Isomers

The strain in cyclic molecules comes from **angle strain** (created by stretching or compressing angles from their normal size), **torsional strain** (from eclipsing conformations), and **nonbonded strain** (from interactions between substituents attached to nonadjacent carbons). Cyclic molecules usually adopt nonplanar shapes to minimize this strain. Substituents attached to cyclohexane can be classified as **axial** (sticking up or down from the plane of the molecule) or **equatorial** (in the plane of the molecule), as shown in Figure 12.6. Axial substituents create more nonbonded strain. In cyclohexane molecules with multiple substituents, the largest substituent usually takes the equatorial position to minimize strain.

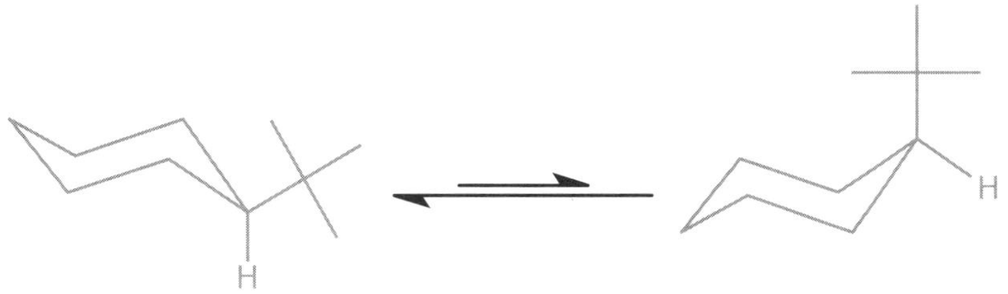

Figure 12.6. Axial and Equatorial Positions in Cyclohexane

Configurational isomers can be interchanged only by breaking and reforming bonds. **Enantiomers** are nonsuperimposable mirror images and thus have opposite stereochemistry at every chiral carbon. They have the same chemical and physical properties except for rotation of plane-polarized light and for reactions in a chiral environment. **Diastereomers** are non-mirror-image stereoisomers. They differ at some, but not all, chiral centers and have different chemical and physical properties. The *cis–trans* isomers are a subtype of diastereomers in which groups differ in position about an immovable bond (such as a double bond or in a cycloalkane). **Chiral centers** have four different groups attached to the central carbon.

Optical activity refers to the ability of a molecule to rotate plane-polarized light: D- or (+) molecules rotate light to the right, and L- or (−) molecules rotate light to the left. **Racemic mixtures**, with equal concentrations of two enantiomers, are not optically active because the two enantiomers' rotations cancel out each other. *Meso* **compounds**, with an internal plane of symmetry, are also optically inactive because the two sides of the molecule cancel out each other.

Relative configuration gives the stereochemistry of a compound in comparison to another molecule, while **absolute configuration** gives the stereochemistry without having to compare to other molecules. Absolute configuration uses the **Cahn-Ingold-Prelog priority rules** in which priority is given by looking at the atoms connected to the chiral carbon or double-bonded carbons; whichever has the highest atomic number gets highest priority. If there is a tie, one moves outward from the chiral carbon or double-bonded carbon until the tie breaks.

An alkene is **Z–** if the highest-priority substituents are on the same side of the double bond and is **E–** if the highest-priority substituents are on opposite sides of the double bond. A stereocenter's configuration is determined by putting the lowest-priority group in the back and drawing a circle from group 1 to 2 to 3 in descending priority. If this circle is clockwise, the stereocenter is **R**; if it is counterclockwise, the stereocenter is **S.**

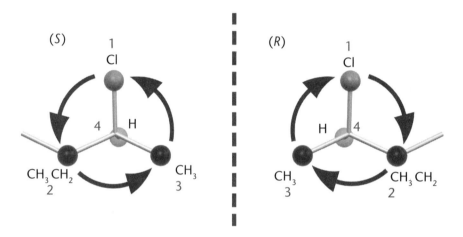

Figure 12.7. Determining Absolute Configuration
Drawing a circle to determine absolute configuration counterclockwise = (S); clockwise = (R)

Vertical lines in **Fischer diagrams** go into the plane of the page (dashes); horizontal lines come out of the plane of the page (wedges). Switching one pair of substituents in a Fischer diagram inverts the stereochemistry of the chiral center. Switching two pairs retains the stereochemistry. Rotating a Fischer diagram 90° inverts the stereochemistry of the chiral center. Rotating 180° retains the stereochemistry. (See Figure 12.8.)

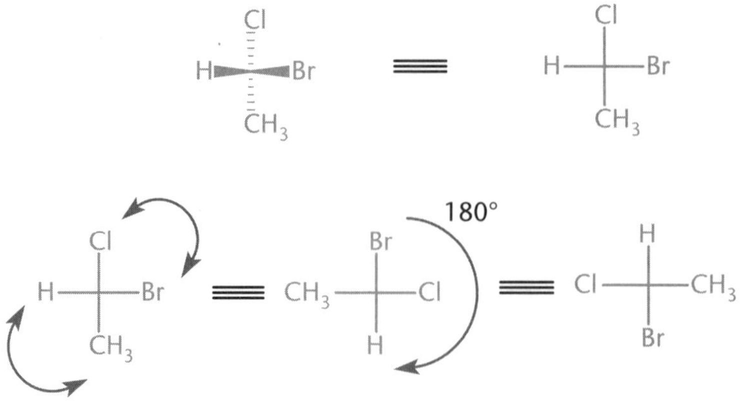

Figure 12.8. Manipulations of Fischer Projections

ORBITALS AND HYBRIDIZATION

Bonding

Quantum numbers describe the size, shape, orientation, and number of **atomic orbitals** an element possesses.

- The **principal quantum number**, n, describes the energy level (shell) in which an electron resides and indicates the distance from the nucleus to the electron. Its possible values range from 1 to ∞.
- The **azimuthal quantum number**, l, determines the subshell in which an electron resides. Its possible values range from 0 to $n - 1$. The subshell is often indicated with a letter: $l = 0$ corresponds to s, 1 is p, 2 is d, and 3 is f.
- The **magnetic quantum number**, m_l, determines the orbital in which an electron resides. Its possible values range from $-l$ to $+l$. Different orbitals have different shapes: s-orbitals are spherical, while p-orbitals are dumbbell shaped and are located on the x-, y-, or z-axis.
- The **spin quantum number**, m_s, describes the spin of an electron. Its possible values are $\pm \dfrac{1}{2}$.

Molecular orbitals are either bonding or antibonding, as shown in Figure 12.9. **Bonding orbitals** are created by head-to-head or tail-to-tail overlap of atomic orbitals of the same sign and are energetically favorable. **Antibonding orbitals** are created by head-to-head or tail-to-tail overlap of atomic orbitals that have opposite signs and are energetically unfavorable.

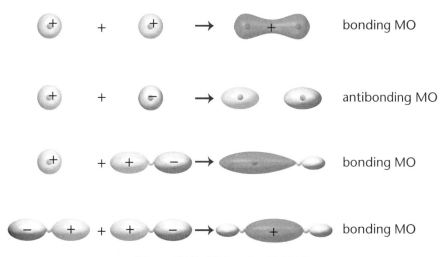

Figure 12.9. Molecular Orbitals

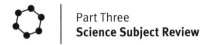

Single bonds are **sigma** (σ) **bonds**, which contain two electrons. **Double bonds** contain one σ bond and one **pi** (π) **bond** (see Figure 12.10). The π bonds are created by the sharing of electrons between two unhybridized p-orbitals that align side by side. **Triple bonds** contain one σ bond and two π bonds. Multiple bonds are less flexible than single bonds because rotation is not permitted in the presence of a π bond. Multiple bonds are shorter and stronger than single bonds, although individual π bonds are weaker than σ bonds.

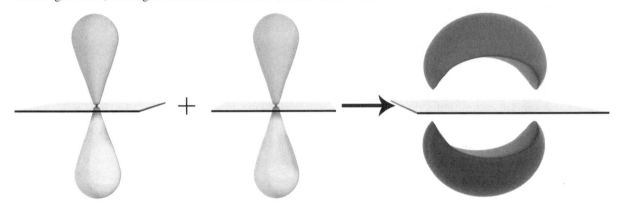

Figure 12.10. Pi (π) Bond

Hybridization

sp^3-hybridized orbitals have 25 percent s character and 75 percent p character. They form tetrahedral geometry with 109.5° bond angles. Carbons with all single bonds are sp^3 hybridized. sp^2-hybridized orbitals have 33 percent s character and 67 percent p character. They form trigonal planar geometry with 120° bond angles. Carbons with one double bond are sp^2 hybridized. sp-hybridized orbitals have 50 percent s character and 50 percent p character. They form linear geometry with 180° bond angles. Carbons with a triple bond, or with two double bonds, are sp hybridized.

Resonance describes the delocalization of electrons in molecules that have conjugated bonds (see Figure 12.11). **Conjugation** occurs when single and multiple bonds alternate, creating a system of unhybridized p-orbitals down the backbone of the molecule through which π electrons can delocalize. Resonance increases the stability of a molecule. The various resonance forms all contribute to the true electron density of the molecule; the more stable the resonance form, the more it contributes to true electron density. Resonance forms are favored if they lack formal charge, form full octets on electronegative atoms, or stabilize charges through induction and aromaticity.

Figure 12.11. Resonance Structure of Ozone

ANALYZING ORGANIC REACTIONS

Lewis acids are electron acceptors; they have vacant orbitals or positively polarized atoms. **Lewis bases** are electron donors; they have a lone pair of electrons and are often anions. **Brønsted-Lowry acids** are proton donors; **Brønsted-Lowry bases** are proton acceptors. **Amphoteric molecules** can act as either acids or bases, depending on reaction conditions. Water is a common example of an amphoteric molecule.

The **acid dissociation constant**, K_a, is a measure of acidity. It is the equilibrium constant corresponding to the dissociation of an acid, HA, into a proton (H^+) and its conjugate base (A^-).

The **pK_a** is the negative logarithm of K_a. A lower (or even negative) pK_a indicates a stronger acid. The pK_a decreases down the periodic table and increases with electronegativity.

Alcohols, aldehydes, ketones, carboxylic acids, and carboxylic acid derivatives are common acidic functional groups. The **α-hydrogens** (hydrogens connected to an **α-carbon**, which is a carbon adjacent to a carbonyl) are acidic. Amines and amides are common basic functional groups.

Nucleophiles are "nucleus loving" and contain lone pairs or π bonds. They have increased electron density and often carry a negative charge. Nucleophilicity is similar to basicity. However, nucleophilicity is a kinetic property, while basicity is thermodynamic. Charge, electronegativity, steric hindrance, and the solvent can all affect nucleophilicity. Amino groups are common organic nucleophiles.

Electrophiles are "electron loving" and either contain a positive charge or are positively polarized. More positive compounds are more electrophilic. Alcohols, aldehydes, ketones, carboxylic acids, and their derivatives can act as electrophiles.

Leaving groups are the molecular fragments that retain the electrons after **heterolysis**. The best leaving groups can stabilize additional charge through resonance or induction. Weak bases (the conjugate bases of strong acids) make good leaving groups. Alkanes and hydrogen ions are almost never leaving groups because they form reactive anions.

Unimolecular nucleophilic substitution (S_N1) reactions proceed in two steps (see Figure 12.12). In the first step, the leaving group leaves, forming a **carbocation**, which is an ion with a positively charged carbon atom. In the second step, the nucleophile attacks the planar carbocation from either side, leading to a racemic mixture of products. S_N1 reactions prefer more substituted carbons because the alkyl groups can donate electron density and stabilize the positive charge of the carbocation. The rate of an S_N1 reaction is dependent on only the concentration of the substrate: rate $= k[R - L]$, where L is the leaving group and R is the rest of the molecule.

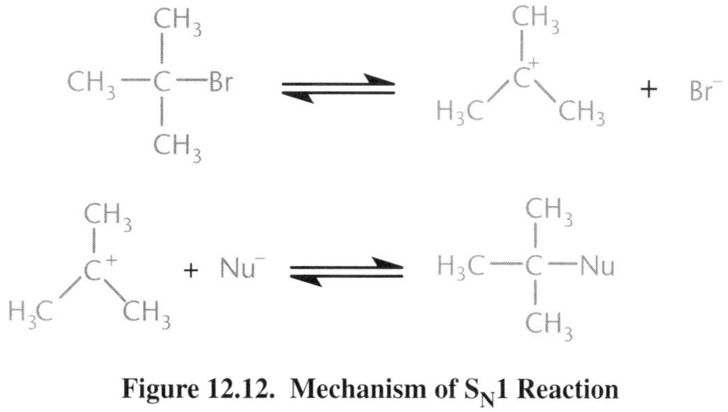

Figure 12.12. Mechanism of S_N1 Reaction

Bimolecular nucleophilic substitution (S_N2) reactions proceed in one concerted step (see Figure 12.13). The nucleophile attacks at the same time as the leaving group leaves. The nucleophile must perform a **backside attack**, which leads to an inversion of stereochemistry. The absolute configuration is changed—from R to S and vice versa—if the incoming nucleophile and the leaving group have the same priority in the molecule. S_N2 reactions prefer less-substituted carbons because the alkyl groups create steric hindrance and inhibit the nucleophile from accessing the electrophilic substrate carbon. The rate of an S_N2 reaction is dependent on the concentrations of both the substrate and the nucleophile: rate $= k[Nu:][R - L]$, where Nu: is the nucleophile, L is the leaving group, and R is the rest of the molecule.

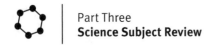
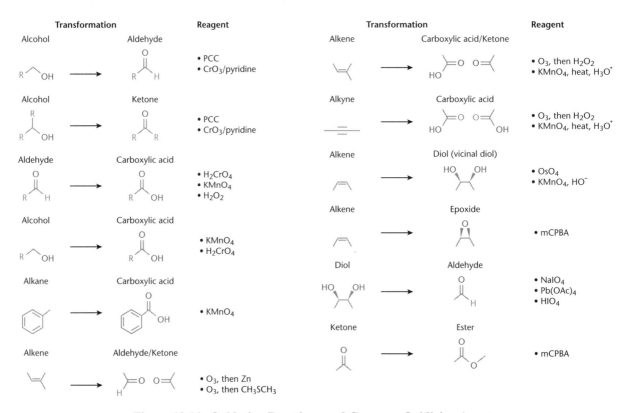

Figure 12.13. Mechanism of S$_N$2 Reaction

The **oxidation state** of an atom is the charge it would have if all its bonds were completely ionic. CH_4 is the lowest oxidation state of carbon (most reduced); CO_2 is the highest (most oxidized). Carboxylic acids and carboxylic acid derivatives are the most oxidized functional groups; followed by aldehydes, ketones, and imines; followed by alcohols, alkyl halides, and amines.

Oxidation is an increase in oxidation state and is assisted by oxidizing agents. **Oxidizing agents** accept electrons and are reduced in the process. (See Figure 12.14.) They have a high affinity for electrons or an unusually high oxidation state. They often contain a metal and a large number of oxygens.

Figure 12.14. Oxidation Reactions and Common Oxidizing Agents

Reduction is a decrease in oxidation state and is assisted by reducing agents. **Reducing agents** donate electrons and are oxidized in the process. They have low electronegativity and ionization energy. They often contain a metal and a large number of hydrides. Aldehydes, ketones, and carboxylic acids can be reduced to alcohols, amides to amines, and esters to a pair of alcohols by lithium aluminum hydride ($LiAlH_4$).

Both nucleophile-electrophile and oxidation-reduction reactions tend to act at the highest-priority (most oxidized) functional group. One can make use of steric hindrance properties to selectively target functional groups that might not primarily react or to protect functional groups. Diols are often used as protecting groups for aldehyde or ketone carbonyls.

ALCOHOLS

Alcohols have the general form ROH and are named with the suffix *–ol*. If they are not the highest priority, they are given the prefix *hydroxy–*. **Phenols** are benzene rings with hydroxyl groups (see Figure 12.15). They are named for the relative positions of the hydroxyl groups: *ortho–* or *o–* (adjacent carbons), *meta–* or *m–* (separated by one carbon), or *para–* or *p–* (on opposite sides of the ring).

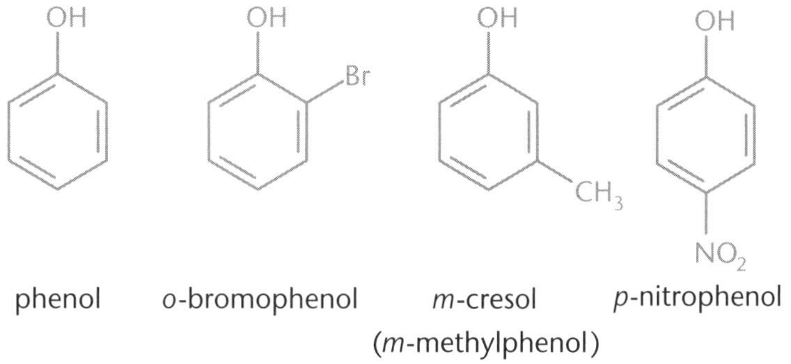

Figure 12.15. Phenols: Aromatic Alcohols

Alcohols can hydrogen bond, thereby raising their boiling and melting points relative to the corresponding alkanes. Hydrogen bonding also increases the solubility of alcohols. Phenols are more acidic than other alcohols because the aromatic ring can delocalize the charge of the conjugate base. Electron-donating groups like alkyl groups decrease acidity because they destabilize negative charges. Electron-withdrawing groups, such as electronegative atoms and aromatic rings, increase acidity because they stabilize negative charges.

Alcohols can be converted to mesylates or tosylates to make them better leaving groups for nucleophilic substitution reactions (see Figure 12.16). **Mesylates** contain the functional group $-SO_3CH_3$, and **tosylates** contain the functional group $-SO_3C_6H_4CH_3$.

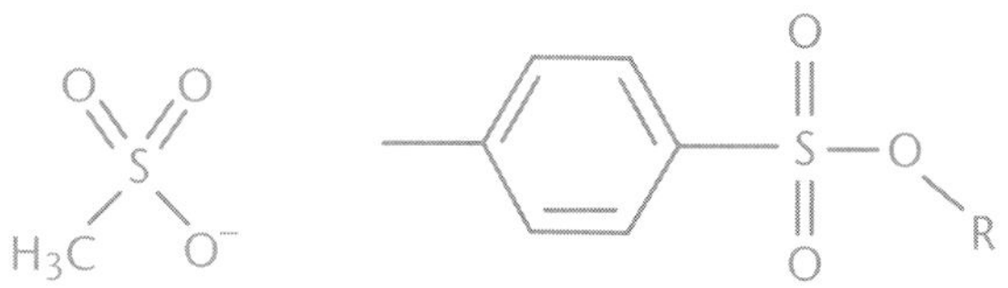

Figure 12.16. Mesylate and Tosylate Ions

Aldehydes or ketones can be protected by converting them into acetals or ketals. Two equivalents of alcohol or a dialcohol are reacted with the carbonyl to form an **acetal** (a primary carbon with two –OR groups and a hydrogen atom) or a **ketal** (a secondary carbon with two –OR groups). Other functional groups in the compound can be reacted (especially by reduction) without effects on the newly formed acetal or ketal. The acetal or ketal can then be converted back to a carbonyl by catalytic acid, which is called **deprotection**.

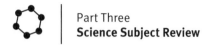

Quinones are resonance-stabilized electrophiles synthesized through oxidation of phenols (see Figure 12.17). **Hydroxyquinones** are produced by oxidation of quinones, which adds a variable number of hydroxyl groups.

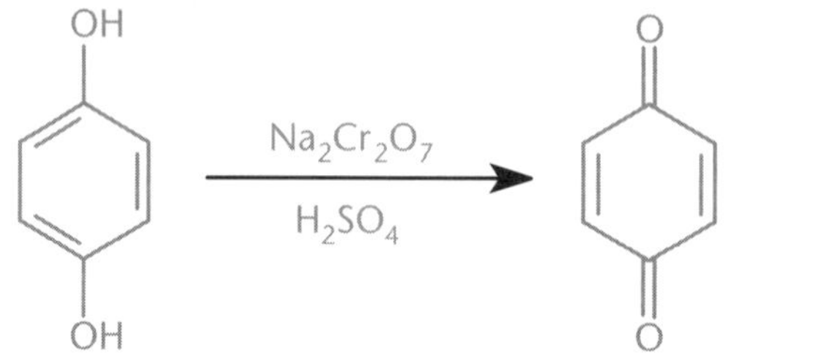

p-benzenediol   1,4-benzoquinone

Figure 12.17. Oxidation of *p*-Benzenediol to a Quinone

ALDEHYDES AND KETONES

Aldehydes are terminal functional groups containing a carbonyl bonded to at least one hydrogen. In nomenclature, they use the suffix *–al* and the prefix *oxo–*. In rings, they are indicated by the suffix *–carbaldehyde*. **Ketones** are internal functional groups containing a carbonyl bonded to two alkyl chains. In nomenclature, they use the suffix *–one* and the prefix *oxo–* or *keto–*.

The reactivity of a **carbonyl** (C=O) is dictated by the polarity of the double bond. The carbon has a partial positive charge and is therefore electrophilic. Carbonyl-containing compounds have higher boiling points than their equivalent alkanes because of dipole interactions. Alcohols have higher boiling points than carbonyls because of hydrogen bonding.

Aldehydes and ketones are commonly produced by oxidation of primary and secondary alcohols, respectively. Weaker, anhydrous oxidizing agents like **pyridinium chlorochromate** (**PCC**) must be used for synthesizing aldehydes or the reaction will continue oxidizing to the level of the carboxylic acid. Various oxidizing agents can be used for ketones, such as dichromate, chromium trioxide, or PCC because ketones are the most oxidized functional group for secondary carbons.

When a nucleophile attacks and forms a bond with a carbonyl carbon, electrons in the π bond are pushed to the oxygen atom. If there is no good leaving group (aldehydes and ketones), the carbonyl remains open and is protonated to form an alcohol (see Figure 12.18). However, if there is a good leaving group (carboxylic acids and derivatives), the carbonyl reforms and kicks off the leaving group.

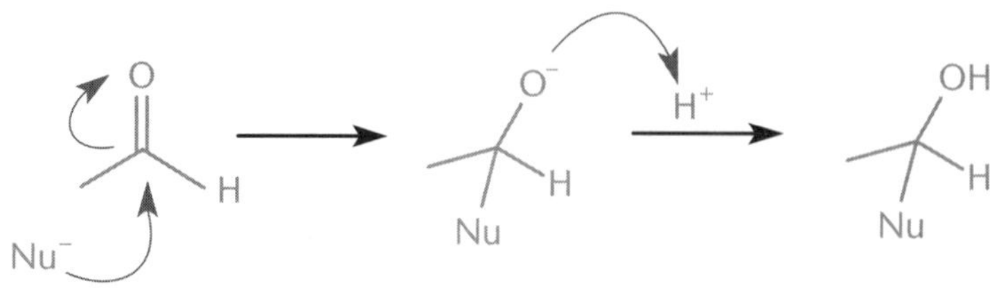

Figure 12.18. Nucleophilic Addition Reaction Mechanism

In **hydration** reactions, water adds to a carbonyl, forming a **geminal diol**. When one equivalent of alcohol reacts with an aldehyde (via nucleophilic addition), a **hemiacetal** is formed. When the same reaction occurs with a ketone, a **hemiketal** is formed. When another equivalent of alcohol reacts with a hemiacetal (via nucleophilic substitution), an **acetal** is formed. When the same reaction occurs with a **hemiketal**, a ketal is formed.

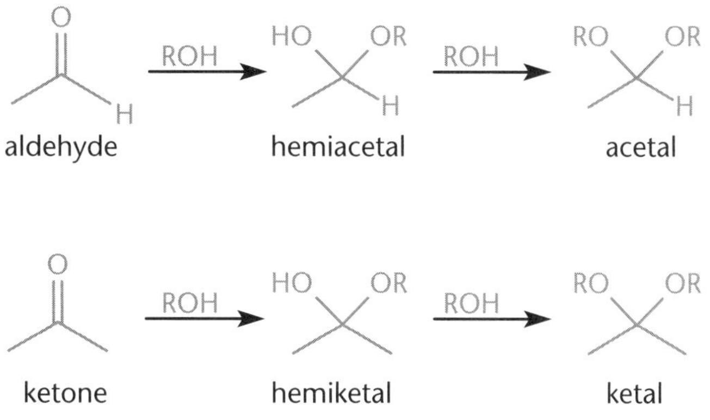

Figure 12.19. Acetal and Ketal Formation

Nitrogen and nitrogen derivatives react with carbonyls to form **imines**, oximes, hydrazones, and semicarbazones. Imines can tautomerize to form **enamines**. Hydrogen cyanide reacts with carbonyls to form **cyanohydrins**.

KEY CONCEPT

Ketones cannot be further oxidized but can be reduced to secondary alcohols using hydride reagents.

Aldehydes can be oxidized to carboxylic acids using an oxidizing agent like $KMnO_4$, CrO_3, Ag_2O, or H_2O_2. They can be reduced to primary alcohols via **hydride reagents** ($LiAlH_4$, $NaBH_4$).

The carbon adjacent to the carbonyl carbon is termed an **α-carbon**; the hydrogens attached to the α-carbon are called **α-hydrogens**. The α-hydrogens are relatively acidic and can be removed by a strong base (see Figure 12.20). The electron-withdrawing oxygen of the carbonyl weakens the C–H bonds on α-carbons. The **enolate** resulting from deprotonation can be stabilized by resonance with the carbonyl.

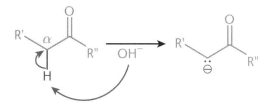

Figure 12.20. Deprotonation of an α-Carbon, Forming a Carbanion

Ketones are less reactive toward nucleophiles because of steric hindrance and α-carbanion destabilization. The presence of an additional alkyl group crowds the transition step and increases its energy. The alkyl group also donates electron density to the carbanion, making the carbanion less stable.

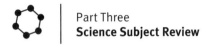

Aldehydes and ketones exist in the traditional **keto form** (C=O) and in the less common **enol form** (*ene + ol =* double bond + hydroxyl group). **Tautomers** are isomers that can be interconverted by moving a hydrogen and a double bond. The keto and enol forms are tautomers of each other (see Figure 12.21). The enol form can be deprotonated to form an **enolate**. Enolates are good nucleophiles.

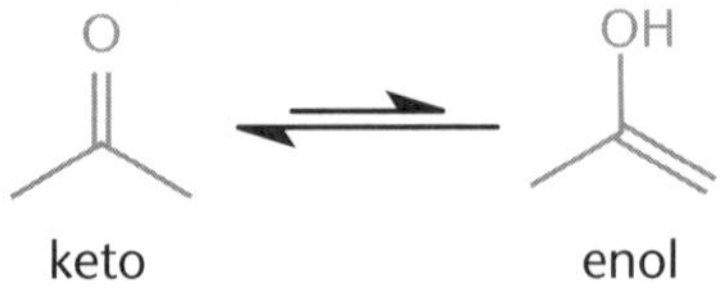

keto   enol

Figure 12.21. Enolization (Tautomerization)

In the **Michael addition**, an enolate attacks an α,β-unsaturated carbonyl, thereby creating a bond. The **kinetic enolate** is favored by fast, irreversible reactions at lower temperatures with strong, sterically hindered bases. The **thermodynamic enolate** is favored by slower, reversible reactions at higher temperatures with weaker, smaller bases. **Enamines** are tautomers of imines. Like enols, enamines are the less common tautomer.

In **aldol condensation**, the aldehyde or ketone acts as both nucleophile and electrophile, resulting in the formation of a carbon–carbon bond in a new molecule called an aldol. An **aldol** contains both aldehyde and alcohol functional groups. The nucleophile is the enolate formed from the deprotonation of the α-carbon, and the electrophile is the aldehyde or ketone in the form of the keto tautomer. First, a **condensation reaction** occurs in which the two molecules come together. After the aldol is formed, a **dehydration reaction** (loss of a water molecule) occurs, resulting in an α,β-unsaturated carbonyl.

Retro-aldol reactions are the reverse of aldol condensations. In these reactions, the bond between an α-carbon and a β-carbon is cleaved. These reactions are catalyzed by heat and a base.

CARBOXYLIC ACIDS

Carboxylic acids contain a carbonyl and a hydroxyl group connected to the same carbon. They are always terminal groups. They are indicated with the suffix *–oic acid*. Salts are named with the suffix *–oate*, and **dicarboxylic acids** are *–dioic acids*.

Carboxylic acids are polar and hydrogen bond very well, resulting in high boiling points. They often exist as **dimers** in solution. The acidity of a carboxylic acid is enhanced by the resonance between its oxygen atoms (see Figure 12.22). Acidity can be further enhanced by substituents that are electron withdrawing and can be further decreased by substituents that are electron donating.

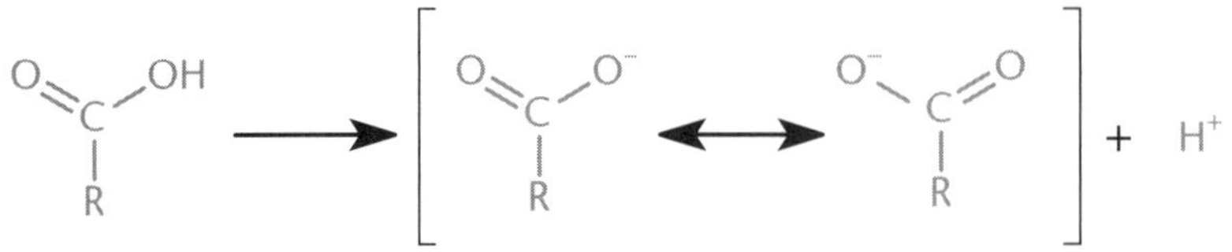

Figure 12.22. Carboxylate Anion Stability

Nucleophilic acyl substitution is a common reaction in carboxylic acids. A nucleophile attacks the electrophilic carbonyl carbon, opening the carbonyl and forming a tetrahedral intermediate. The carbonyl reforms, kicking off the leaving group.

- If the nucleophile is ammonia or an amine, an **amide** is formed. Amides are given the suffix *–amide*. Cyclic amides are called **lactams.**
- If the nucleophile is an alcohol, an **ester** is formed. Esters are given the suffix *–oate*. Cyclic esters are called **lactones.**
- If the nucleophile is another carboxylic acid, an **anhydride** is formed. Both linear and cyclic anhydrides are given the suffix *anhydride.*

Carboxylic acids can be reduced to a primary alcohol with a strong reducing agent like lithium aluminum hydride ($LiAlH_4$). Aldehyde intermediates are formed but are also reduced to primary alcohols. Sodium borohydride ($NaBH_4$) is a common reducing agent for other organic reactions but is not strong enough to reduce a carboxylic acid.

Mixing long-chain carboxylic acids (fatty acids) with a strong base results in the formation of a salt we call **soap**. This process is called **saponification.** Soaps contain hydrophilic carboxylate heads and hydrophobic alkyl chain tails. Soaps organize in hydrophilic environments to form **micelles.** A micelle dissolves nonpolar organic molecules in its interior and can be solvated with water due to its exterior shell of hydrophilic groups.

CARBOXYLIC ACID DERIVATIVES

Amides are the condensation products of carboxylic acids and ammonia or amines. They are given the suffix *–amide*. The alkyl groups on a substituted amide are written at the beginning of the name with the prefix *N–*. Cyclic amides are called **lactams.**

Esters are the condensation products of carboxylic acids with alcohols. This is called **Fischer esterification**, as seen in Figure 12.23. Esters are given the suffix *–oate*. The **esterifying group** is written as a substituent, without a number. Cyclic esters are called **lactones.**

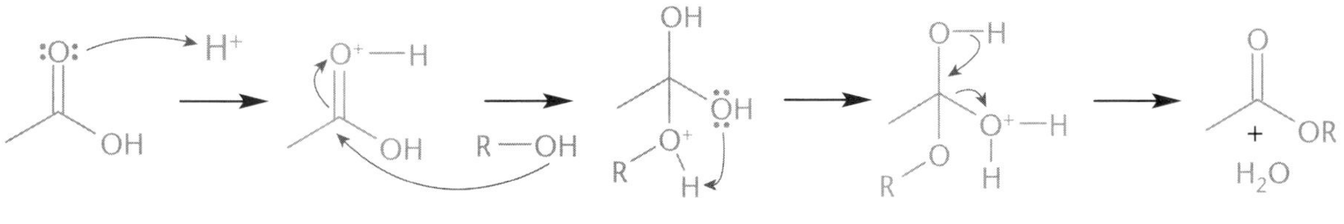

Figure 12.23. Fischer Esterification

Triacylglycerols, which are a form of fat storage, include three ester bonds between glycerol and fatty acids. **Saponification** is the breakdown of fat using a strong base to form **soap** (salts of long-chain carboxylic acids).

Anhydrides are the condensation dimers of carboxylic acids (see Figure 12.24). Symmetric anhydrides are named for the parent carboxylic acid, followed by *anhydride.* Asymmetric anhydrides are named by listing the parent carboxylic acids alphabetically, followed by *anhydride.* Some cyclic anhydrides can be synthesized by heating dioic acids. Five- or six-membered rings are generally stable.

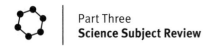

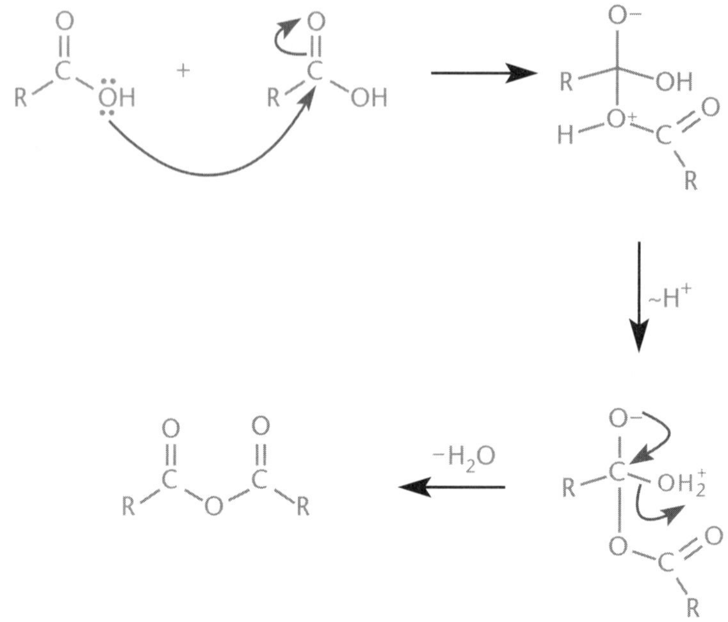

Figure 12.24. Synthesis of an Anhydride via Carboxylic Acid Condensation

In nucleophilic substitution reactions, anhydrides are more reactive than esters, which are more reactive than amides. **Steric hindrance** describes when a reaction cannot proceed (or significantly slows) because of substituents crowding the reactive site. **Protecting groups**, such as acetals, can be used to increase steric hindrance or otherwise decrease the reactivity of a particular portion of a molecule.

Induction refers to an uneven distribution of charge across a σ bond because of differences in electronegativity. The more electronegative groups in a carbonyl-containing compound, the greater the compound's reactivity. **Conjugation** refers to the presence of alternating single and multiple bonds, which creates delocalized π electron clouds above and below the plane of the molecule. (See Figure 12.25.) Electrons experience **resonance** through the unhybridized *p*-orbitals, increasing stability. Conjugated carbonyl-containing compounds are more reactive because they can stabilize their transition states.

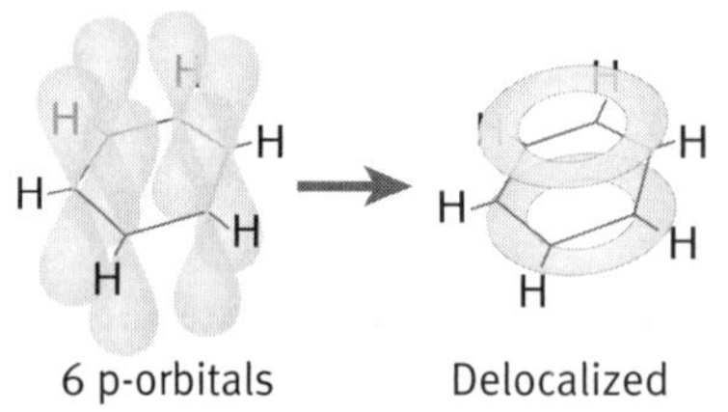

6 p-orbitals   Delocalized

Figure 12.25. Conjugation in Benzene

Increased strain in a molecule can make it more reactive. The β-**lactams** are prone to hydrolysis because they have significant ring strain. **Ring strain** is due to torsional strain from eclipsing interactions and angle strain from compressing bond angles below 109.5°.

All carboxylic acid derivatives can undergo nucleophilic substitution reactions. The rates at which they do so are determined by their relative reactivities.

Anhydrides can be **cleaved** by the addition of a nucleophile. Addition of ammonia or an amine results in an amide and a carboxylic acid. Addition of an alcohol results in an ester and a carboxylic acid. Addition of water results in two carboxylic acids.

Transesterification is the exchange of one esterifying group for another on an ester. The attacking nucleophile is an alcohol. **Amides** can be hydrolyzed to carboxylic acids under strongly acidic or basic conditions. The attacking nucleophile is water or the hydroxide anion.

NITROGEN- AND PHOSPHORUS-CONTAINING COMPOUNDS

The α-carbon of an amino acid is attached to four groups: an amino group, a carboxyl group, a hydrogen atom, and an **R-group**. It is a chiral stereocenter in all amino acids except **glycine**. All amino acids in eukaryotes are L-amino acids. They all have S stereochemistry except **cysteine**, which is R.

Amino acids are **amphoteric**, meaning they can act as acids or bases. Amino acids get their acidic characteristics from carboxylic acids and their basic characteristics from amino groups. In neutral solution, amino acids tend to exist as **zwitterions** (dipolar ions).

Amino acids can be classified by their R-groups.

- **Nonpolar nonaromatic amino acids** include alanine, valine, leucine, isoleucine, glycine, proline, and methionine.
- **Aromatic amino acids** include tryptophan, phenylalanine, and tyrosine. Both nonpolar nonaromatic and aromatic amino acids tend to be hydrophobic and reside in the interior of proteins.
- **Polar amino acids** include serine, threonine, asparagine, glutamine, and cysteine.
- **Negatively charged amino acids** contain carboxylic acids in their R-groups and include aspartic acid and glutamic acid.
- **Positively charged amino acids** contain amines in their R-groups and include arginine, lysine, and histidine.

KEY CONCEPT

Nonpolar nonaromatic and aromatic amino acids tend to be hydrophobic and reside in the interior of proteins. Polar, negatively charged (acidic), and polar, positively charged (basic) amino acids tend to be hydrophilic and reside on the surface of proteins, making hydrogen bonds with the aqueous environment.

Peptide bonds form by condensation reactions and can be cleaved hydrolytically. **Polypeptides** are made up of multiple amino acids linked by peptide bonds.

Biologically, amino acids are synthesized in many ways. In the lab, certain standardized mechanisms are used. Via the **Strecker synthesis**, an aldehyde is mixed with ammonium chloride (NH_4Cl) and potassium cyanide. The ammonia attacks the carbonyl carbon, generating an imine. The imine is then attacked by the cyanide, generating an aminonitrile. The aminonitrile is hydrolyzed by two equivalents of water, generating an amino acid.

The **Gabriel synthesis** also generates an amino acid. Phthalimide attacks the diethyl bromomalonate, generating a phthalimidomalonic ester. The phthalimidomalonic ester attacks an alkyl halide, adding an alkyl group to the ester. The product is then hydrolyzed, creating phthalic acid (with two carboxyl groups) and converting the esters into carboxylic acids. One carboxylic acid of the resulting 1,3-dicarbonyl is removed by decarboxylation.

KEY CONCEPT

Resonance of the peptide bond restricts motion about the C–N bond, which takes on partial double-bond character. Either a strong acid or a strong base is needed to cleave a peptide bond.

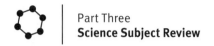

KEY CONCEPT

Phosphate bonds are high energy because of large negative charges in adjacent phosphate groups and resonance stabilization of phosphates.

Phosphorus is found in **inorganic phosphate** (P_i), a buffered mixture of hydrogen phosphate (HPO_4^{2-}) and dihydrogen phosphate ($H_2PO_4^-$). Phosphorus is also found in the backbone of DNA, which uses **phosphodiester bonds.** In forming these bonds, a **pyrophosphate** (PP_i, $P_2O_7^{4-}$) is released. Pyrophosphate can then be hydrolyzed to two inorganic phosphates. **Organic phosphates** are carbon-containing compounds that also have phosphate groups.

The most notable examples are nucleotide triphosphates (such as ATP or GTP) and DNA. Phosphoric acid has three hydrogens, each with a unique pK_a. This wide variety in pK_a values allows phosphoric acid to act as a buffer over a large range of pH values.

SPECTROSCOPY

Infrared (IR) spectroscopy measures **absorption** of infrared light, which causes molecular vibration (stretching, bending, twisting, and folding). IR spectra are generally plotted as **percent transmittance** *vs.* **wave number** (1λ). The normal range of a spectrum is 4,000 to 400 cm^{-1}, and the **fingerprint region** is between 1,500 and 400 cm^{-1}. An IR spectrum contains a number of peaks that can be used by experts to identify a compound. To appear on an IR spectrum, vibration of a bond must change the bond dipole moment. Certain bonds have characteristic absorption frequencies, which allow us to infer the presence (or absence) of particular functional groups (see Table 12.3).

Functional Group	Wavenumber (cm^{-1})	Vibration
Alkanes	2,800–3,000 1,200	C—H C—C
Alkenes	3,080–3,140 1,645	=C—H C=C
Alkynes	3,300 2,200	≡C—H C≡C
Aromatic	2,900–3,100 1,475–1,625	C—H C—C
Alcohols	3,100–3,500	O—H (broad)
Ethers	1,050–1,150	C—O
Aldehydes	2,700–2,900 1,700–1,750	(O)C—H C=O
Ketones	1,700–1,750	C=O
Carboxylic Acids	1,700–1,750 2,800–3,200	C=O O—H (broad)
Amines	3,100–3,500	N–H (sharp)

Table 12.3. Absorption Frequencies

Ultraviolet (UV) spectroscopy measures absorption of ultraviolet light, which causes movement of electrons between molecular orbitals. UV spectra are generally plotted as percent transmittance or absorbance *vs.* wavelength. To appear on a UV spectrum, a molecule must have a small enough energy difference between its **highest occupied molecular orbital (HOMO)** and its **lowest unoccupied molecular orbital (LUMO)** to permit an electron to move from one orbital to the other. The smaller the difference between HOMO and LUMO, the longer the wavelengths a molecule can absorb. **Conjugation** occurs in molecules with unhybridized *p*-orbitals. Conjugation shifts the spectrum to higher maximum wavelengths (lower frequencies).

Nuclear magnetic resonance (NMR) spectroscopy measures alignment of nuclear spin with an applied magnetic field, which depends on the magnetic environment of the nucleus itself. It is useful for determining the structure (connectivity) of a compound, including functional groups.

NMR spectra are generally plotted as frequency *vs.* absorption of energy. They are standardized by using **chemical shift (δ)**, measured in parts per million (ppm) of spectrophotometer frequency. Higher chemical shifts are located to the left (**downfield**); lower chemical shifts are located to the right (**upfield**).

Proton (^{1}H) NMR is the most common (see Figure 12.26). The **integration** (area under the curve) of this peak is proportional to the number of protons contained under the peak. **Deshielding** of protons occurs when electron-withdrawing groups pull electron density away from the nucleus, allowing it to be more easily affected by the magnetic field. Deshielding moves a peak further downfield.

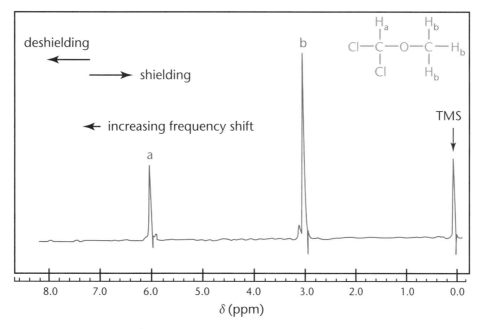

Figure 12.26. ^{1}H–NMR Spectrum of Dichloromethyl Methyl Ether
Peak a: dichloromethyl proton;
peak b: methyl protons

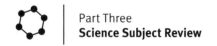
When hydrogens are on adjacent atoms, they interfere with each other's magnetic environment, causing **spin-spin coupling (splitting)**. A proton's (or group of protons') peak is split into $n + 1$ subpeaks, where n is the number of protons that are three bonds away from the proton of interest. Splitting patterns include **doublets**, **triplets**, and **multiplets.**

- Protons on sp^3-hybridized carbons are usually in the 0 to 3 ppm range (but higher if electron-withdrawing groups are present).
- Protons on sp^2-hybridized carbons are usually in the 4.6 to 6.0 ppm range.
- Protons on sp-hybridized carbons are usually in the 2.0 to 3.0 ppm range.
- Aldehydic hydrogens tend to appear between 9 and 10 ppm.
- Carboxylic acid hydrogens tend to appear between 10.5 and 12 ppm.
- Aromatic hydrogens appear between 6.0 and 8.5 ppm.

SEPARATIONS AND PURIFICATIONS High-Yield

Extraction combines two immiscible liquids, one of which easily dissolves the compound of interest. The polar (water) layer is called the **aqueous phase** and dissolves compounds with hydrogen bonding or polarity. The nonpolar layer is called the **organic phase** and dissolves nonpolar compounds. Extraction is carried out in a separatory funnel. One phase is collected, and the solvent is then evaporated. A **wash** is the reverse of extraction, in which a small amount of solute that dissolves impurities is run over the compound of interest.

KEY CONCEPT

Like dissolves like. *Polar* solutes have a preference for *polar* solvents, and *nonpolar* solutes have a preference for *nonpolar* solvents.

Filtration isolates a solid (**residue**) from a liquid (**filtrate**). **Gravity filtration** is used when the product of interest is in the filtrate. Hot solvent is used to maintain solubility. **Vacuum filtration** is used when the product of interest is the solid. A vacuum is connected to the flask to pull the solvent through more quickly.

In **recrystallization**, the product is dissolved in a minimum amount of hot solvent. If the impurities are more soluble, the crystals reform while the flask cools, excluding the impurities.

Distillation separates liquids according to differences in their boiling points; the liquid with the lowest boiling point vaporizes first and is collected as the **distillate. Simple distillation** can be used if the boiling points are under 150°C and are at least 25°C apart. **Vacuum distillation** should be used if the boiling points are over 150°C to prevent degradation of the product. **Fractional distillation** should be used if the boiling points are less than 25°C apart because it allows more refined separation of liquids by boiling point.

KEY CONCEPT

All forms of **chromatography** use two phases to separate compounds based on physical or chemical properties.

In chromatography, the **stationary phase** or **adsorbent** is usually a polar solid. The **mobile phase** runs through the stationary phase and is usually a liquid or gas. This **elutes** the sample through the stationary phase. Compounds with higher affinity for the stationary phase have smaller **retardation factors** and take longer to pass through, if at all; compounds with higher affinity for the mobile phase elute through more quickly. Compounds therefore get separated from each other, called **partitioning**.

Thin-layer and **paper chromatography** are used to identify a sample. The stationary phase is a polar material, such as silica, alumina, or paper. The mobile phase is a nonpolar solvent, which climbs the card through capillary action. The card is **spotted** and **developed**; R_f values can be calculated and compared to reference values. **Reverse-phase chromatography** uses a nonpolar card with a polar solvent.

Column chromatography utilizes polarity, size, or affinity to separate compounds based on their physical or chemical properties. The stationary phase is a column containing silica or alumina beads. The mobile phase is a nonpolar solvent, which travels through the column by gravity. In **ion-exchange chromatography**, the beads are coated with charged substances to bind compounds with opposite charge. In **size-exclusion chromatography**, the beads have small pores that trap smaller compounds and allow larger compounds to travel through faster. In **affinity chromatography**, the column is made to have high affinity for a compound by coating the beads with a receptor or an antibody to the compound.

Gas chromatography separates vaporizable compounds according to how well they adhere to the adsorbent in the column. The stationary phase is a coil of crushed metal or a polymer. The mobile phase is a nonreactive gas. Gas chromatography may be combined in sequence with **mass spectrometry**, which ionizes and fragments molecules and passes these fragments through a magnetic field to determine molecular weight or structure.

High-performance liquid chromatography (HPLC) is similar to column chromatography but uses sophisticated computer-mediated solvent and temperature gradients. It is used if the sample size is small or if forces such as capillary action will affect results. It was formerly called high-pressure liquid chromatography.

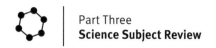

12.5 Organic Chemistry Worked Examples

The following steps will walk you through the following passage using the Kaplan Passage Strategy.

PREVIEW FOR DIFFICULTY

A quick Preview of the passage shows peptides and amino acids. The text refers to enzymes, and there are two "pathways" to go along with the two figures. This passage is likely to start with an introduction to enzymes followed by the specifics of each pathway. Let your comfort with organic chemistry and enzymes determine whether this is a now or later passage for you.

CHOOSE YOUR APPROACH

As found in our Preview step, the passage includes mechanisms, pathways, and figures. As this is a densely packed information passage, choose **Outlining.**

READ AND DISTILL

P1: The first paragraph reads like a textbook. It's relatively familiar content, although it introduces the idea that enzymes don't always directly stabilize the transition state.
Outline: Enzyme functions: bond strain

MCAT EXPERTISE

After looking at the figures involving reactions, it's tempting to work out the exact mechanism of each step. However, this is almost always a bad idea. It's unlikely that an MCAT question requires such comprehensive understanding. You are generally asked about a specific step of a reaction or the role of a particular reagent. For information passages like this, save the figure analysis until a question requires it.

P2: The second paragraph picks up where the first one left off and still reads like a text-book. This time the topics include entropy, mechanisms, and bonding. Not until the last two sentences do we get the introduction to the figures that we have been anticipating. Unfortunately, that introduction doesn't provide much more information than the figure captions.
Outline: Enzyme functions: reduce entropy, acid-base, transient bonding

F1/F2: When presented with multiple versions of the same general concept, we should be looking for similarities and differences. In this case, both pathways involve an attack by an activated water molecule. However, in Pathway 1 the enzyme attacks first, whereas in Pathway 2, details of the enzyme's role aren't explicitly given.
Outline:
F1. Serine protease: Pathway 1
F2. Aspartic protease: Pathway 2

PASSAGE I: REACTION MECHANISMS

The mechanisms by which enzymes increase reaction rates are varied. Enzymes can induce bond strain in substrates by favoring the conformation of the transition state over that of the substrate. In this way, the substrates are destabilized, thereby decreasing the potential energy difference between the substrate and the transition state. It is important to recognize that enzymes, with this mechanism, do not directly stabilize the transition state.

Acidic and basic residues of enzymes can activate nucleophiles or electrophiles through protonation or deprotonation. Leaving groups also can be stabilized by these residues. Enzymes can form either transient ionic or covalent bonds with the substrate. However, these bonds must be broken to regenerate the enzyme. The hydrolysis of protein requires the presence of proteases to catalyze the process. Generally, proteins are hydrolyzed by one of two pathways:

Pathway 1: A nucleophilic residue of an enzyme attacks the substrate protein to form an acyl-enzyme intermediate. An activated water molecule attacks, causing the release of half of the product and regeneration of the enzyme, as shown in Figure 1.

Pathway 2: An activated water molecule performs nucleophilic attack on the peptide bond to hydrolyze it, as shown in Figure 2.

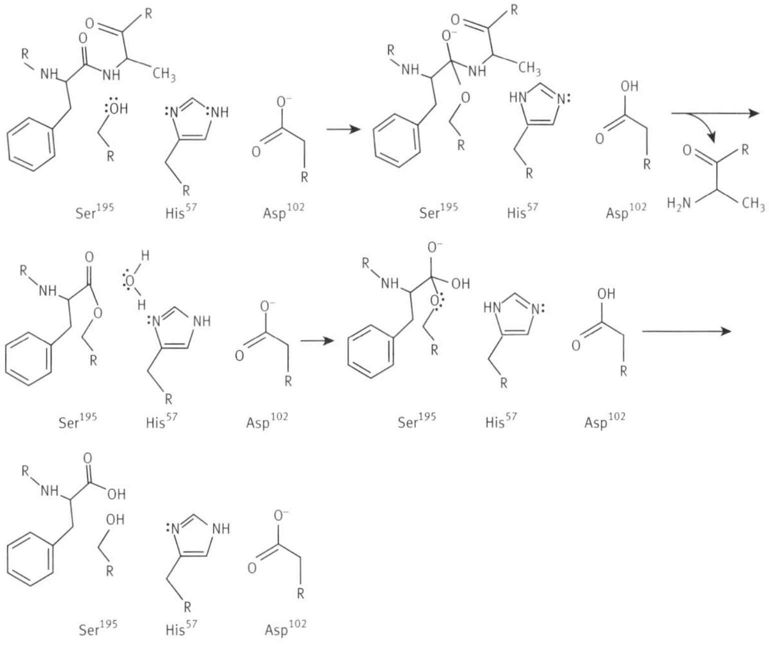

Figure 1. Mechanism of protein breakdown by a serine protease

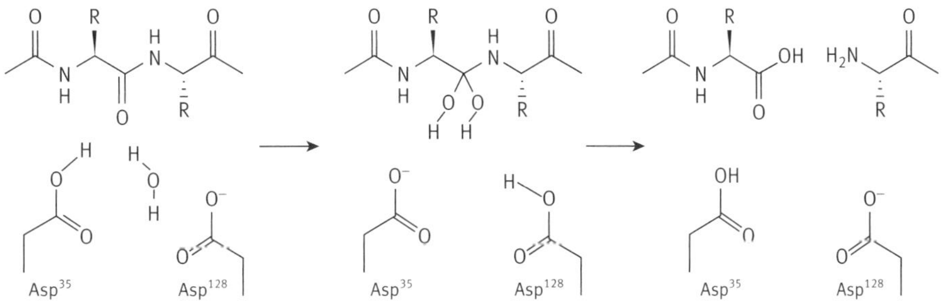

Figure 2. Mechanism of protein breakdown by an aspartic protease

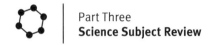

1. How does aspartate contribute to the first step of the mechanism illustrated in Figure 1?

    A. It directly increases the nucleophilicity of the serine residue through deprotonation.

    B. It functions to maintain an acidic environment for optimal enzymatic activity.

    C. It increases the pK_a of histidine through electrostatic interactions.

    D. It serves to increase the basicity of histidine by protecting its aromaticity.

❶ Type the question

The question stem limits the scope of the question to Figure 1. Because the passage does not directly address how serine proteases hydrolyze proteins, it is not necessary to refer to the text. Therefore, only the mechanism must be analyzed.

❷ Rephrase the question stem

The question requires us to understand aspartate's role in Figure 1. However, a quick glance at the first step of the mechanism shows that aspartic acid (Asp), along with histidine (His), are not directly interacting with serine (Ser), which is where the nucleophilic attack takes place. Therefore, we must consider how both histidine and aspartate influence the reaction between serine and the protease. This question stem can be Rephrased as, *What are the roles of His and Asp in Figure 1?*

❸ Investigate potential solutions

To determine the role of aspartate, it is essential to look at both the reactants and the products following the first step. As is the case with most organic chemistry problems, begin by identifying relevant nucleophiles and electrophiles and then form a prediction.

Serine is deprotonated and then performs a nucleophilic attack on the carbonyl carbon of the substrate. At the same time, histidine appears to be not only protonated (left side) but also deprotonated (right side), and the aspartic acid residue is protonated. Each residue interacts with the adjacent residue. In this case, aspartic acid is removing a proton from histidine. Removing the proton allows histidine to pick up a proton on its other nitrogen, removing a proton from serine and activating the serine residue as a nucleophile. Because histidine is extracting a proton from serine, histidine is behaving as a base. Thus aspartic acid must be increasing the basicity of histidine.

❹ Match your prediction to an answer choice

(C) states that aspartic acid increases the pK_a of histidine through electrostatic interactions. This is equivalent to stating that aspartic acid increases the basicity of histidine through the interaction of positive and negative charges. Hence, **(C)** is correct.

Aspartic acid does not deprotonate serine directly as stated in (**A**); it deprotonates histidine, which deprotonates serine. Histidine contains both protonated and deprotonated nitrogen atoms. If the environment was acidic, as described in (**B**), these nitrogen atoms would both be protonated. (**D**) can be eliminated because although aspartic acid does increase the basicity of histidine, it does not do so by protecting histidine's aromaticity. The aromaticity of histidine is not in jeopardy. If it was, histidine would not react regardless of aspartic acid's presence.

---

2. In Figure 1, activated water can perform nucleophilic attack only after half of the substrate has been cleaved off. Which of the following best explains why this is so?

    A. Histidine will preferentially extract a proton from serine before it will activate water.

    B. Steric hindrance prevented water from performing nucleophilic attack.

    C. The carbonyl carbon of the amide was initially not sufficiently electrophilic.

    D. The deprotonated serine is a less effective leaving group than the substrate fragment.

KEY CONCEPT

Nucleophilic reaction in carboxylic acid derivatives

1 Type the question

This question requires identifying the best explanation for a scientific phenomenon. From a content perspective, this question tests nucleophilic substitution. Given the critical thinking involved in answering this question, it is a good candidate to save for later in the passage set.

2 Rephrase the question stem

The question stem specifically asks about the role of water in Figure 1. The question can be Rephrased as, *Why can't water attack the carbonyl carbon initially?*

3 Investigate potential solutions

Recognizing the difference between the original substrate structure and substrate structure after half of it is cleaved off is essential. Activation of the water is irrelevant because water could be activated at any point in the mechanism.

For water to perform nucleophilic attack, the carbonyl carbon must be sufficiently electrophilic. At the beginning of the mechanism, the carbonyl group is part of an amide, whereas later it is part of an ester. Because amide groups have greater double-bond character, they are more stable than esters. In addition, the nitrogen of the amide is more electron donating compared to the oxygen of the ester; this makes the ester more subject to nucleophilic attack. Let the distinction between amides and esters serve as your prediction.

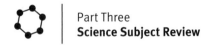
④ Match your prediction to an answer choice

Evaluating each answer choice should Match to **(C)**, as it is synonymous with the prediction.

There are a couple of ways that water could be activated (aspartic acid could do this). Therefore, histidine's preferred target does not explain why activated water cannot perform nucleophilic attack until the substrate is cleaved in **(A)**.

(B) can be eliminated because water is a small molecule, so steric hindrance would not be a major factor here. **(D)** is incorrect because the deprotonated serine is a better leaving group than the substrate fragment.

KEY CONCEPT
_____

Hydrolysis

> **3.** Why can aspartic proteases hydrolyze peptide bonds in fewer steps than can serine proteases?
>
> **A.** Aspartic proteases hydrogen bond with the carbonyl oxygen, but serine proteases do not.
>
> **B.** The aspartic acid in serine proteases is located too far from the peptide bond.
>
> **C.** Histidine is not a strong enough base to deprotonate water.
>
> **D.** Aspartic proteases are able to stabilize tetrahedral intermediates.

① Type the question

The question stem asks for a comparison between aspartic proteases and serine proteases. Figures 1 and 2 must be compared. Thus, this is a passage-based question, but it should require only information from the figures.

② Rephrase the question stem

The phrasing of the question stem is relatively clear, but it can be Rephrased into an actionable task. The main difference between the mechanism in Figures 1 and the mechanism in Figure 2 is when water performs nucleophilic attack. Rephrase the question stem: *Why can water attack earlier in Figure 2 compared to Figure 1?*

③ Investigate potential solutions

Water can perform nucleophilic attack earlier in the aspartic protease mechanism because the carbonyl carbon is especially electrophilic. The additional aspartic acid residue can hydrogen bond with the carbonyl oxygen. As a result, the carbonyl oxygen becomes relatively more electronegative. The carbonyl oxygen will sap negative charge from the carbonyl carbon so that it becomes relatively electropositive. Water can then attack earlier with aspartic proteases (Figure 2) versus serine proteases (Figure 1).

4 Match your prediction to an answer choice

(**A**) matches the prediction and is the correct answer.

(**B**) is incorrect because the enzymes are folded such that all of the amino acid residues are located within close proximity of each other. Histidine deprotonates water later in the mechanism, so (**C**) is not true. Both serine proteases and aspartic proteases are able to stabilize tetrahedral intermediates sufficiently. If this was not the case, as described in (**D**), they would not be able to catalyze proteolysis effectively.

---

4. Based on the mechanism illustrated in Figure 2, what must be true of the active site of aspartic proteases?

    A. It binds to hydrophobic proteins more readily than to hydrophilic proteins.
    B. It binds to bulky proteins more readily than to smaller proteins.
    C. It is kept relatively acidic.
    D. It is kept relatively basic.

KEY CONCEPT

Amino acid chemistry

1 Type the question

The question stem asks for a generalization about the aspartic protease's active site, and the answers are related to reactivity.

2 Rephrase the question stem

This question stem doesn't provide much direction, so our Rephrase is on par: *What must be true of aspartic proteases' active site based on Figure 2?*

3 Investigate potential solutions

It is important to recognize that Figure 2 is only a snapshot of a portion of the active site of aspartic proteases. Therefore, only a limited number of conclusions can be drawn.

Upon analyzing the mechanism in Figure 2, it is apparent that one of the aspartic acid residues is protonated. Because carboxylic acids are acidic and lose a proton at a neutral pH, the microenvironment of aspartic proteases must be acidic.

4 Match your prediction to an answer choice

(**C**) matches the prediction.

Many other relevant amino acids are not illustrated in Figure 2. Hence, (**A**) and (**B**) cannot be determined with the information that is available. If the microenvironment of the active site was basic, as stated in (**D**), then both the aspartic acid residues would be deprotonated.

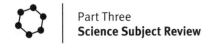

> 5. Why is water necessary to carry out proteolysis instead of simply using an amino acid residue already found on the enzyme?
>
>   **A.** Water is ubiquitous and therefore maximally increases reaction kinetics.
>   **B.** Water is a small molecule that can easily perform nucleophilic attack without significant steric hindrance.
>   **C.** Water can be activated by basic amino acid residues, making it the most nucleophilic entity in the microenvironment of the active site.
>   **D.** Water allows for the recycling of the enzyme in proteolysis.

❶ Type the question

This question beings with a *why* and demands that we explain the need for a third-party molecule of water for proteolysis to occur as opposed to another amino acid residue. As this is a Skill 2 (scientific reasoning) question, it may be worthwhile to save for later.

❷ Rephrase the question stem

The question implies two situations: (1) water carrying out proteolysis or (2) the enzyme's amino acid residue carrying out proteolysis. To answer this question, we need an answer that explains why the first scenario must be true or why the second cannot be. As such, we can Rephrase this question as, *Why must water be used for proteolysis?* or *Why can't the enzyme itself be used for proteolysis?*

❸ Investigate potential solutions

Investigate the solution on two fronts. First let's consider water's role. Water acts the nucleophile attacking the electrophilic carbon and gets incorporated into the products as a hydroxyl group. Next, consider why the enzyme itself cannot be used for this purpose. If the amino acid residues of an enzyme were to attack the substrate, a small piece of the enzyme would be lost during each reaction. Because an enzyme must be regenerated during the course of a reaction, this cannot occur.

Let this train of thought serve as a general prediction, and evaluate the answer choices.

❹ Match your prediction to an answer choice

(D) matches the prediction.

Water is everywhere and thus is a solid option for enzyme catalysis. However, water's viability as an option in **(A)** does not explain why a third-party molecule is essential. In addition, the extreme phrasing of *maximally* is too strong. For **(B)**, many amino acid residues with side chains are potentially much more nucleophilic and would not be dramatically impacted by steric hindrance. Thus, **(B)** cannot be correct. Water is not necessarily the most nucleophilic entity in the microenvironment of the active site, as stated by **(C)**, even after being activated.

> **6.** The amino acid residues of serine proteases, Gly-193 and Ser-195, form an oxyanion hole, which hydrogen bonds to the substrate. When will the oxyanion hole be particularly important?
>
> **A.** After the substrate has entered the active site but before hydrolysis has begun
> **B.** When serine performs nucleophilic attack on the substrate
> **C.** When the substrate exhibits tetrahedral geometry
> **D.** When water performs nucleophilic attack on the substrate

❶ Type the question

The question stem mentions serine proteases and thus is a passage-based question centering around Figure 1. The answers appear to be key points in the reaction.

❷ Rephrase the question stem

Asking *when* a specific feature of a system is *particularly important* provides insight on how to Rephrase this question. Hydrogen bonding is particularly useful in providing stability during unstable transition states. Thus, we can Rephrase this question as, *Which steps in the reaction are particularly unstable and require hydrogen bonding?*

❸ Investigate potential solutions

The most unstable steps illustrated in Figure 1 are those that include intermediates. In Figure 1, the intermediates all exhibit tetrahedral geometry. Another way to approach this problem is to use the information in the passage. The passage explains that enzymes catalyze reactions by inducing strain in the substrate by "favoring the conformation of the transition state." This phrase essentially means that the enzymes interact most favorably with the substrate when it is in the transition state.

❹ Match your prediction to an answer choice

(C) matches the prediction.

If the substrate was stabilized too much, the reaction would not proceed forward. In **(A)**, the substrate is held in place by the enzyme but not much more than that. The amino acid residues of serine proteases work together to facilitate nucleophilic attack on the substrate, as described in **(B)**. However, there is no need to provide extra stability to the substrate. **(D)** can be eliminated because the substrate is relatively stable at this point. It is not carrying any charges and would not require additional stability.

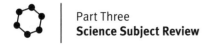
ORGANIC CHEMISTRY PASSAGE II: ALDEHYDES AND KETONES

Amphetamines are a class of potent nervous system stimulants popularized as performance and cognitive enhancers; in some cases, they are used recreationally as aphrodisiacs or euphoriants. Amphetamines diffuse across the blood-brain barrier as well as the placental barrier, making unwanted side effects a serious concern. To mitigate adverse effects, medical dosage and availability are strictly controlled. Although debate persists over amphetamines' neurotoxicity in humans, there appears to be evidence that amphetamine metabolism increases the concentration of reactive oxygen species (ROS).

Amphetamines are legally and illicitly synthesized in a variety of ways. Figure 1 outlines the production of racemic amphetamines via two different intermediates.

Figure 1. Synthesis of methamphetamine via arrangement

Because the biological activity of amphetamines is stereospecific and amphetamine is often produced as a racemic mixture, it is generally necessary to isolate the biologically active enantiomer. Figure 2 outlines the resolution of racemic amphetamine via hot, basic tartaric acid. In addition, Figure 2 shows a stereospecific synthetic pathway.

Figure 2. Stereoselective production of D-amphetamine

Amphetamines have biological analogs termed *trace amines*. Trace amines are structurally and metabolically related to traditional monoamine neurotransmitters, such as dopamine and norepinephrine, and are so named because they are found only in trace amounts.

1. Epinephrine, shown below, is not able to cross the blood-brain barrier. Which of the following best explains why amphetamines can do so and epinephrine cannot?

   A. Amphetamines are mostly lipid soluble because of their aromatic ring and relative lack of polar protic groups.
   B. The methyl group of amphetamines provides stereospecificity for trace amine receptors.
   C. ROS species produced by amphetamines facilitate membrane transfer.
   D. The polarity of the hydroxyl groups reduces affinity for plasma membrane transporters.

2. What is the most likely reason why methamphetamine (a secondary amine and amphetamine analog) can elicit sympathetic responses similar to epinephrine despite differences in their chemical makeup?

   A. Metabolites of methamphetamine structurally resemble epinephrine receptors.
   B. Methamphetamine inhibits epinephrine reuptake mechanisms.
   C. Methamphetamine is a configurational isomer of epinephrine and reacts similarly.
   D. Epinephrine receptors have a high affinity for the benzene ring of both molecules.

3. What is the primary difficulty in synthetically producing trace amine compounds from ketone intermediates?

   A. Carbonyls are prone to ring-closing mechanisms and thus create intermediates unfavorable to amination.
   B. Carbonyl compounds, particularly ketones, are relatively unreactive to amines.
   C. There are a number of side products possible from carbonyl compounds.
   D. Addition to the carbonyl carbon is reversible, and synthesis is subject to equilibrium constraints.

4. A student wishing to resolve optically pure amphetamine uses mesotartaric acid, a diastereomer of D-tartaric acid. Is the student likely to be successful?

   A. Yes; mesotartaric acid will combine with each enantiomer to form a pair of diastereomers, which can be separated by physical means.
   B. Yes; the enantiomer of D-tartaric acid will react with the racemates to form distinct salts that can be separated by physical means.
   C. No; D-tartaric acid is necessary to form a pair of diastereomers that can be separated.
   D. No; mesotartaric acid will react with the mixture to form distinct salts that are mirror images.

5. Which of the following statements best describes the rearrangements in Figure 1?

   A. In the Hofmann rearrangement, primary amides are converted to derivatives by the action of halohydroxides or halogens in alkaline solution. Excess base generates a conjugate acid of the product.
   B. In the Curtius rearrangement, an acyl azide is prepared by reacting an acyl chloride with diazonium followed by treatment with cold nitrous acid. Subsequent heating results in decomposition.
   C. Both the Hofmann and Curtius rearrangements involve acyl nitrenes that quickly rearrange to isocyanate isomers, which are isolated or reacted in acidic solvents.
   D. Both the Hofmann and Curtius rearrangements involve the addition of water to isocyanates to produce an unstable carbamic acid that decomposes to an amine and CO_2.

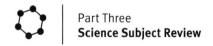
MCAT EXPERTISE

When presented with complex molecules or reactions, look for recognizable functional groups or reaction conditions.

USING THE KAPLAN METHOD

Preview the passage: At a glance, this is an organic chemistry passage with synthesis reactions in the figures. In addition, most paragraphs are very short, with the exception of the first. However, paragraph 1 appears to provide background knowledge. This is a light on detail information passage.

Choose your approach: Highlight

Read and Distill:

P1: This paragraph provides background information on amphetamines and their effects, which is unlikely to be tested in an organic chemistry passage. However, the final sentence describes a testable trend, amphetamine metabolism increases ROS.
Highlight: "Amphetamine metabolism increases"

P2: Describes Figure 1, which is the production of methamphetamine via two pathways.
Highlight: "Racemic"

P3: Describes an issue with the racemic production and presents the solution to select for the active enantiomer.
Highlight: "Isolate the biologically active enantiomer"

P4: Defines trace amines.
Highlight: *"Trace amines"*

---

1. Epinephrine, shown below, is not able to cross the blood-brain barrier. Which of the following best explains why amphetamines can do so and epinephrine cannot?

   A. Amphetamines are mostly lipid soluble because of their aromatic ring and relative lack of polar protic groups.
   B. The methyl group of amphetamines provides stereospecificity for trace amine receptors.
   C. ROS species produced by amphetamines facilitate membrane transfer.
   D. The polarity of the hydroxyl groups reduces affinity for plasma membrane transporters.

① Type the question

This question demands knowledge of the blood-brain barrier and being able to compare two compounds. The topics tested are chemical structure analysis and membrane diffusion.

② Rephrase the question stem

To answer this question, it is necessary to focus on the differences between the two molecules. Those differences combined with new information from the passage and required outside knowledge will be enough to find the correct answer. Epinephrine is structurally similar to amphetamines, with the addition of several hydroxyl groups. We can Rephrase this question as, *How do the additional hydroxyl groups prevent epinephrine from crossing the blood-brain barrier?*

③ Investigate potential solutions

Paragraph 1 indicates that amphetamines can diffuse across the blood-brain barrier. The blood-brain barrier is primarily lipid or small nonpolar molecule soluble. Thus, the hydrocarbon structure, including the aromatic ring, allows amphetamine to diffuse, whereas the polar, hydroxyl groups in epinephrine prevent its diffusion. Let this serve as a prediction.

④ Match your prediction to an answer choice

(A) matches this prediction, addressing both components: amphetamines being lipid soluble and implying that epinephrine has polar groups.

(B) is perhaps true, but it does not address why one molecule is able to cross and another is not—so it cannot be the correct answer (to this question). **(C)** recalls another fact from the passage; even though ROS may damage cells and thereby compromise the integrity of the blood-brain barrier, ROS does not facilitate membrane transfer. Hydrophobicity, which is a consequence of molecular structure, facilitates membrane transfer.

The most tempting wrong answer is **(D)**. It addresses a key difference between the two molecules (the hydroxyl groups) and is generally aligned with our prediction. However, it incorrectly references membrane transporters rather than diffusion. Although membrane transporters are present in the blood-brain barrier, the passage explicitly states that amphetamines cross the barrier via diffusion.

TAKEAWAYS

When asked to explain a difference in function, look for a difference in structure.

THINGS TO WATCH OUT FOR

Be aware of answer choices that bring up unrelated facts about one molecule or another.

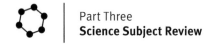

KEY CONCEPT

Form dictates function.

> 2. What is the most likely reason why methamphetamine (a secondary amine and amphetamine analog) can elicit sympathetic responses similar to epinephrine despite differences in their chemical makeup?
>
> A. Metabolites of methamphetamine structurally resemble epinephrine receptors.
>
> B. Methamphetamine inhibits epinephrine reuptake mechanisms.
>
> C. Methamphetamine is a configurational isomer of epinephrine and reacts similarly.
>
> D. Epinephrine receptors have a high affinity for the benzene ring of both molecules.

1 Type the question

Much like the previous question, to answer question 2, it will be necessary to explain an observation about two molecules. Unlike its predecessor, the correct answer to this question must address a similarity in function despite a difference in form.

2 Rephrase the question stem

The phrasing of this question is relatively clear, but we can shorten it: *Considering the similarities between the two compounds, explain how methamphetamine can activate the sympathetic response.*

3 Investigate potential solutions

It's best to make a few predictions and then use the process of elimination. There are a few notable differences between the two molecules and one notable similarity. The similarity is a good place to start. To elicit a response from the sympathetic nervous system, there must be stimulation of the appropriate receptors. Although it is uncertain how methamphetamine works, it's likely one of a few common mechanisms. The molecule could mimic epinephrine and bind to epinephrine receptors. It also could prevent the degradation or reuptake of epinephrine. There are other, more obscure mechanisms. However, their validity should be addressed on an individual basis using passage information, outside knowledge, and logic.

4 Match your prediction to an answer choice

While keeping the general prediction from your Investigate step in mind, evaluate each answer choice.

(A) may be tempting because it provides a possible explanation that takes into account structural differences; however, the last portion of this answer is not plausible. The correct answer would indicate that the metabolites are structurally similar to epinephrine, not the epinephrine receptor.

(**B**) matches a likely mechanism from our Investigate step.

(**C**) states that methamphetamine and epinephrine are configurational isomers; this is incorrect. Furthermore, configurational isomers can react very differently. So this is not the best answer.

(**D**) provides a possible explanation for the similarity; it focuses on a common element of both molecules. However, given the stereospecificity of amphetamine receptors and the fact that methamphetamine is an analog, it's unlikely that the achiral benzene ring is sufficient to stimulate a sympathetic response. In addition, many compounds have benzene rings. Therefore, it is unlikely that the benzene ring alone is sufficient to allow binding.

Through the process of elimination, we eliminated (**A**), (**C**), and (**D**), indicating that (**B**) is the correct answer.

TAKEAWAYS

Consider what needs to be found in the correct answer, but remain open to unconsidered explanations that are in line with passage information and outside knowledge.

THINGS TO WATCH OUT FOR

Commonly, wrong answers address the question but contradict information from the passage.

MCAT EXPERTISE

The MCAT blurs the lines between organic chemistry, general chemistry, biochemistry, and biology.

---

3. What is the primary difficulty in synthetically producing trace amine compounds from ketone intermediates?

   A. Carbonyls are prone to ring-closing mechanisms and thus create intermediates unfavorable to amination.

   B. Carbonyl compounds, particularly ketones, are relatively unreactive to amines.

   C. There are a number of side products possible from carbonyl compounds.

   D. Addition to the carbonyl carbon is reversible, and synthesis is subject to equilibrium constraints.

---

① Type the question

This question requests the primary difficulty experienced during a synthesis and therefore tests critical reasoning regarding what may go wrong during the given reaction.

② Rephrase the question stem

It's possible to make some predictions based on the compounds in question. Ultimately, finding the answer requires eliminating those answers that are less problematic. We can Rephrase this question as, *Why can't ketone intermediates be used to produce trace amines?*

③ Investigate potential solutions

Carbonyl groups undergo a wide variety of reactions—a preliminary prediction. Furthermore, many of the intermediates are also reactive. There is also an example of amphetamine production from a ketone (the second reaction in Figure 2) that can be used for reference. In the reaction, the amine attacks the carbonyl carbon, forming an alcohol intermediate. Then dehydration of the alcohol forms the imine intermediate.

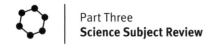
④ Match your prediction to an answer choice

It is unlikely that a focused prediction will be generated for this question type. Therefore use the process of elimination while keeping the general predictions from your Investigate step in mind.

(**A**) may seem reasonable. However, it references the creation of ring structures, which are not part of any of the synthesis pathways shown.

TAKEAWAYS

When presented with multiple answer choices each containing factual information, eliminate those that are least relevant to the question.

THINGS TO WATCH OUT FOR

When asked for a primary difficulty, consider all answer choices before making a selection.

(**B**) indicates that carbonyl groups are unreactive, which is untrue. Carbonyl groups, including ketones, undergo a wide variety of reactions.

(**C**) is a true statement and it addresses a fundamental problem when working with reactive species.

(**D**) must be eliminated because, although this answer choice is true, equilibrium reactions can be coerced via application of Le Châtelier's principle. Therefore, it is unlikely that equilibrium constraints would be the primary difficulty of concern.

Thorough reasoning dictates that the best of these choices is (**C**). In fact, synthetic routes for almost all pharmaceuticals suffer from some form of yield issues due to competing reactions and the formation of side products.

MCAT EXPERTISE

The carbonyl is a favorite reaction point on the MCAT; be familiar with its common mechanisms.

> 4. A student wishing to resolve optically pure amphetamine uses mesotartaric acid, a diastereomer of D-tartaric acid. Is the student likely to be successful?
>
>   **A.** Yes; mesotartaric acid will combine with each enantiomer to form a pair of diastereomers, which can be separated by physical means.
>
>   **B.** Yes; the enantiomer of D-tartaric acid will react with the racemates to form distinct salts that can be separated by physical means.
>
>   **C.** No; D-tartaric acid is necessary to form a pair of diastereomers that can be separated.
>
>   **D.** No; mesotartaric acid will react with the mixture to form distinct salts that are mirror images.

① Type the question

This question asks about the reasoning behind the experimental design. The answers are Yes/No followed by a brief explanation. As this is a challenging Skill 3 question, consider waiting until later in the passage set to work the problem.

② Rephrase the question stem

The question stem introduces a mesotartaric acid, a diastereomer of D-tartaric acid. Notice the prefix *meso–* in mesotartaric acid. This tells us it's a *meso* compound. You can confirm this by looking at D-tartaric acid in Figure 2 and deducing the structure of its diastereomer. Thus, this question stem can be Rephrased as, *Can a* meso *compound be used to resolve enantiomers?*

③ Investigate potential solutions

It's best to approach the answers with a prediction in mind. Once a prediction is made, attack the answer. The correct answer will not only answer the question but will also have sound reasoning. If unsure about the content, focus on the reasoning within the answer.

To resolve a racemic mixture into optically pure enantiomers, the mixture must be reacted with another optically active reagent. Commonly, acid-base properties are exploited to form salts. The salts thus formed are diastereomers of each other.

Mesotartaric acid is a *meso* compound and, as such, is optically inactive. Therefore, it is incapable of resolving a racemic mixture.

④ Match your prediction to an answer choice

While armed with this prediction, Match to (**D**).

(**A**) and (**B**) can be eliminated because the resolution does not work. Furthermore, (**B**) claims that the enantiomer of D-tartaric acid reacts when the question stem clearly identifies meso-tartaric acid as a diastereomer (the two terms are mutually exclusive).

(**C**) has the first part correct; however, it distorts the second half. D-tartaric acid is useful, but it is not necessary. Many other optically active resolving agents could be used, including L-tartaric acid.

(**D**) must be correct and matches the prediction. Distinct molecules that are mirror images are enantiomers, which is what would result from a reaction of a racemic mixture and an optically inactive reagent. Enantiomers cannot be separated by physical means, so the student's procedure would not work.

MCAT EXPERTISE

Diastereomers have different physical properties and can be separated by physical means. (Crystallization is common with amines.)

TAKEAWAYS

To resolve a racemic mixture, an optically active reagent must be used.

THINGS TO WATCH OUT FOR

Expect to see the same concept mentioned in different terms; the test makers commonly employ synonyms.

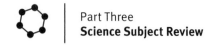
5. Which of the following statements best describes the rearrangements in Figure 1?

    A. In the Hofmann rearrangement, primary amides are converted to derivatives by the action of halohydroxides or halogens in alkaline solution. Excess base generates a conjugate acid of the product.

    B. In the Curtius rearrangement, an acyl azide is prepared by reacting an acyl chloride with diazonium followed by treatment with cold nitrous acid. Subsequent heating results in decomposition.

    C. Both the Hofmann and Curtius rearrangements involve acyl nitrenes that quickly rearrange to isocyanate isomers, which are isolated or reacted in acidic solvents.

    D. Both the Hofmann and Curtius rearrangements involve the addition of water to isocyanates to produce an unstable carbamic acid that decomposes to an amine and CO_2.

① Type the question

The question stem is fairly vague, indicating an understanding of Figure 1 is needed. Glancing at the answer choices indicates that they contain specific steps of Figure 1 and specific functional groups. This realization can provide direction during our Rephrase and Investigate steps.

② Rephrase the question stem

Based on the answer choices, the question stem can be Rephrased as, *Which answer choice correctly describes the events of the Hofmann and Curtius rearrangement?*

③ Investigate potential solutions

Investigating the differences and similarities between the two rearrangements leads us to Figure 1. The Hofmann rearrangement begins with an amide, while the Curtius rearrangement begins with a acyl azide. Both rearrangements results in methamphetamine. Although this is a very general prediction and therefore won't likely Match to an exact answer, it does provide enough insight to evaluate each answer choice.

4 Match your prediction to an answer choice

Due to the fairly vague question stem, making a focused prediction is not possible. Instead, evaluate each answer choice.

Starting with (**A**) and following the narrative, everything is consistent except the last statement that the conjugate acid is produced—eliminate (**A**).

(**B**) requires careful analysis and deduction regarding the Curtius pathway. The answer mentions a diazonium when, in fact, the reactant is an azide. This can be deduced either by the names of the reactants (diazonium compounds contain the $R-N_2^+$ functional group) or by looking at the name of the product (an azide).

(**C**) can be eliminated because the Hofmann rearrangement involves a basic workup. So although the workup for the Curtius rearrangement is unknown, the fact that this answer says *both* makes it incorrect.

At this point, the process of elimination shows that the correct response is (**D**). No evidence directly refutes this answer; it must, therefore, be chosen. Furthermore, based on the reaction in Figure 1, the process described in (**D**) seems plausible. A decarboxylation reaction occurs to produce an amine, and CO_2 would be an additional product.

Using our prediction to eliminate (**A**), (**B**), and (**C**), we deduced that the correct answer must be (**D**).

TAKEAWAYS

High-difficulty problems may require one to deduce unstated steps of a reaction.

THINGS TO WATCH OUT FOR

Refer to the passage to double-check for consistency.

MCAT EXPERTISE

Mechanisms are viable topics for analysis on the MCAT. Be sure to understand the reactants and products of every reaction. Also extend your analysis to side reactions that the intermediates may be involved in.

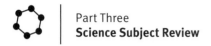

12.6 **Organic Chemistry on Your Own**

ORGANIC CHEMISTRY PASSAGE III (QUESTIONS 1–6)

Humans can synthesize only 11 of the proteogenic amino acids. Nine others are known as *essential amino acids* and must be supplied through one's diet—although some essential amino acids may be interconverted (the sulfur-containing and aromatic amino acids are interchangeable in the body).

De novo synthesis of amino acids usually starts with the nonessential amino acid glutamate (the conjugate base of glutamic acid). Glutamate is formed from the molecule α-ketoglutarate, a product of the Krebs cycle. In amino acid synthesis, α-ketoglutarate is aminated by ammonium to form glutamate. Glutamate can then be used to transaminate a number of different precursors into their respective amino acids. The transamination converts glutamate to α-ketoglutarate. For example, pyruvate, shown in Figure 1, can be aminated by glutamate to form alanine.

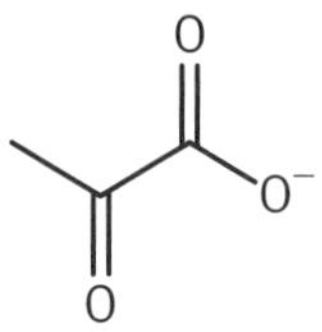

Figure 1. Pyruvate

Amino acid synthesis in the lab follows a variety of other pathways, using molecules not usually found in the human body. The Strecker synthesis starts with a carefully chosen aldehyde. The aldehyde is reacted with ammonium ions, leading to an iminium intermediate. The iminium intermediate is then attacked by a cyanide ion that forms an aminonitrile. Subsequently, this aminonitrile is converted to a carboxylic acid by the addition of water and acid, proceeding through a 1,2-diamino diol intermediate.

Amino acids have unique isoelectric points (pI), a pH where the amino acid will have a net neutral charge. The pI is determined by the appropriate pK_a of each functional group. The pI can be found for individual amino acids or for a polypeptide chain. In a polypeptide chain, most of the carboxylic acid and amino groups are bound and thus have no charge. Therefore the charge and, subsequently, the pI are influenced most significantly by the side chains in the polypeptide.

1. Which of the following amino acids will be negatively charged at physiological pH?

    A. Glutamic acid
    B. Arginine
    C. Valine
    D. Phenylalanine

2. The following structure shows an ionized form of tyrosine and its pK_a values. Based on this information, what is tyrosine's pI?

    A. 5.64
    B. 6.17
    C. 9.04
    D. 9.57

3. Which of the following is a significant disadvantage of using Strecker amino acid synthesis to create amino acids for the body?

    A. The ammonium ion causes the reaction to proceed too quickly to control.
    B. The nucleophile used can also attack side chains with carbonyls.
    C. The nucleophilic attack on the carbonyl causes racemization.
    D. All amino acids formed from this synthesis are useless biologically.

4. Given the structure of L-alanine and α-ketoglutaric acid, what is the structure of L-glutamic acid?

    A.

    B.

    C.

    D.

5. Suppose a portion of a peptide chain contains a large amount of phenylalanine, alanine, and valine residues. If the peptide is part of an enzyme that is dissolved in the cytoplasm, where on the enzyme is this region likely to be located?

    A. In the active site of the enzyme
    B. In the allosteric site of the enzyme
    C. In the interior of the enzyme
    D. On the exterior of the enzyme

6. Which of the following setups would be most appropriate for isoelectric focusing of protein molecules?

    A. A pH gradient (0–14) from left to right, with the anode on the left and the cathode on the right
    B. A pH gradient (0–14) from right to left, with the anode on the left and the cathode on the right
    C. A pH gradient (0–14) from bottom to top, with the anode on the right and the cathode on the left
    D. A pH gradient (0–14) from top to bottom, with the anode on the right and the cathode on the left

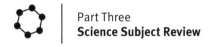
Organic Chemistry Practice Passage Explanations

1. (A)

At physiological pH, the carboxylic acid and the amino group of an amino acid have a negative charge and positive charge, respectively. This implies that if a molecule is to be negatively charged at physiological pH, the side chain must carry a negative charge. Based on this prediction, look for an amino acid with an acidic side chain. A match is found with an *acid* in **(A)**.

2. (A)

When calculating the pI for an amino acid, the side chain must be considered. In this case, the side chain is a relatively unreactive phenol group—which will remain uncharged until it donates a proton, requiring the pH to be near or above its pK_a. At a low pH, the amine group will be protonated and the carboxylic acid group will be neutral (as shown). At a pH equal to the pK_a of the carboxylic acid, approximately half of the carboxylic acids will be deprotonated and carry a negative charge. As the pH nears the pK_a of the protonated amino group, approximately half the amino groups will lose their proton and become neutral while the other half remains positively charged. The pH between these two pK_a values is where the number of ionized carboxyl groups and ionized amine groups is the same. This is the pI, which is calculated as the average of the two pK_a values: $pI = \dfrac{(2.24 + 9.04)}{2} = 5.64$ or **(A)**.

3. (C)

In the Strecker synthesis, before the ammonium attacks the aldehyde, the carbonyl carbon is sp^2 hybridized. This means the electrophile is planar, so the nucleophile can attack from either the top or the bottom. This implies that there will be a racemic mixture of amino acids (for all amino acids except glycine). D-amino acids are not useful biologically because essentially all amino acids in the body are of the L- form. This means that approximately half of the amino acids produced will not be useful, thus potentiating a disadvantage to Strecker synthesis, or **(C)**.

4. (B)

The correct form of glutamic acid is similar in chirality to the alanine shown in the question. This means that the configuration at the α-carbon should be *S*. The passage provides a few clues that can elucidate the molecular formula for glutamic acid. The second paragraph states that pyruvate can be aminated by glutamate to form alanine; in the process, glutamate is deaminated to α-ketoglutarate (pyruvate + glutamate alanine + α-ketoglutarate). Therefore, there must be five carbons in glutamate and its conjugate acid, glutamic acid. This rules out **(C)**. **(D)** can be eliminated because it lacks an amine group and is therefore not an amino acid. Between the remaining answers, **(B)** correctly matches the chirality shown in alanine.

5. (C)

The location of a certain section of a polypeptide chain depends on the types of amino acids contained in that chain. The chain in this question contains nonpolar amino acids, which are also known as hydrophobic amino acids. Interactions between these residues and water are energetically unfavorable, and hydrophobic amino acids will group together in a nonpolar environment. This means that they are unlikely to be located on any part of the enzyme that is exposed to water, so **(C)** is the correct answer.

6. (A)

This question asks how isoelectric focusing works in agar. The idea behind isoelectric focusing is that at a certain pH, the molecules are neutral; at other pH levels, the molecules have charges. Charged particles abide by Coulomb's law: they experience a force from other charges from the anode or cathode and accelerate. In an electrolytic cell, the anode is the source of positive charge and the cathode is the source of negative charge. Positively charged molecules migrate toward the cathode, and negatively charged molecules migrate toward the anode. Molecules become more positive as the conditions become more acidic. This means that the cathode should be on the opposite side of the gel from the acidic side so that when the protein is in acidic conditions and has a net positive charge, it will travel toward the basic side (the cathode). As the protein moves toward the cathode, the pH increases and the molecule begins to lose its positive charge. Once it has lost its charge, the protein will no longer experience a force from other charges and will stop moving. This matches **(A)**.

CHAPTER 13

Physics

Many students approach MCAT physics as a series of equations to memorize. However, the MCAT doesn't award points for simply recalling formulas. In addition, the majority of physics passages and questions on the exam are related to life sciences. What does this mean for you? It means that although you may not face questions about a watermelon shot out of a cannon, you likely will instead be expected to answer questions about things like laminar blood flow within the vasculature, using your knowledge of basic principles such as fluid dynamics.

It is no mystery that physics is one of the most dreaded content areas tested on the MCAT. However, understanding the fundamental concepts and having the ability to apply those concepts can separate the average test taker from an elite test taker. MCAT physics is not like an undergraduate course in physics. The MCAT focuses on conceptual understanding as well as the ability to choose the correct mathematical process. Many of the questions involve living systems and require outside knowledge. The better prepared you are for what you are going to see, the more confident you will feel on Test Day.

In this chapter, we will explore how the MCAT tests physics and what you need to know to maximize your score.

13.1 Reading the Passage

One of the worst things you can do as a test taker is to approach a physics passage with an attitude such as the following: "I'm going to read this entire passage, memorizing all of the details and data points as I go along, so that I won't need to waste time referring to the passage while I answer the questions." This approach results in a tremendous amount of time lost. No points are granted on the MCAT for reading and memorizing the passage. Trust the questions to dictate what details you need from the passage beyond the major takeaways. The passage will always contain information that appears testable but is simply not tested. Remember, the MCAT is asking you to apply what you know to the topic at hand. For some questions, the topic of the passage won't even be important; you'll simply need to apply your knowledge.

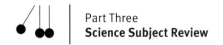

PASSAGE TYPES

The MCAT features two types of passages in the physics section as described in Table 13.1. Identifying the type of passage you are reading helps you to predict what is going to be important for the questions.

Information Passages

- Read like a textbook or journal article.
- Usually describe natural or synthetic phenomena.
- Often provide definitions of new terms.
- Commonly include diagrams of an apparatus.

Experiment Passages

- Consist of an experiment or multiple experiments conducted.
- Generally a variable is manipulated, a parameter is measured, and a conclusion is formed.
- A table or graph with data from the experiment may be presented, and you will likely be asked to interpret the data.
- When multiple experiments are performed, the similarities and differences between the experiments are likely to be tested.
- If making a small change to an experiment creates a radically different result, expect a question that requires you to interpret the results.

As you prepare for the MCAT, remember that your skill at identifying and absorbing what is important within a passage and skimming over what is not important directly translates into time saved and more points on Test Day.

	Information Passages	**Experiment Passages**
Goal	To present information	To summarize an experiment performed
Contents	Information about some phenomena, information presented in a predictable way, a new equation, considerable detail that may or may not be important	A hypothesis, a procedure, data (often in the form of charts and/or tables), a new equation; may consist of two or more experiments
How to read passages	Quickly identify where the details are located but no need to memorize; get the gist of each paragraph and move on to the next	Pay attention to the hypothesis behind the experiment, the procedure, and the outcome; if two experiments are conducted with drastically different results, pay attention to the differences between the experiments
Similar to	Textbook, journal article	Lab report

Table 13.1. MCAT Physics—Passage Types

READING AND DISTILLING THE PASSAGE

Regardless of how the passages in this section differ from those found in the other sections, the same Kaplan Method should be applied across all sciences. Read the passage quickly and efficiently; apply the Distill method best suited to the kind of information being conveyed.

- **Preview** for difficulty
  - Note the structure of the passage, the location of the paragraphs, and any figures such as charts, graphs, tables, or diagrams.
  - Determine whether the passage is an *experiment* or an *information* passage.
  - Determine the topic and the degree of difficulty.
  - Identify whether this passage requires a large time investment.
  - Decide whether this passage is one to do now or later.

- **Choose** your approach
  - Using information from the Preview step, Choose an appropriate Distill approach for the passage (Interrogate, Outline, or Highlight).
  - **Interrogation** should be chosen for experiment passages.
  - **Outlining** should be chosen for information passages that are dense or detail heavy.
  - **Highlighting** should be chosen for information passages that are light on details.

- **Read and Distill** key themes
  - While reading the passage, your aim is to distill the major takeaway of each paragraph and identify testable information using one of the following approaches.
  - **Interrogate:** Thoroughly examine the experiment passage by identifying the key components of experimental design and interrogating *why* specific procedures were done and *how* they connect to the overall purpose of the experiment.
  - **Outline:** Create a brief label for each paragraph that summarizes the contents of the paragraph, allowing you to return quickly to the passage when demanded by a question.
  - **Highlight:** Highlight one to three terms per paragraph that can pull your attention back to testable information when demanded by a question.

MCAT EXPERTISE

Physics passages often have paragraphs that describe equations. If there is an equation, determine its purpose as part of your Read and Distill step. This will allow you to return to it when needed. You can find the purpose of equations by asking, *What does this allow me to solve for?* In addition, if there is a paragraph that describes only variables, make a note of this as you will likely need this information later.

13.2 Answering the Questions

Physics questions on the MCAT have the same underlying demand: the test taker must have a solid foundation in physics. There are a few basic content questions in MCAT physics, but most of the questions require a higher level of conceptual thinking and integration with life sciences concepts. Therefore, well-developed critical-thinking skills are an essential requirement for attaining a high score on Test Day, especially with regard to physics.

As discussed previously, four types of questions appear in the science sections of the MCAT. Let's see how these four types of questions connect to MCAT physics.

- **Discrete questions**
  - Do not accompany a passage.
  - Always preceded by a warning such as, "Questions 12–15 do not refer to a passage and are independent of each other."
  - Invariably requires a thorough understanding of the science behind the question.
  - With a solid foundation in physics, these questions can be easy points on Test Day.
  - All of the information required is in the question stem, the answer choices, and your own outside knowledge.

- **Questions that stand alone from the passage**
  - Found in the question set after a passage, but the passage is not required to determine the correct answer.
  - These questions are really discrete questions hidden within the passage-based questions.
  - May be thematically related to the passage but require no further information from the passage.
  - In physics, these questions are very common.

- **Questions that require data from the passage**
  - Require data from the passage, but an understanding of the passage as a whole is not required.
  - To answer the question, you have to find the information in the passage and apply that information to determine the answer.
  - You have to know how to apply information from the passage to arrive at the correct answer.
  - The information in the passage is usually in the form of a variable or known quantity that must be used to find the answer.

- **Questions that require the goal of the passage**
  - This question type is most likely to appear following an experiment passage.
  - Cannot be answered solely by outside knowledge; an understanding of at least a portion of the passage is necessary.
  - A methodical approach and critical-reading skills, such as the Kaplan Method, are essential for correctly answering these questions.

ATTACKING THE QUESTIONS

Many test takers regularly misread questions or miss an important detail that drastically changes an answer. Furthermore, many test takers misinterpret the answer choices or misread a correct answer choice. The best way to avoid these mistakes is to adopt a systematic method for answering questions and to use this method on every single question. As a reminder, the Kaplan Method consists of four steps.

- **Type** the question
  - Read the question; peek at the answer choices for patterns, but don't analyze closely.
  - Assess the topic and the degree of difficulty.
  - Identify the level of time involvement: is this question likely to take a tremendous amount of time to identify the answer? If so, skip it and come back after you do the other questions in the passage set.
  - Good questions to do now are those that stand alone from the passage because these are generally quicker and require no passage research.

- **Rephrase** the question stem
  - Rephrase the question, focusing on the task(s) to be accomplished.
  - Simplify the phrasing of the original question stem.
  - Translate the question into a specific set of tasks to be accomplished using the passage and your background knowledge.

- **Investigate** potential solutions
  - Complete the task(s) identified in your Rephrase step.
  - Analyze the data; evaluate the experimental design; locate the information required; and connect the information, data, and experimental design with the information you already know.
  - Predict what you can about the answer.
  - Be flexible if your initial approach fails.

- **Match** your prediction to an answer choice
  - Search the answer choices for a response that is synonymous with your prediction, or eliminate answers that are not correct.
  - Select an answer and move on.
  - If you cannot find a match to your prediction, eliminate wrong answers, then select a response from the remaining choices and move on.

13.3 **Getting the Edge in Physics**

Obtaining an elite score on Test Day requires you not only to understand the fundamental concepts of physics but also to have the ability to apply these concepts and perform the required mathematical or critical-thinking operations. This ability starts with your foundation in physics. Memorizing the equations and hoping that the section will be all "plug and chug" is not enough. You need to know the equations and have a conceptual understanding of the physics behind the equations.

On Test Day, there will be two types of physics passages: information and experiment passages. On an information passage, the questions mostly focus on the information in the passage. You are likely to see many questions that do not require information from the passage. On experiment passages, a complete understanding of the experiment is required; this includes the hypothesis tested by the experiment, the details of how the experiment was done, and how to interpret the data obtained from the experiment. The questions accompanying an experiment passage likely require you to use information found in the passage as well as draw conclusions and make predictions based on the data provided.

A systematic method for answering questions is required to maximize your points on Test Day. In physics, the Kaplan Method helps you avoid making unnecessary mistakes while also maximizing your potential. Remember that correct answer choices match the appropriate sign and units for that particular vector or scalar quantity.

13.4 Preparing for the MCAT: Physics

The following presents the physics content you are likely to see on Test Day. Physics is one of the least commonly tested topics on the MCAT. The High-Yield badges will direct you to the specific physics topics that are tested most frequently.

KINEMATICS AND DYNAMICS

The MCAT tests the **SI units** that are related to the metric system, as shown in Table 13.2. The SI units include meter, kilogram, second, ampere, mole, kelvin, and candela.

Quantity	Unit	Symbol
Length	meter	m
Mass (*not weight*)	kilogram	kg
Time	second	a
Current	ampere (coulomb/second)	A
Amount of substance	mole	mol
Temperature	kelvin	K
Luminous intensity	candela	cd

Table 13.2. SI Units

Vectors are physical quantities that have both magnitude and direction. Vector quantities include displacement, velocity, acceleration, and force, among others. **Scalars** are quantities without direction. Scalar quantities may be the magnitude of vectors, like speed, or may be dimensionless, like coefficients of friction.

Vector addition may be accomplished using the tip-to-tail method or by breaking a vector into its components and using the Pythagorean theorem. Vector subtraction is accomplished by changing the direction of the subtracted vector and then following the procedures for vector addition. Multiplying a vector by a scalar changes the vector's magnitude. If the scalar is negative, then scalar multiplication will also reverse the vector's direction.

Multiplying two vectors using the **dot product** results in a scalar quantity. The dot product is the product of the vectors' magnitudes and the cosine of the angle between the vectors. In contrast, multiplying two vectors using the **cross product** results in a vector quantity. The cross product is the product of the vectors' magnitudes and the sine of the angle between the vectors. The right-hand rule is used to determine the resultant vector's direction.

Displacement is the vector representation of a change in position. It is path independent and is equivalent to the straight-line distance between the start and end locations. **Distance** is a scalar quantity that records the total length of the path traveled.

KEY CONCEPT

Dot product: $\mathbf{A} \cdot \mathbf{B} = |A|\,|B|\cos\theta$
Cross product: $\mathbf{A} \times \mathbf{B} = |A|\,|B|\sin\theta$

Velocity is the vector representation of the change in displacement with respect to time. **Average velocity** is the total displacement divided by the total time. **Average speed** is the total distance traveled divided by the total time. **Instantaneous velocity** is the limit of the change in displacement over time as the change in time approaches zero. **Instantaneous speed** is the magnitude of the instantaneous velocity vector. **Acceleration** is the vector representation of the change in velocity over time. Similar to velocity, either average or instantaneous acceleration may be considered.

KEY CONCEPT

$$F_g = \frac{Gm_1m_2}{r^2}$$

A **force** is any push or pull that has the potential to result in an acceleration. **Gravity** is the attractive force between two objects as a result of their masses.

Friction is a force that opposes motion. It results from electrostatic interactions at the surfaces of two objects in contact. **Static friction** exists between two objects that are not in motion relative to each other. **Kinetic friction** exists between two objects that are in motion relative to each other. The magnitude of static friction can take on any value, up to some maximum, and always cancels applied force in order to keep the object stationary. By contrast, once an object is in motion, the magnitude of kinetic friction is constant. The **coefficient of friction** depends on the two materials in contact. The coefficient of static friction is always higher than the coefficient of kinetic friction.

KEY CONCEPT

$$f_k = \mu_k N$$
$$f_s = \mu_s N$$
$$F_g = m\mathbf{g}$$

Mass and weight are not synonymous. **Mass** is a measure of the inertia of an object—its amount of material. **Weight** is the force experienced by a given mass due to its gravitational attraction to the earth.

KEY CONCEPT

$$F_{g,\parallel} = m\mathbf{g} \sin\theta$$
$$F_{g,\perp} = m\mathbf{g} \cos\theta$$

KEY CONCEPT

$$F_{net} = m\mathbf{a} = 0$$
$$F_{net} = m\mathbf{a}$$
$$F_{AB} = -F_{BA}$$

Newton's first law, or the **law of inertia**, states that an object remains at rest or remains in motion with a constant velocity if there is no net force acting on the object.

Newton's second law states that any acceleration is the result of the sum of the forces acting on the object and its mass.

Newton's third law states that any two objects interacting with one another experience equal and opposite forces as a result of their interaction.

KEY CONCEPT

$$\mathbf{v} = \mathbf{v}_0 + \mathbf{a}t$$
$$\mathbf{x} = \mathbf{v}_0 t + \frac{\mathbf{a}t^2}{2}$$
$$\mathbf{v}^2 = \mathbf{v}_0^2 + 2\mathbf{a}\mathbf{x}$$
$$\mathbf{x} = \bar{\mathbf{v}}t$$

Linear motion includes **free fall** and motion in which the velocity and acceleration vectors are parallel or antiparallel, whereas **projectile motion** contains both an *x*- and a *y*-component. Assuming negligible air resistance, the only force acting on the object is gravity. **Inclined planes** are another example of two-dimensional movement. It is often easiest to consider the dimensions as being parallel and perpendicular to the surface of the plane.

KEY CONCEPT

$$F_c = \frac{mv^2}{r}$$

Circular motion is best thought of as having both radial and tangential dimensions. In **uniform circular motion**, the only force is the **centripetal force**, pointing radially inward. The instantaneous velocity vector always points tangentially.

KEY CONCEPT

$$\tau = \mathbf{r} \times \mathbf{F} = rF \sin\theta$$

Free-body diagrams are representations of the forces acting on an object. They are useful for equilibrium and dynamics problems. **Translational equilibrium** occurs in the absence of any net forces acting on an object. An object in translational equilibrium has a constant velocity and may or may not also be in rotational equilibrium. **Rotational equilibrium** occurs in the absence of any net **torques** acting on an object. Rotational motion may consider any pivot point, but the center of mass is most commonly used. An object in rotational equilibrium has a constant angular velocity; on the MCAT, the angular velocity is usually zero.

WORK AND ENERGY

High-Yield

Energy is the property of a system that enables it to do something or to make something happen, including the capacity to do work. The SI units for all forms of energy are joules (J). **Kinetic energy** is energy associated with the movement of objects. It depends on mass and speed squared (not velocity).

Potential energy is energy stored within a system. It exists in gravitational, elastic, electrical, and chemical forms. **Gravitational potential energy** is related to the mass of an object and its height above a zero point, called a **datum.** **Elastic potential energy** is related to the **spring constant** (a measure of the stiffness of a spring) and the degree of stretch or compression of a spring squared. Additionally, **electrical potential energy** exists between charged particles. **Chemical potential energy** is stored in the bonds of compounds. The total **mechanical energy** of a system is the sum of its kinetic and potential energies.

Conservative forces are path independent and do not dissipate the mechanical energy of a system. If only conservative forces act on an object, then the total mechanical energy is conserved. Examples of conservative forces include gravity and electrostatic forces. Elastic forces, such as those created by springs, are nearly conservative.

Nonconservative forces are path dependent and cause dissipation of mechanical energy from a system. Although total energy is conserved, some mechanical energy is lost as thermal or chemical energy. Examples of nonconservative forces include friction, air resistance and viscous drag.

Work is a process by which energy is transferred from one system to another. It is often expressed as the dot product of force and displacement, which is calculated by multiplying the magnitudes of these two vectors and the cosine of the angle between them. Work may also be expressed as the area under a **pressure-volume (P-V) curve**, as shown in Figure 13.1.

KEY CONCEPT

$K = \frac{1}{2}mv^2$

KEY CONCEPT

$U = mgh$

$U = \frac{1}{2}kx^2$

KEY CONCEPT

$W = \mathbf{F} \cdot \mathbf{d} = Fd\cos\theta$

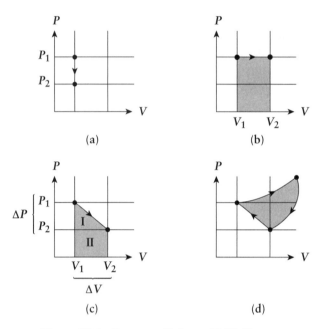

Figure 13.1. Pressure-Volume (P-V) Curves

KEY CONCEPT

$$P = \frac{W}{t} = \frac{\Delta E}{t}$$

Power is the rate at which work is done or energy is transferred. The SI unit for power is the watt (W). **The work-energy theorem** states that when net work is done on or by a system, the system's kinetic energy changes by the same amount. In more general applications, the work done on or by a system can be transferred to other forms of energy as well.

Mechanical advantage is the factor by which a simple machine multiplies the input force to accomplish work. The six **simple machines** are the inclined plane, wedge, wheel and axle, lever, pulley, and screw. Mechanical advantage makes it easier to accomplish a given amount of work because the input force necessary to accomplish the work is reduced. The distance through which the reduced input force must be applied, however, is increased by the same factor (assuming 100% efficiency).

The **load** is the output force of a simple machine, which acts over a given **load distance** to determine the work output of the simple machine. The effort is the input force of a simple machine, which acts over a given **effort distance** to determine the work input of the simple machine. **Efficiency** is the ratio of the machine's work output to work input when nonconservative forces are taken into account.

THERMODYNAMICS

High-Yield

The **zeroth law of thermodynamics** states that objects are in thermal equilibrium when they are at the same temperature. These objects therefore experience no net exchange of heat energy. **Temperature** is a qualitative measure of how hot or how cold an object is; quantitatively, temperature is related to the average kinetic energy of the particles that make up a substance.

A thermodynamic **system** is the portion of the universe that we are interested in observing, whereas the **surroundings** include everything that is not part of the system. **Isolated systems** do not exchange matter or energy with the surroundings. **Closed systems** exchange energy but not matter with their surroundings. **Open systems** exchange both energy and matter with their surroundings.

State functions like pressure, density, temperature, volume, enthalpy, internal energy, Gibbs free energy, and entropy are properties of a system that depend only on the difference between the system's initial and final state, and not on the pathway taken between initial and final state. By contrast, **process functions**, like work and heat, describe the pathway from one equilibrium state to another.

The **first law of thermodynamics** is a statement of conservation of energy: the total energy in the universe can never decrease nor increase. For a closed system, the total internal energy is equal to the heat flow into the system minus the work done by the system.

KEY CONCEPT

$\Delta U = q - W$

Heat is the process of energy transfer between two objects at different temperatures that occurs until the two objects come into thermal equilibrium. **Specific heat** is the amount of energy necessary to raise one gram of a substance by 1 degree Celsius or by 1 kelvin.

KEY CONCEPT

$q = mc\Delta T$

There are four special types of thermodynamic systems in which a given variable is held constant.

- For **isothermal processes**, the temperature is constant; the change in internal energy is therefore 0.
- For **adiabatic processes**, no heat is exchanged.
- For **isobaric processes**, the pressure is held constant.
- For **isovolumetric (isochoric) processes**, the volume is held constant and the work done by or on the system is 0.

The second law of thermodynamics states that in a closed system (up to and including the entire universe), energy will spontaneously and irreversibly go from being localized to being spread out (dispersed). **Entropy** is a measure of how spread out energy has become. On a statistical level, as the number of available **microstates** increases, the potential energy of a molecule is distributed over that larger number of microstates, thereby increasing entropy.

Of note, every **natural process** is ultimately **irreversible.** Under highly controlled conditions, certain equilibrium processes such as phase changes can be treated as essentially **reversible.**

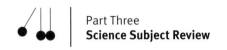

FLUIDS

High-Yield

Fluids are substances that have the ability to flow and conform to the shape of their containers. They can exert perpendicular forces, but not shear forces. Liquids and gases are both forms of fluids. **Solids** do not flow and they retain their shape regardless of their containers.

KEY CONCEPT

$$\rho = \frac{m}{V}$$

$$P = \frac{F}{A}$$

Density is the mass per unit volume of a substance (fluid or solid). **Pressure** is defined as a measure of force per unit area; it is exerted by a fluid on the walls of its container and on objects placed into the fluid. It is a scalar quantity and therefore has magnitude only, no direction. The pressure exerted by a gas against the walls of its container is always perpendicular (normal) to the container walls.

Absolute pressure is the sum of all pressures at a certain point within a fluid; it is equal to the pressure at the surface of the fluid (usually atmospheric pressure) plus the pressure due to the fluid itself. **Gauge pressure** is the name for the difference between absolute pressure and atmospheric pressure. In liquids, gauge pressure is caused by the weight of the liquid above the point of measurement.

KEY CONCEPT

$$P = \frac{F_1}{A_1} = \frac{F_2}{A_2}$$

$$F_2 = F_1\left(\frac{A_2}{A_1}\right)$$

Pascal's principle states that a pressure applied to an incompressible fluid will be distributed undiminished throughout the entire volume of the fluid, as shown in Figure 13.2. **Hydraulic machines** apply Pascal's principle to generate mechanical advantage.

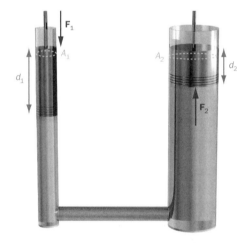

Figure 13.2. Hydraulic Lift
According to Pascal's principle, a force applied to an incompressible fluid adds pressure throughout. That pressure can magnify the original force if the pressure is applied to a greater area. Conservation of (displaced) volume means the larger force is applied over a shorter distance (energy is conserved in the process).

KEY CONCEPT

$$F_{buoy} = \rho_{fluid}V_{fluid\ displaced}g$$

$$F_{buoy} = \rho_{fluid}V_{submerged}g$$

Archimedes' principle governs the buoyant force. When an object is placed into a fluid, the fluid generates a **buoyant force** against the object that is equal to the weight of the fluid displaced by the object. Thus the direction of the buoyant force is always opposite to the direction of gravity. If the maximum buoyant force is larger than the force of gravity on the object, the object floats, and this occurs whenever the object is less dense than the fluid it is in. When the maximum buoyant force is smaller than the force of gravity on the object, the object sinks, and this occurs whenever the object is more dense than the fluid it is in. Fluids experience **cohesive** forces with other molecules of the same fluid and **adhesive** forces with other materials; cohesive forces give rise to **surface tension**.

Fluid dynamics is a set of principles regarding actively flowing fluids. **Viscosity** is a measurement of a fluid's internal friction, while **viscous drag** is a nonconservative force generated by viscosity. Fluids can move with either **laminar flow** or **turbulent flow**. On the MCAT, incompressible fluids are assumed to have laminar flow and very low viscosity while flowing, allowing us to assume conservation of energy.

The **continuity equation** is a statement of the conservation of mass as applied to fluid dynamics. This equation explains that flow rate is the product of linear speed and cross-sectional area. Because flow rate is constant, fluid moves more quickly through narrow spaces.

KEY CONCEPT

$$Q = v_1 A_1 = v_2 A_2$$

Bernoulli's equation is an expression of conservation of energy for a flowing fluid. This equation states that the sum of the **static pressure** and the **dynamic pressure** is constant between any two points in a closed system. For a horizontal flow, there is an inverse relationship between pressure and speed. In a closed system, there is a direct relationship between cross-sectional area and pressure exerted on the walls of the tube known as the **Venturi effect** (see Figure 13.3).

KEY CONCEPT

$$P_1 + \frac{1}{2}\rho v_1^2 + \rho g h_1 = P_2 + \frac{1}{2}\rho v_2^2 + \rho g h_2$$

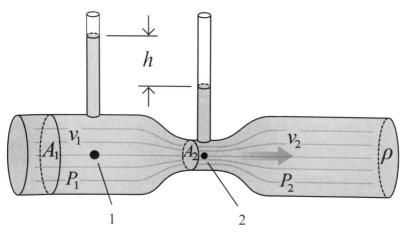

Figure 13.3. Venturi Flow Meter
According to the Venturi effect, where fluid speed is greater (in the narrower portion of the meter) the pressure is lower. Hence the fluid height above point 2 is lower than above point 1.

The circulatory system behaves as a closed system with nonconstant flow powered by the pumping heart. Arterial circulation is motivated by the heart. Venous circulation, with three times the blood volume of arterial circulation, is motivated by skeletal musculature and expansion of the heart. Blood vessels vary in diameter, and resistance decreases as the total cross-sectional area increases (such as at the aorta). Additionally, inspiration and expiration create a pressure gradient for the circulatory system as well.

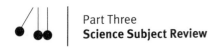
ELECTROSTATICS AND MAGNETISM

The SI unit of charge is the **coulomb**, and both protons and electrons possess the fundamental unit of charge ($e = 1.60 \times 10^{-19}$ C). Protons have greater mass and a positive charge, while electrons have negligible mass and a negative charge. These opposite charges exert **attractive** forces, while like charges exert **repulsive** forces.

Conductors allow the free and uniform passage of electrons when charged. In contrast, **insulators** resist the movement of charge and have localized areas of charge that do not distribute over the surface of the material.

KEY CONCEPT

$$F_e = \frac{kq_1q_2}{r^2}$$

Coulomb's law gives the magnitude of the electrostatic force vector between two charges, which always points along the line connecting the centers of the two charges. Every charge generates an **electric field**, which can exert forces on other charges. This electric field is the ratio of the force that is exerted on a test charge to the magnitude of that charge. Electric field vectors can be represented as **field lines**, which radiate outward from positive source charges and inward toward negative source charges. Positive test charges move in the direction of the field lines, and negative test charges move in the direction opposite of the field lines.

KEY CONCEPT

$$E = \frac{F_e}{q} = \frac{kQ}{r^2}$$

KEY CONCEPT

$$U = \frac{kQq}{r}$$

Electric potential energy is the amount of work required to bring the test charge from infinitely far away to a given position in the vicinity of a source charge. The electric potential energy of a system increases when two like charges move toward each other or when two opposite charges move farther apart. On the contrary, the electric potential energy of a system decreases when two opposite charges move toward each other or when two like charges move farther apart.

KEY CONCEPT

$$V = \frac{U}{q}$$
$$V = \frac{kQ}{r}$$

Electric potential is the electric potential energy per unit charge. Potential difference (**voltage**) is the change in electric potential that accompanies the movement of a test charge from one position to another. Potential difference is path independent and depends on only the initial and final positions of the test charge.

Test charges move spontaneously in whichever direction results in a decrease in their electric potential energy. Thus, positive test charges move spontaneously from high potential to low potential, while negative test charges move spontaneously from low potential to high potential.

Equipotential lines designate the set of points around a source charge or multiple source charges that have the same electric potential; these lines are always perpendicular to electric field lines. Work is done when a charge is moved from one equipotential line to another; however, the work is independent of the pathway taken between the lines. No work is done when a charge moves from a point on an equipotential line to another point on the same equipotential line.

KEY CONCEPT

$$\tau = pE \sin \theta$$

Two charges of opposite sign separated by a fixed distance d generate an **electric dipole** (see Figure 13.4). In an external electric field, an electric dipole experiences a net torque until it is aligned with the electric field vector. The electric field does not induce any translational motion in the dipole regardless of its orientation with respect to the electric field vector.

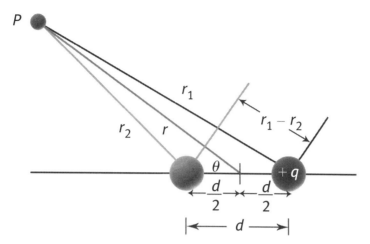

Figure 13.4. A Generic Dipole

Magnetic fields are created by magnets and moving charges; the SI unit for the magnetic field is the **tesla** (**T**; 1 T = 10,000 gauss). There are several forms of magnetic materials with variable properties. **Diamagnetic materials** possess no unpaired electrons and are slightly repelled by a magnet. **Paramagnetic materials** possess some unpaired electrons and become weakly magnetic in an external magnetic field. **Ferromagnetic materials** possess some unpaired electrons and become strongly magnetic in an external magnetic field.

Magnets have a north and a south pole as well as field lines that point from the north to the south pole. Current-carrying wires create magnetic fields in the shape of concentric circles surrounding the wire. The magnetic field for an infinitely long, straight, current-carrying wire is calculated differently from the magnetic field of a current-carrying circular loop.

External magnetic fields exert forces on charges moving in any direction except parallel or antiparallel to the field. Point charges may undergo uniform circular motion in a uniform magnetic field wherein the centripetal force is the magnetic force acting on the point charge. The direction of the magnetic force on a moving charge or a current-carrying wire is determined using the right-hand rule. The **Lorentz force** is the sum of the electrostatic and magnetic forces acting on a body.

KEY CONCEPT

$F_B = qv\mathbf{B} \sin\theta$

$F_B = Il\mathbf{B} \sin\theta$

CIRCUITS

Current is the movement of charge that occurs between two points of different electrical potentials. By convention, current is defined as the movement of positive charge from the high-potential end of a voltage source to the low-potential end. In many real-world circuits, the charge carriers are negative electrons, which actually move in the circuit from low potential to high potential.

Current flows only in **conductive materials**. **Metallic conduction** relies on uniform movement of free electrons in metallic bonds, while **electrolytic conduction** relies on the ion concentration of a solution. **Insulators** are materials that do not conduct a current.

KEY CONCEPT

$I = \frac{Q}{\Delta t}$

KEY CONCEPT

$I_{\text{into junction}} = I_{\text{leaving junction}}$

$V_{\text{source}} = V_{\text{drop}}$

Kirchhoff's laws express conservation of charge and energy. **Kirchhoff's junction rule** states that the sum of currents directed into a point within a circuit equals the sum of the currents directed away from that point. **Kirchhoff's loop rule** states that in a closed loop, the sum of voltage sources is always equal to the sum of voltage drops.

KEY CONCEPT

$R = \frac{\rho L}{A}$

Resistance is opposition to the movement of electrons through a material. Resistors are generally conductive materials with a moderate amount of resistance that slow down electrons without stopping them. Resistance is calculated using the resistivity, length, and cross-sectional area of the material in question.

KEY CONCEPT

$V = IR$

Ohm's law states that for a given resistance, the magnitude of the current through a resistor is proportional to the voltage drop across the resistor. Resistors in circuits can be combined to calculate the equivalent resistance of a full or partial circuit. Resistors in **series** (see Figure 13.5) are additive and sum together to create the total resistance of a circuit.

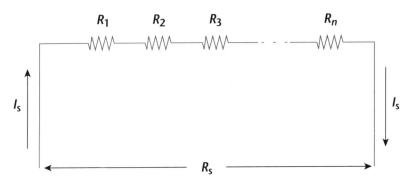

KEY CONCEPT

$R_s = R_1 + R_2 + R_3 + \cdots + Rn$

Figure 13.5. Resistors in Series

Resistors in **parallel** cause a decrease in equivalent resistance of a circuit. (See Figure 13.6.)

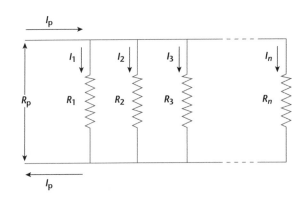

KEY CONCEPT

$\frac{1}{R_p} = \frac{1}{R_1} + \frac{1}{R_2} + \frac{1}{R_3} + \cdots + \frac{1}{R_n}$

Figure 13.6. Resistors in Parallel

KEY CONCEPT

$P = IV = I^2R = \frac{V^2}{R}$

Across each resistor in a circuit, a certain amount of power is dissipated, which is dependent on the current through the resistor and the voltage drop across the resistor.

Capacitors have the ability to store and discharge electrical potential energy. **Capacitance** in parallel plate capacitors is determined by the area of the plates and the distance between the plates. Capacitors in series (see Figure 13.7) cause a decrease in the equivalent capacitance of a circuit.

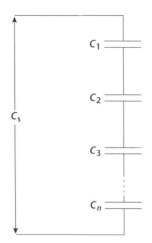

Figure 13.7. Capacitors in Series

KEY CONCEPT

$$\frac{1}{C_s} = \frac{1}{C_1} + \frac{1}{C_2} + \frac{1}{C_3} + \cdots + \frac{1}{C_n}$$

Capacitors in parallel (see Figure 13.8) sum together to create a larger equivalent capacitance.

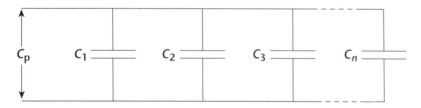

Figure 13.8. Capacitors in Parallel

KEY CONCEPT

$$C_p = C_1 + C_2 + C_3 + \cdots + C_n$$

Dielectric materials are insulators placed between the plates of a capacitor that increase capacitance by a factor equal to the material's **dielectric constant, κ.**

KEY CONCEPT

$C' = \kappa C$

Ammeters are inserted in series in a circuit to measure current; they have negligible resistance. **Voltmeters** are inserted in parallel in a circuit to measure a voltage drop; they have very large resistances and thus cannot be ignored when calculating the resistance of the complete circuit. **Ohmmeters** are inserted around a resistive element to measure resistance; they are self-powered and have negligible resistance.

WAVES AND SOUND

High-Yield

Sinusoidal waves may be either transverse or longitudinal (see Figure 13.9). During **transverse waves**, the material oscillates in a direction perpendicular to the direction of wave **propagation** (for example, electromagnetic waves). During **longitudinal waves**, the material oscillates in a direction parallel to the direction of wave propagation (for example, sound waves).

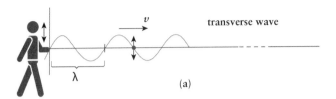

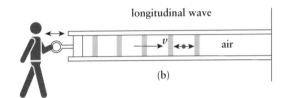

Figure 13.9. Wave Types

Displacement (x) in a wave refers to how far a point displaced by the wave is from the the point's **equilibrium position**, expressed as a vector quantity. The **amplitude** (A) of a wave is the magnitude of its maximal displacement. Similarly, the maximum point of a wave (point of most positive displacement) is called a **crest**, and the minimum point of a wave (point of most negative displacement) is called a **trough.** The **wavelength** (λ) of a wave is the distance between two crests or two troughs. (See Figure 13.10.)

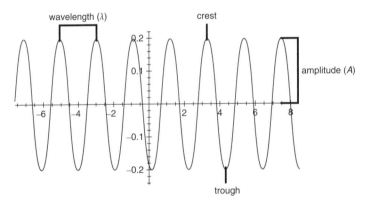

Figure 13.10. Anatomy of a Wave

KEY CONCEPT

$\omega = 2\pi f = \frac{2\pi}{T}$

$T = \frac{1}{f}$

The **frequency** (f) of a wave, measured in **hertz (Hz)**, is the number of cycles the wave makes per second. The **angular frequency** (ω) is another way of expressing frequency and is expressed in radians per second. The **period** (T) of a wave is the number of seconds required to complete a cycle; period is the inverse of frequency.

Interference describes the ways in which waves interact in space to form a **resultant wave** (see Figure 13.11). **Constructive interference** occurs when waves are exactly **in phase** with each other. The amplitude of the resultant wave is equal to the sum of the amplitudes of the two interfering waves. On the contrary, **destructive interference** occurs when waves are exactly **out of phase** with each other. The amplitude of the resultant wave is equal to the difference in amplitude between the two interfering waves. Interference does not always occur in absolutes; **partially constructive interference** and **partially destructive interference** occur when two waves are not quite perfectly in or out of phase with each other. The displacement of the resultant wave is equal to the sum of the displacements of the two interfering waves.

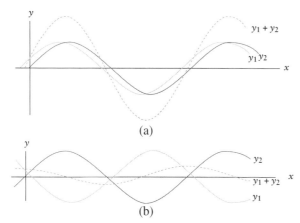

Figure 13.11. Phase Difference

Traveling waves have continuously shifting points of maximum and minimum displacement. **Standing waves** are produced by the constructive and destructive interference of two waves of the same frequency traveling in opposite directions in the same space. Such waves feature **nodes** (points where there is no oscillation) as well as **antinodes** (points of maximum oscillation).

Resonance is the increase in amplitude that occurs when a periodic force is applied at the **natural (resonant) frequency** of an object. The opposite of this effect is **damping**, which is a decrease in amplitude caused by an applied or a nonconservative force.

Sound is produced by mechanical disturbance of a material that creates an oscillation of the molecules in the material. These waves propagate through all forms of matter (but not in a vacuum). They move fastest through solids, followed by liquids, and slowest through gases. Within a medium, as density increases, the speed of sound decreases. The **pitch** of a sound is determined by the frequency of the wave.

The **Doppler effect** is a shift in the perceived frequency of a sound compared to the actual frequency of the emitted sound when the source of the sound and its detector are moving relative to one another. The apparent frequency is higher than the emitted frequency when the source and detector are moving toward each other. The apparent frequency is lower than the emitted frequency when the source and detector are moving away from each other. The apparent frequency can be higher, lower, or equal to the emitted frequency when the two objects are moving in the same direction, depending on their relative speeds. When the source is moving at or above the speed of sound, **shock waves** (**sonic booms**) can form.

MCAT EXPERTISE

The subtopic of sound is an MCAT favorite!

KEY CONCEPT

$$f' = f\frac{(v \pm v_D)}{(v \mp v_S)}$$

KEY CONCEPT

$$I = \frac{P}{A}$$

Loudness or volume of sound (**sound level**) is related to the sound's **intensity.** Intensity decreases over distance as some energy is lost to **attenuation** (damping) from frictional forces.

Strings and **open pipes** (open at both ends) support standing waves, and the length of the string or pipe is equal to some multiple of half-wavelengths. **Closed pipes** (closed at one end) also support standing waves, and the length of the pipe is equal to some odd multiple of quarter-wavelengths.

LIGHT AND OPTICS

Electromagnetic waves are transverse waves that consist of both an oscillating electric field and an oscillating magnetic field. These two fields are perpendicular to each other and to the direction of propagation of the wave.

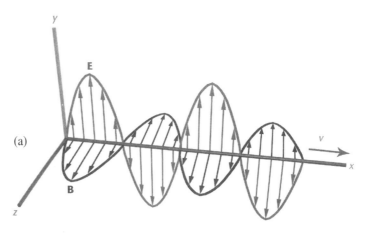

Figure 13.12. Electromagnetic Wave

The **electromagnetic (EM) spectrum** is the range of frequencies and wavelengths found in EM waves. These EM waves include, from lowest to highest energy, **radio waves, microwaves, infrared light**, visible light, **ultraviolet light, X-rays**, and **γ-rays** (gamma rays). The **visible spectrum** runs from approximately 400 nm (violet) to 700 nm (red).

KEY CONCEPT

$$\frac{1}{f} = \frac{1}{o} + \frac{1}{i} = \frac{2}{r}$$

Reflection is the rebounding of incident light waves at the boundary of a medium. The **law of reflection** states that the incident angle equals the angle of reflection, as measured from the normal. **Spherical mirrors** have **centers** and **radii of curvature** as well as **focal points**.

Concave mirrors are **converging** systems and can produce **real, inverted** images or **virtual, upright** images, depending on the placement of the object relative to the focal point. **Convex** mirrors are **diverging** systems and produce only virtual, upright images. (See Table 13.3.)

Plane mirrors also produce virtual, upright images; these images are always the same size as the object. They may be thought of as spherical mirrors with infinite radii of curvature.

Symbol	Positive	Negative
o	Object is in front of mirror	Object is behind mirror (extremely rare)
i	Image is in front of mirror (real)	Image is behind mirror (virtual)
r	Mirror is concave (converging)	Mirror is convex (diverging)
f	Mirror is concave (converging)	Mirror is convex (diverging)
m	Image is upright (erect)	Image is inverted

Table 13.3. Sign Convention for a Single Mirror

Refraction is the bending of light as it passes from one medium to another. The speed of light changes depending on the index of refraction of the medium, thereby causing refraction. The amount of refraction depends on the wavelength of the light involved; this behavior causes **dispersion** of light through a prism.

Snell's law (the law of refraction) states that there is an inverse relationship between the index of refraction and the sine of the angle of refraction (measured from the normal). **Total internal reflection** occurs when light cannot be refracted out of a medium and is instead reflected back inside the medium, as shown in Figure 13.13. This happens when light moves from a medium with a higher index of refraction to a medium with a lower index of refraction with a high incident angle. The minimum incident angle at which total internal reflection occurs is called the **critical angle.**

KEY CONCEPT

$n = \frac{c}{v}$

$n_1 \sin \theta_1 = n_2 \sin \theta_2$

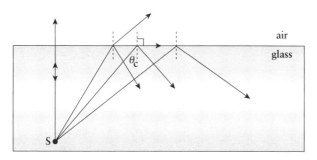

Figure 13.13. Total Internal Reflection

Lenses refract light to form images of objects. (See Table 13.4.) Thin symmetrical lenses have focal points on each side. Convex lenses are converging systems and can produce either real, inverted images or virtual, upright images. Concave lenses are diverging systems and produce only virtual, upright images.

Symbol	Positive	Negative
o	Object is on same side of lens as light source	Object is on opposite side of lens from light source (extremely rare)
i	Image is on opposite side of lens from light source (real)	Image is on same side of lens as light source (virtual)
r	Lens is convex (converging)	Lens is concave (diverging)
f	Lens is convex (converging)	Lens is concave (diverging)
m	Image is upright (erect)	Image is inverted

Table 13.4. Sign Convention For a Single Lens

Table 13.5 summarizes image creation in converging and diverging systems for both mirrors and lenses.

	Converging Systems					Diverging Systems
o relative to *f*	$o > 2f$	$o = 2f$	$2f > o > f$	$o = f$	$o < f$	all object distances
image	real, inverted, reduced	real, inverted, same	real, inverted, magnified	no image	virtual, upright, magnified	virtual, inverted, reduced

Table 13.5. Image Creation in Converging and Diverging Mirrors and Lenses

Diffraction is the bending and spreading out of light waves as they pass through a narrow slit, often producing a large central light fringe surrounded by alternating light and dark fringes with the addition of a lens. **Young's double-slit experiment** (see Figure 13.14) shows the constructive and destructive interference of waves that occur as light passes through parallel slits, resulting in minima (dark fringes) and maxima (bright fringes) of intensity.

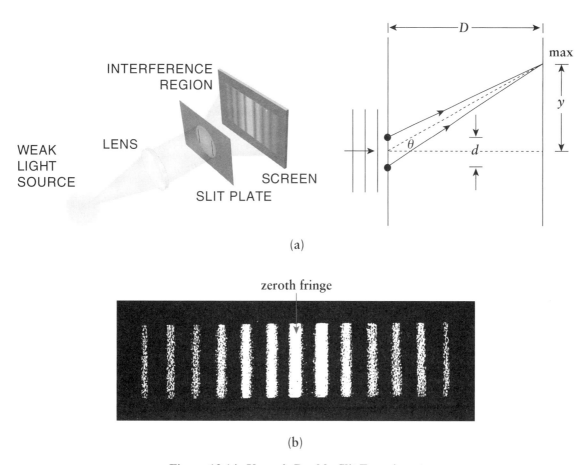

(a)

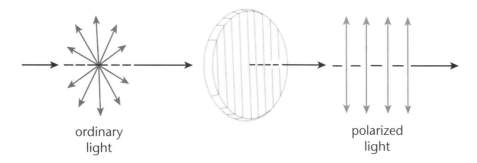

(b)

Figure 13.14. Young's Double-Slit Experiment

In **plane-polarized light**, all of the light rays have electric fields with parallel orientation. Plane-polarized light is created by passing unpolarized light through a **polarizer**, as shown in Figure 13.15.

ordinary
light

polarized
light

Figure 13.15. Plane-Polarized Light

In **circularly polarized light**, all of the light rays have electric fields with equal intensity but constantly rotating direction. Circularly polarized light is created by exposing unpolarized light to special pigments or filters.

ATOMIC AND NUCLEAR PHENOMENA

The **photoelectric effect** describes the ejection of an electron from the surface of a metal in response to a minimum light frequency known as the **threshold frequency.** The **work function** is the minimum energy necessary to eject an electron from a given metal. Its value depends on the metal used and can be calculated by multiplying the threshold frequency by **Planck's constant.** The greater the energy of the incident photon above the work function, the more kinetic energy each ejected electron can possess. Once ejected, electrons create a current proportional to the intensity of the incident beam of light.

The **Bohr model of the atom** states that electron energy levels are stable and discrete and that they correspond to specific orbits. An electron can jump from a lower-energy orbit to a higher-energy orbit by **absorbing** a photon of light of the same energy as the energy difference between the orbits. An electron can fall from a higher-energy to a lower-energy orbit, **emitting** a photon of light of the same energy as the energy difference between the orbits.

Absorption spectra may be impacted by small changes in molecular structure. **Fluorescence** occurs when a species absorbs high-frequency light and then returns to its **ground state** in multiple steps. Each step has less energy than the absorbed light and is within the visible range of the electromagnetic spectrum.

Nuclear binding energy is the amount of energy released when **nucleons** (protons and neutrons) bind together. The more binding energy per nucleon released, the more stable the nucleus is. The four fundamental forces of nature are the **strong** and **weak nuclear forces,** which contribute to the stability of the nucleus, the electromagnetic force, and gravitation.

The **mass defect** is the difference between the mass of the unbonded nucleons and the mass of the bonded nucleons within the nucleus. The unbonded constituents have more mass than the bonded constituents. Upon binding, some mass is converted into energy and released. So the mass defect accounts for the amount of mass converted to energy during nuclear fusion.

Fusion occurs when small nuclei combine into larger nuclei; **fission** occurs when a large nucleus splits into smaller nuclei. Energy is released in both fusion and fission because the nuclei formed in both processes are more stable than the starting nuclei.

Radioactive decay is the loss of small particles from the nucleus.

- During **alpha** (α) **decay**, an alpha particle (α, $^4_2\alpha$, $^4_2$He) is emitted. An alpha particle is a helium nucleus (two protons and two neutrons with zero electrons).
- **Beta-negative** (β^-) **decay** is the decay of a neutron into a proton, with emission of an electron (e^-, β^-) and an antineutrino (ν^-).
- **Beta-positive** (β^+) **decay**, also called **positron emission**, is the decay of a proton into a neutron, with emission of a **positron** (e^+, β^+) and a neutrino (ν).
- **Gamma** (γ) **decay** is the emission of a gamma ray, which converts a high-energy nucleus into a more stable nucleus.
- **Electron capture** is the absorption of an electron from the inner shell that combines with a proton in the nucleus to form a neutron.

Half-life is the amount of time required for half of a sample of radioactive nuclei to decay. In **exponential decay**, as shown in Figure 13.16, the rate at which radioactive nuclei decay is proportional to the number of nuclei that remain.

MCAT EXPERTISE

The subtopic of nuclear reactions is an MCAT favorite!

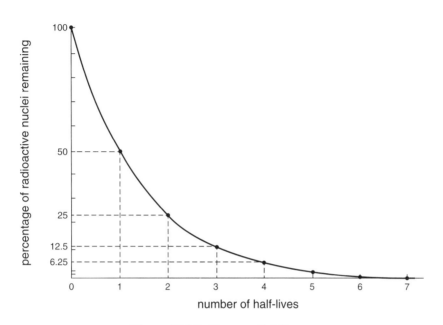

Figure 13.16. Exponential Decay

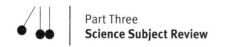
13.5 Physics Worked Examples

The following steps will walk you through the following passage using the Kaplan Passage Strategy.

PREVIEW FOR DIFFICULTY

The predominant feature of this passage is a pressure versus flow graph. Several lines on the graph show various degrees of stenosis, indicating this passage discusses the physics of cardiovascular disease. In addition, glancing at the first few words of each paragraph reveals the structure of the passage. The first paragraph discusses cardiovascular disease, the second discusses stenosis, and the third describes the experiment and accompanying graph. Let your comfort with the cardiovascular system and fluid dynamics determine whether this is a now or later passage for you.

CHOOSE YOUR APPROACH

Although this passage has two information paragraphs, the presence of the experiment and accompanying data makes this an experimental passage. As such, **Interrogation** should be chosen. With this choice in mind, still aim to read this passage efficiently; note test-worthy material and avoid getting caught up in the finer details.

READ AND DISTILL

P1: While reading the first paragraph, ask yourself: what is the purpose of this paragraph and how can this be tested on the MCAT? This paragraph describes atherosclerosis, which results in the narrowing or blockage. How can the MCAT test these concepts? Think Bernoulli, continuity, and Poiseuille!

P2: The second paragraph describes a relationship among stenosis, blood flow, and vascular pressure. From a content perspective, these variables are paralleled in circuitry by resistance, current, and voltage, respectively. Therefore, think Ohm's law! Finally, given our quick glance at the figure in the Preview step, this relationship is likely explored in the third paragraph.

P3: The third paragraph describes the experimental setup and accompanying data. The experiment manipulates the degree of stenosis while measuring the resulting change in pressure and flow. The paragraph also introduces terms: "PFLA," "normalized PFLA," and "loop slope." Interrogate by asking, *why would the author include these new terms?* They must be introduced to help the reader understand the data and outcomes, meaning test questions on these terms should be expected.

F1: Interrogation of Figure 1 should focus on identifying the key trends in the data. Begin with the accompanying legend: the graph shows five degrees of stenosis. This is the independent variable (IV). Relate any changes to the independent variable to changes in the dependent variables (DV). As the degree of stenosis increases, the PFLA (pressure-flow loop area) increases, as does the loop slope.

Armed with this interrogation, you should know what each paragraph contains and how each may be tested. In addition, you should have a general understanding of the experiment IVs, DVs, and the trends that connect them.

PHYSICS PASSAGE I: FLUID DYNAMICS

Cardiovascular disease is the leading cause of death in the world. It is primarily caused by atherosclerosis, which is characterized by thickening and hardening of the arterial walls resulting from the deposition of cholesterol, triglycerides, and other substances. The accumulation of cholesterol plaques within arteries causes stenosis, or narrowing, which in severe cases can drastically reduce the blood supply to downstream tissues and result in ischemia.

At low levels of stenosis, increasing stenosis causes dilation of the arteries to preserve flow up to the point where the vascular bed is maximally dilated. Further stenosis increases impedance to blood flow to the point where the blood flow starts to drop and becomes dependent on vascular pressure. Thus, at high levels of stenosis, increasing stenosis causes an increase in vascular pressure but a decrease in flow.

An experiment was performed to determine the relationship among the severity of stenosis, vascular blood pressure, and volumetric flow rate of blood. Controlled, artificial stenoses were induced in the femoral artery of a dog using an external balloon catheter. Vascular pressure and flow rate were measured simultaneously just proximal to the stenoses. The resulting pressure waves were plotted against the flow waves in the form of pressure-flow loop areas (PFLAs), as shown in Figure 1. Each loop in the figure is the sum of ten cardiac cycles and corresponds to a specific degree of stenosis. PFLA is sometimes expressed as normalized PFLA, the ratio of PFLA at a given degree of stenosis to the maximum PFLA observed at any degree of stenosis. The *loop slope*, which can be defined as the slope of the line passing through the lowest and highest points on the loop, corresponds to the relative increase in pressure required to increase the flow rate.

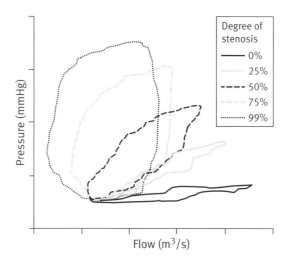

Figure 1. Pressure-flow loops corresponding to different stenosis levels

1. Based on the results of the experiment, which of the following graphs correctly depicts the relationship between normalized PFLA and the degree of stenosis?

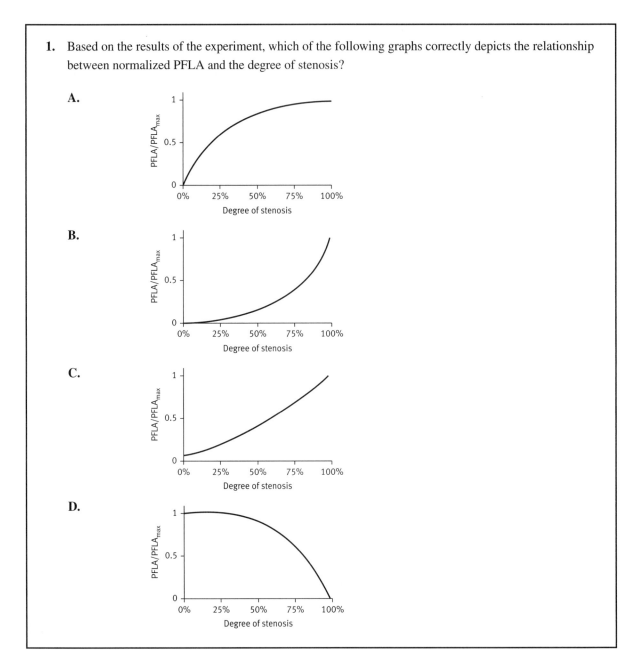

A.

B.

C.

D.

1 Type the question

The answer choices are graphs with stenosis and normalized PFLA along the *x*-axis and *y*-axis, respectively. Thus, this is a Skill 4 (Data and Statistical Analysis) question that tests the information presented in Figure 1. Take a moment to notice key differences among the answer choices. Choices **(A)**, **(B)**, and **(C)** all show a direct relationship but differ in the rate of increase and *y*-intercept.

② Rephrase the question stem

The answer choice patterns noted above allow us to Rephrase the question to, *How do normalized PFLA and stenosis relate?* In addition, differences between the answer choices direct us to pay close attention to the slopes and *y*-intercepts of the data.

③ Investigate potential solutions

First investigate PFLA and normalized PFLA in the third paragraph. The passage states that PFLA is the loop area—the amount of space inside each loop on the graph. Figure 1 shows that as the degree of stenosis increases, the PFLA increases. Thus we can predict a positive correlation between these two variables. Look at the *y*-intercept. When stenosis is 0 percent, the loop area is nonzero, which means the correct answer should have a positive *y*-intercept.

④ Match your prediction to an answer choice

Look at the answer choices. (**D**) has a negative correlation, so eliminate it. In the remaining answer choices, (**A**) and (**B**) have their *y*-intercepts at zero, so we can eliminate them. That leaves (**C**) as the correct answer. The graph in (**C**) shows a positive, almost linear correlation between normalized PFLA and degree of stenosis, which matches the data in Figure 1.

---

2. Which of the following statements about the variables described in the experiment in the passage is correct?

    A. Pressure and flow are independent variables, whereas degree of stenosis is the dependent variable.

    B. Degree of stenosis is the independent variable, whereas pressure and flow are dependent variables.

    C. Degree of stenosis, pressure, and flow are all independent variables.

    D. Degree of stenosis, pressure, and flow are all dependent variables.

---

① Type the question

The question and answer choices focus on passage-specific content in the form of experimental variables, specifically the independent and dependent variables. Thus, this question is a Skill 3 (Experimental and Research Design) question.

② Rephrase the question stem

The question stem can be Rephrased as, *What are the independent and dependent variables in the experiment?* Based on the answer choices, we need to determine the role of pressure, flow, and the degree of stenosis in the experiment.

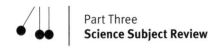
③ Investigate potential solutions

An independent variable is a causative factor in an experiment—a variable the researcher manipulates. A dependent variable is an output or effect of the experiment—a variable the researcher measures.

Paragraph 3 states that controlled, artificial stenoses are produced by a catheter. This degree of stenosis influences the vascular pressure and rate of blood flow, which are measured just proximal to the stenosis. Thus, the degree of stenosis is controlled by the researcher and, hence, is an independent variable. Pressure and flow, though, are effects of the stenosis and, hence, are dependent variables. Note that if you interrogated the passage as your Distill step, you would be ready to answer this question with very little investigation!

④ Match your prediction to an answer choice

Our prediction matches **(B)**.

---

3. The velocity of blood in a supine patient is 40 cm/s immediately proximal to a stenosis and 80 cm/s immediately distal to it. Assuming that the density of blood equals the density of water, how would the vascular pressures compare at those two points?

   A. The pressure at the proximal point is 240 Pa greater than the pressure at the distal point.
   B. The pressure at the distal point is 240 Pa greater than the pressure at the proximal point.
   C. The pressure at the proximal point is 480 Pa greater than the pressure at the distal point.
   D. Additional information is required to answer this question.

---

① Type the question

The question stem and associated answer choices indicate that an equation needs to be applied to a novel situation, specifically a clinical situation. This question appears to be focused on the physics topic area of fluids. Therefore, this question is a Skill 2 (Critical Thinking) question. No information from the passage is required to answer this question.

② Rephrase the question stem

The values and variables mentioned in the question stem and answer choices indicate that we should use Bernoulli's principle. Thus we can Rephrase this question as, *Apply Bernoulli's principle to find the difference between vascular pressures.*

3 Investigate potential solutions

Write the expression for Bernoulli's principle at the two points of interest. For this problem, the two points are the locations immediately proximal and distal to the stenosis. Hence, Bernoulli's equation for this problem can be written as follows:

$$P_p + \frac{1}{2}\rho v_p^2 + \rho g h_p = P_d + \frac{1}{2}\rho v_d^2 + \rho g h_d$$

Because the question stem states that the patient is supine, we can assume that $h_p \approx h_d$. This approximation cancels out the third term on both sides of the equation:

$$P_p + \frac{1}{2}\rho v_p^2 = P_d + \frac{1}{2}\rho v_d^2$$

The question stem provides the proximal and distal velocities and states that we should use the density of water, 1,000 kg/m^3, for the density of blood. By plugging these values into the above equation, we can determine the difference between the two pressures, $P_p - P_d$.

$$P_p + \frac{1}{2}\left(1{,}000\,\frac{kg}{m^3}\right)\left(0.4\,\frac{m}{s}\right)^2 = P_d + \frac{1}{2}\left(1{,}000\,\frac{kg}{m^3}\right)\left(0.8\,\frac{m}{s}\right)^2$$

$$P_p - P_d = 500\left(0.8^2 - 0.4^2\right)Pa = 500\left(0.64 - 0.16\right)Pa = 500\left(0.48\right)Pa$$

$$P_p - P_d = 240\,Pa$$

4 Match your prediction to an answer choice

Because $P_p - P_d$ is positive, the proximal vascular pressure exceeds the distal vascular pressure by 240 Pa. This matches **(A)**.

---

4. To transport blood efficiently throughout the body, blood vessels must run in parallel to one another. When analyzing a single blood vessel, which of the following statements about the volumetric rate of blood flow in the body is FALSE?

  A. Flow rate is directly proportional to the cross-sectional area of the blood vessel.
  B. Flow rate is directly proportional to the pressure drop along a blood vessel.
  C. Flow rate is inversely proportional to the viscosity of blood.
  D. Flow rate is directly proportional to the length of the blood vessel.

---

1 Type the question

The question stem describes the parallel "circuitry" of the cardiovascular system but specifically asks about volumetric blood flow. Though the question mentions concepts we associate with biology, the topic here seems to be fluid dynamics. The mention of parallel flow indicates circuits may also be an important topic area to consider. Because we will have to connect these ideas, this question is a Skill 2 (Critical Thinking) question.

2 Rephrase the question stem

A quick glance at the answer choices tells us that we need to consider flow rate carefully. In circuits, flow rate is analogous to current. In addition, recall that the current in parallel loops of a circuit can differ. Thus, we can Rephrase this question as, *How does flow rate connect the variables in the answer choices if flow rate is nonconstant?*

3 Investigate potential solutions

The variables in the answer choices (cross-sectional area, pressure drop, viscosity, length of blood vessel) and flow rate itself can be connected via Poiseuille's law:

$$\text{flow rate} = \frac{\pi(\Delta P)r^4}{8L\eta}$$

where ΔP is the pressure drop across the vessel, r is the radius of the vessel, L is the length of the vessel, and η is the viscosity of the fluid.

Avoid using the continuity equation in this situation as it assumes a constant flow rate, which is not the case in this scenario.

Let the recall of Poiseuille's law serve as your prediction. We can look at the answer choices and find the one that contradicts it.

4 Match your prediction to an answer choice

Look at **(A)**; although cross-sectional area is not explicitly stated in Poiseuille's law, it can be inferred from the radius. Flow rate would increase as radius increases, so **(A)** is true and can be eliminated. Similarly, both **(B)** and **(C)** are consistent with Poiseuille's law: flow rate is directly proportional to ΔP and inversely proportional to η. Therefore, we can eliminate these answers as well, leaving **(D)** as the only possible answer. According to Poiseuille's law, flow rate is inversely proportional to length, not directly proportional.

---

5. Based on information in the passage, when the degree of stenosis increases:
    A. PFLA increases and the loop slope decreases.
    B. PFLA increases and the loop slope increases.
    C. PFLA decreases and the loop slope increases.
    D. PFLA decreases and the loop slope decreases.

---

1 Type the question

The mention of *stenosis* in the question stem and of both *PFLA* and *loop slop* in the answer choices indicates analysis of Figure 1. Thus, this question is another Skill 4 (Data and Statistical Analysis) question. Because several other questions in this question set have also relied upon Figure 1, the Rephrase and Investigate steps are likely to be relatively quick: we know Figure 1 pretty well by this point!

② Rephrase the question stem

Using the structure of the answer choices, this question can be Rephrased as, *What is the relationship between the independent variable, degree of stenosis, and the dependent variables—PFLA and loop slope?* To answer this question, we need to know how the degree of stenosis influences PFLA and the loop slope.

③ Investigate potential solutions

If your Interrogation of the passage already yielded the trends between the IVs and DVs, let those trends serve as your prediction. If not, look at the graph in Figure 1 to determine the relationship among PFLA, the loop slope (which is defined in paragraph 3), and the degree of stenosis. Because the loops change incrementally from one extreme to another, we can use the loops at the two extremes to determine the effects of the degree of stenosis.

With zero stenosis, the loop area is the smallest and the line between the lowest and highest points is nearly horizontal (that is, close to zero). At the other extreme, 99 percent stenosis, the loop area gets larger and larger, so PFLA increases. The loop slope is much higher because the line between the lowest and highest points is nearly vertical. So both PFLA and loop slope should increase.

④ Match your prediction to an answer choice

Once we know that PFLA increases, we can eliminate **(C)** and **(D)**. Knowing that loop slope also increases makes **(B)** the correct answer.

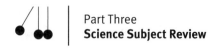

PHYSICS PASSAGE II: THERMODYNAMICS

Normal respiratory function is an autonomic nervous system process regulated by the pons and the medulla oblongata. However, injury or disease may impact this function such that a patient's own system cannot sustain itself with adequate respiration. Patients in these circumstances must receive outside assistance through mechanical ventilation. This assistance, meant to supplement or replace normal spontaneous breathing, can be accomplished through either a negative pressure system or a positive pressure system.

Several early ventilators, including the "iron lung," use *negative pressure* ventilation. This mechanism simulates the normal function of the respiratory system. In an iron lung, the patient's entire body, except the head and neck, is enclosed within a large chamber. To simulate inhalation, the iron lung removes air from the chamber, decreasing the pressure below that within the lungs, creating a pressure gradient. As a result, the lungs expand, which causes air from the environment to be sucked into the lungs. A typical iron lung might create a pressure gradient of -3 mmHg between the lungs and the outside air to generate an inspiration of 0.5 L.

Most modern ventilators, however, rely on *positive pressure* ventilation. Such a machine pressurizes the air slightly before delivering it to the patient, who often is intubated. In both mechanisms, expiration is facilitated when the ventilator ceases its pressure generation. This allows the thoracic cavity to return to initial pressure and volume as the natural elasticity of the chest wall pushes air out. The expiration happens quickly enough that it can be considered an adiabatic process.

1. For a patient on positive pressure mechanical ventilation, which of the following must necessarily be true regarding the air expired during one breath?

   A. No work is done.

   B. No overall change in internal energy takes place.

   C. The magnitude of work done is equal to the overall change in internal energy that takes place.

   D. The heat energy transferred is equal to the overall change in internal energy that takes place.

2. For the iron lung described in the passage, how much work does air do in inflating the patient's lungs? (Note: 1 mmHg = 133 Pa; 1 L = 10^{-3} m^3; $R = 0.0821 \dfrac{\text{L·atm}}{\text{mol·K}}$ or $8.31 \dfrac{\text{J}}{\text{mol·K}}$.)

   A. 50.46 J

   B. 0.49 J

   C. −0.49 J

   D. −50.46 J

3. A pulmonologist wants to conduct an experiment to determine if inspiration is an adiabatic process. To answer this question, which of these sets of quantities would he need to be able to measure?

   I. Pressure changes within the lung

   II. Temperature changes within the lung

   III. Volume changes within the lung

   A. I only

   B. II only

   C. II and III only

   D. I, II, and III

4. Suppose a mechanical ventilator existed that used the stepwise process illustrated here.

   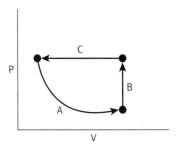

   Which of the following must be FALSE for this process?

   A. Temperature increases during step C.

   B. Internal energy increases during step B.

   C. No work is done during step B.

   D. Temperature remains constant during step A.

5. For a patient on negative pressure ventilation, the process of inhalation, with respect to the gas within the lungs, can best be described as:

   A. spontaneous, with entropy increasing.

   B. spontaneous, with entropy decreasing.

   C. nonspontaneous, with entropy increasing.

   D. nonspontaneous, with entropy decreasing.

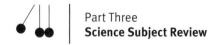
KEY CONCEPT

First law of thermodynamics
Gas laws
Thermodynamics
Respiratory system

USING THE KAPLAN METHOD

Preview the passage: At a glance, this passage is informational and fairly light on content specifics.

Choose your approach: Highlight

Read and Distill:

P1: Discusses the need for mechanical ventilation and the distinction between positive and negative pressure systems.
   Highlight: "Negative pressure system or a positive pressure system"

P2: Discusses negative pressure ventilation and explains the specifics of inhalation using negative pressure ventilation.
   Highlight: "*Negative pressure* ventilation" and "simulate inhalation"

P3: Briefly describes positive pressure ventilation but, more importantly, describes the exhalation process of both types of ventilation systems. Finally, we Highlight "adiabatic" because it is highly testable.
   Highlight: "*Positive pressure* ventilation," "in both mechanisms, expiration," and "adiabatic"

---

1. For a patient on positive pressure mechanical ventilation, which of the following must necessarily be true regarding the air expired during one breath?

   A. No work is done.

   B. No overall change in internal energy takes place.

   C. The magnitude of work done is equal to the overall change in internal energy that takes place.

   D. The heat energy transferred is equal to the overall change in internal energy that takes place.

---

① Type the question

Here we're asked to find a true statement about positive pressure ventilation. Look at the answer choices; our answer involves work and internal energy. Thus, this question is a thermodynamics question.

② Rephrase the question stem

All the answer choices contain terms found in the first law of thermodynamics, $\Delta U = Q - W_{\text{by the system}}$. The question can be Rephrased as, *What must be true when applying the first law of thermodynamics to exhalation?*

③ Investigation potential solutions

Positive pressure ventilation is described in paragraph 3, in particular in the last sentence. We are told that we can assume that expiration can be considered an adiabatic process. By definition, the heat exchanged in an adiabatic process is zero. Because no heat is transferred, $Q = 0$. So according to the first law of thermodynamics, $\Delta U = -W$. This is our prediction.

④ Match your prediction to an answer choice

By looking at the answer choices one at a time, we can eliminate **(A)** because work is done. Similarly, because work is done, there is a change in internal energy, so **(B)** is false. **(D)** is incorrect because no heat is transferred in an adiabatic process. **(C)**, though, matches our conclusion exactly; so it must be the correct answer.

KEY CONCEPT

Work
Gas laws

---

2. For the iron lung described in the passage, how much work does air do in inflating the patient's lungs? (Note: 1 mmHg = 133 Pa; 1 L = 10^{-3} m^3; $R = 0.0821 \dfrac{\text{L·atm}}{\text{mol·K}}$ or $8.31 \dfrac{\text{J}}{\text{mol·K}}$.)

   A. 50.46 J
   B. 0.49 J
   C. −0.49 J
   D. −50.46 J

---

① Type the question

The question stem tells us that we're going to calculate the work done in inflating the lungs. A quick look at the answer choices tells us that the magnitude and sign of the answer are more important than the exact value. In addition, although the units in the answer choices and provided constants indicate the topic is thermodynamics, these terms also indicate the need to do unit conversions.

② Rephrase the question stem

Recall that the iron lung is an example of negative pressure. Therefore, this question can be Rephrased as, *What is the work done by the air in a negative pressure system?*

THINGS TO WATCH OUT FOR

Noticing differing units and other answer choice patterns during the Type step can help you avoid careless errors and trap answers in your Investigate and Match steps.

---

3 Investigate potential solutions

THINGS TO WATCH OUT FOR

If you recognize that a problem is going to involve a multi-step calculation, consider triaging the problem for later.

Because paragraph 2 describes the iron lung and gives us information on pressure and volume, the work formula we'll need is $W = P\Delta V$. The key question here is what value to use for P. The −3 mmHg in paragraph 2 is the gradient formed, not the actual pressure involved. Because 1 atm ≈ 760 mmHg, 3 mmHg is a small enough number that we can ignore it; so we can assume the actual pressure is 1 atm. Now we can use our work formula:

$$W = P\Delta V = (1\text{ atm})(0.5\text{ L}) = 0.5\text{ L·atm}$$

This result gives us a work value in L·atm, but the answer choices are all in joules. We can use the two values of R provided to make this conversion. Because the denominators are the same, it follows that 8.314 J = 0.0821 L·atm. Use that ratio to convert the work to joules:

$$0.5\text{ L·atm} \times \frac{8.31\text{ J}}{0.0821\text{ L·atm}} \approx 0.5\text{ L·atm} \times 100\ \frac{\text{J}}{\text{L·atm}} = 50\text{ J}$$

4 Match your prediction to an answer choice

Based on the magnitude of our estimate, we can eliminate (**B**) and (**C**). Here, the tissue of the lungs is stretched outward by the air as the air expands the lungs, implying that the tissue gains energy and the air loses energy. A loss of energy indicates positive work, so the air does positive work as the air inflates the lungs. Thus the correct answer is (**A**).

---

3. A pulmonologist wants to conduct an experiment to determine if inspiration is an adiabatic process. To answer this question, which of these quantities would need to be monitored during the experiment?

   I. Pressure within the lung

   II. Temperature within the lung

   III. Volume within the lung

  A. I only

  B. II only

  C. II and III only

  D. I, II, and III

---

1 Type the question

This question is a Roman numeral question asking which quantities—pressure, temperature, and/or volume—would need to be measured to determine if a process is adiabatic. Roman numeral questions offer extra opportunities to eliminate and are often a good choice to work now.

2 Rephrase the question stem

Because this question focuses solely on the definition of adiabatic processes, it doesn't require any information from the passage. This question can be Rephrased as, *What is an adiabatic process and how can it be identified?*

3 Investigate potential solutions

By definition, in an adiabatic process, $Q = 0$ because no heat flows into or out of the system. Therefore, the change in internal energy equals the work done: $\Delta U = -W_{\text{by the system}}$. So to determine whether the process is adiabatic, we need to be able to calculate the work done as well as the internal energy of the system and then determine if the two quantities are equal. Now we can further simplify the question to, *What quantities do we need to know to measure ΔU and $-W_{\text{by the system}}$?*

4 Match your prediction to an answer choice

Look at our answer choices. Item II, temperature, comes up in three choices. If it's wrong, three answers will be eliminated and only one will be possible. However, internal energy is $U = \frac{3}{2}nRT$, so we need temperature. Thus, item II is correct, and we can eliminate **(A)**.

We can eliminate the two remaining wrong answers by considering the definition of thermodynamic work, $W = P\Delta V$. Thus, measuring the work would require knowing both temperature and volume. The correct answer is **(D)**; we need all three quantities.

THINGS TO WATCH OUT FOR

Sometimes trap answers are answers that would be correct for a slightly different question. For example, in this question, **(B)** would be correct if the question were asking about an isothermal process.

KEY CONCEPT

First law of thermodynamics
P-V diagram
Work

---

4. Suppose a mechanical ventilator existed that used the stepwise process illustrated here.

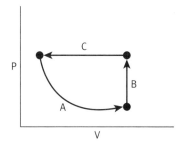

Which of the following must be FALSE for this process?

A. Temperature increases during step C.
B. Internal energy increases during step B.
C. No work is done during step B.
D. Temperature remains constant during step A.

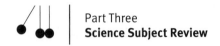

① Type the question

This question is asking for a false statement about the process shown in the pressure-volume diagram. Because this question gives us a new diagram to study, it's unlikely we will need any information from the passage. We do, however, need our knowledge of thermodynamics, especially the types of processes depicted in the diagram. As this is a FALSE question, it is a good option to triage for later in the passage set.

② Rephrase the question stem

Because the question stem is already simplified, we can Rephrase it to an actionable step, *Consider the changes in pressure and volume in each step to evaluate the answer choices.*

③ Investigate potential solutions

Step B is isovolumetric (or isochoric): the pressure increases, but volume remains constant. Pressure-volume work is given by $P\Delta V$, so no work is done. From the ideal gas law, $PV = nRT$, we can also conclude that if V is constant, temperature is proportional to pressure; so the temperature will increase as well. If temperature increases, internal energy also increases. **(B)** and **(C)** both agree with these statements, so neither of them is the answer we seek.

In step C, pressure is constant while volume decreases. Using $PV = nRT$ once more, we can conclude that if pressure is constant and volume decreases, T will decrease as well.

④ Match your prediction to an answer choice

MCAT EXPERTISE

If a question asks for what "must be" or "is necessarily" true/false, then what "could be" true/false is never good enough.

(A) says that temperature increases during step C when it should decrease; because **(A)** is a false statement, it's the answer we're looking for.

As for step A, because we don't have enough information to determine whether PV remains constant or changes, we can't definitively conclude whether **(D)** is true or false. The question stem keeps us from worrying about that, however. The question asks for a statement that *must* be false, not one that could possibly be false.

5. For a patient on negative pressure ventilation, the process of inhalation, with respect to the gas within the lungs, can best be described as:

    A. spontaneous, with entropy increasing.
    B. spontaneous, with entropy decreasing.
    C. nonspontaneous, with entropy increasing.
    D. nonspontaneous, with entropy decreasing.

❶ Type the question

This question asks us to consider inhalation in negative pressure ventilation and determine (1) whether inhalation is a spontaneous process and (2) whether we would expect entropy to increase or decrease.

❷ Rephrase the question stem

To answer this question, we need the description from paragraph 2 of how negative pressure ventilation works. We also need our knowledge of spontaneous processes and entropy. Thus, we can Rephrase the question stem as, *Is the flow of gas into the lungs spontaneous in negative pressure ventilation?*

❸ Investigate potential solutions

Paragraph 2 tells us that in negative pressure ventilation, "the iron lung removes air from the chamber, decreasing the pressure below that within the lungs, creating a pressure gradient." The movement of gas from areas of higher pressure to areas of lower pressure occurs naturally and should proceed without any outside forces. So the expansion should be considered spontaneous.

What happens, though, to the entropy? Entropy is a measure of dispersion of energy, often viewed as randomness; it is proportional to the number of gas particles in a system. Because air enters the lungs during inhalation, the number of moles of gas in the lungs tends to increase. Therefore, the entropy should increase as well.

❹ Match your prediction to an answer choice

Once we know the process is spontaneous, we can eliminate (**C**) and (**D**). Determining that the entropy in the lungs must increase allows us to eliminate (**B**) and select (**A**) as the correct answer.

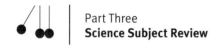

13.6 **Physics on Your Own**

PHYSICS PASSAGE (QUESTIONS 1–5)

The rhythmic contraction of the heart is initiated by the firing of myogenic electrical impulses at the sinoatrial node located in the wall of the right atrium. Any deviation from the normal range of 60–100 rhythmic heartbeats/minute in adults is classified as cardiac dysrhythmia, a potentially fatal condition. Defibrillators can reset the heart and reestablish the normal functioning of the sinoatrial node by delivering therapeutic doses of electrical energy to the heart. A circuit diagram of a defibrillator is shown in Figure 1.

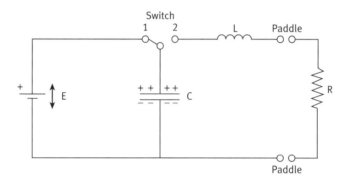

Figure 1. Circuit diagram of a defibrillator with paddle electrodes

A typical defibrillator consists of a capacitor (C), an inductor (L), and a power supply. When the switch is in position 1, the defibrillator is in charging mode, and the power supply E is used to store charges across the plates of the capacitor. The work done to charge the capacitor is stored as potential energy U in the capacitor and can be calculated as follows:

$$U = \frac{1}{2} A \kappa \varepsilon_0 E^2 d$$

where A is the area of the capacitor plates, κ is the dielectric constant, ε_0 is the permittivity of free space, and d is the distance between the capacitor plates.

When the switch is in position 2, the defibrillator is in discharging mode and the circuit is completed by the patient, who is represented as a resistor R in the circuit diagram. Metal paddles with insulated handles are held on the patient's skin with about 25 pounds of force to deliver the stored electrical energy of the capacitor to the patient. To prevent the capacitor from discharging and delivering its stored energy too quickly, the inductor is used to prolong the duration of current flow.

1. A defibrillator consisting of a 5 mF capacitor with a distance of 10 mm between its plates is powered by a step-up transformer that supplies peak voltages of 10,000 V. What is the maximum electrical energy that can be delivered by this capacitor to a patient?

   A. 25×10^{-3} J
   B. 0.5 J
   C. 25 J
   D. 50 J

2. Many standard defibrillators exhibit a type of defibrillation waveform known as a biphasic waveform, as depicted here.

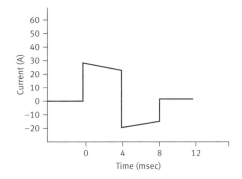

   What is the magnitude of the total charge delivered in a single biphasic current pulse of such a defibrillator?

   A. 85 μC
   B. 170 μC
   C. 85 mC
   D. 170 mC

3. The following diagram shows the raw electrocardiograph (ECG) data of a person with a healthy heart. The graph shows superimposed noise from the 60 Hz power supply and motion artifacts from breathing. Given the standard ECG wave here, what are the heart rate and respiratory rate, respectively, for this individual?

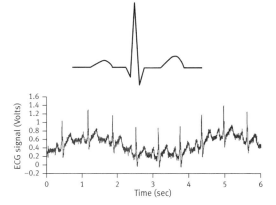

   A. 1.5 Hz, 0.25 Hz
   B. 25 Hz, 5 Hz
   C. 60 Hz, 12 Hz
   D. 80 Hz, 20 Hz

4. A defibrillator is used to deliver 50 J of energy to a patient over a period of 20 msec. If the current flowing through the inductor component of the defibrillator is 2 A, what is the effective resistance of the electrical pathway through the patient?

   A. 250 Ω
   B. 625 Ω
   C. 850 Ω
   D. 1,250 Ω

5. Gel is applied to the skin where the electrodes of a defibrillator will be placed. This is most likely done to:

   A. minimize electrical conductance of the body and reduce the possibility of serious burns to the skin.
   B. maximize electrical conductance of the body and reduce the possibility of serious burns to the skin.
   C. minimize electrical conductance of the body and ensure that a sufficiently high amount of electrical energy is delivered to the myocardial tissue
   D. maximize electrical resistance of the body and ensure that a sufficiently high amount of electrical energy is delivered to the myocardial tissue.

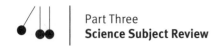

Physics Practice Passage Explanations

1. (C)

The first step is to set up an equation for energy stored by a capacitor. The maximum electrical energy that can be delivered by a capacitor is equal to the energy stored by the capacitor, which, according to the passage, is given as follows:

$$U = \frac{1}{2} A \kappa \varepsilon_0 E^2 d$$

However, because the question stem provides us with only the values for E, C, and d, we need to rewrite the equation in terms of those variables. It is necessary to know that $C = \dfrac{A \kappa \varepsilon_0}{d}$, which rearranges to give $A \kappa \varepsilon_0 = Cd$. Hence, the equation for potential energy can be written as follows:

$$U = \frac{1}{2} C E^2 d^2$$

The second step is to plug in the values for E, C, and d, taking into account the conversion of units to standard SI units:

$$U = \frac{1}{2}\left(5 \times 10^{-3}\ \text{F}\right)\left(10 \times 10^{-3}\ \text{m}\right)^2 \left(10^4\ \text{V}\right)^2 = 25\ \text{J}$$

Hence, the correct answer is **(C)**, 25 J.

2. (D)

The first step is to calculate the area under the pulse from 0 to 4 msec. That portion of the graph can be divided into a triangle and a rectangle. The triangular portion has a height of about 5 A, so the area of the triangle is $\frac{1}{2}(5\ \text{A})(4\ \text{msec}) = \frac{1}{2} \times 5\ \text{A} \times 4\ \text{msec} = 10\ \text{mC}$. The rectangular portion has a height of about 25 A, so the area of the rectangle is $25\ \text{A} \times 4\ \text{msec} = 100\ \text{mC}$. Hence, the total charge delivered by this portion of the biphasic waveform is 110 mC.

The next step is to calculate the area under the pulse from 4 to 8 msec. The triangular portion in this area of the graph has a height of 5 A, so the area of the triangle is 10 mC, like in step 1. However, the rectangular portion

here has a height of about 15 A (remember to consider only magnitude), so the area of the rectangle is 15 A × 4 msec = 60 mC. Thus, the total charge delivered by this portion of the biphasic waveform is 70 mC.

The final step is to calculate the total charge delivered by the biphasic pulse. The total charge delivered by a single biphasic current pulse is simply the sum of the two calculations: 110 mC + 70 mC = 180 mC. This is closest to **(D)**, which is the correct answer.

3. (A)

The first step is to calculate the heart rate. A single heartbeat translates into an ECG signal that looks like the following waveform, which is known as the PQRST signal.

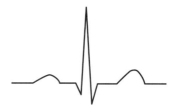

The ECG data in the question stem shows that nine cycles are completed in 6 seconds; this gives 9 cycles/6 s = 1.5 Hz for the heart rate. At this point, we have sufficient information to answer the question.

However, let's look at calculating the respiratory rate as well. The PQRST signal looks like it is superimposed on a slower wave in the ECG data shown in the question stem. The slower wave must be the motion artifact from breathing because the power supply line has a relatively high frequency of 60 Hz. This completes slightly less than 2 cycles in 6 seconds, giving a frequency of slightly less than 2/6 Hz, or less than 0.33 Hz. This is closest to **(A)**, which is the correct answer. **(B)** is off by about a magnitude of ten for each rate. **(C)** is the lower end of the range for the heart rate and respiratory rate when measuring the beats and breaths per minute. **(D)** is the upper end of the range for the heart rate and respiratory rate when measuring the beats and breaths per minute.

4. (B)

The question describes the defibrillator in the discharging mode—that is, the switch is in position 2. First, calculate the power delivered by the defibrillator:

$$P = \frac{\Delta E}{\Delta t} = \frac{50 \text{ J}}{20 \times 10^{-3} \text{ s}} = 2,500 \text{ W}$$

Next, calculate the resistance offered by the patient. Because the inductor and the effective resistance of the patient are in series, the current flowing through the inductor is the same as that flowing through the resistance. The power of this effective resistance is given by $P = I^2R$, which can be rearranged to solve for R. By plugging in the values for I and P, we get:

$$R = \frac{P}{I^2} = \frac{2,500 \text{ W}}{(2 \text{ A})^2} = \frac{2,500}{4} \, \Omega = 625 \, \Omega$$

Hence, the resistance of the electrical pathway through the patient is 625 Ω, which is **(B)**.

5. (B)

Gel acts as a conductor and ensures a better connection between the paddles and skin. This reduces the electrical resistance and thus increases the conductance offered by the patient to the discharging defibrillator. If the resistance offered by the skin was too high, the power delivered to the patient's skin by the defibrillator would be too high because $P = I^2R$. Higher resistance on the skin therefore would transfer dangerously high amounts of energy to the skin, which could result in skin burns. **(B)** is the correct answer. **(A)** is the opposite of the correct answer choice. **(C)** is opposite, as application of gel maximizes electrical conductance of the body. **(D)** actually makes the same claim as **(C)**. Resistance is the reciprocal of conductance. So maximizing resistance equals minimizing conductance. Therefore **(D)** is wrong for the same reason as **(C)**.

PART FOUR

Critical Analysis and Reasoning Skills

CHAPTER 14

Arguments and Formal Logic

The MCAT is ultimately a test of critical thinking. As such, the ability to characterize, understand, and assess arguments plays an important role. The use of formal logic is an important tool in working with arguments as they appear on the MCAT. Mastery of arguments and understanding formal logic allow for deeper understanding of the stated information and will be essential to obtaining a high score on Test Day. Of all the CARS questions, 30 percent involve Reasoning Within the Text and 40 percent require Reasoning Beyond the Text. You can expect more than three-quarters of your points on the CARS questions to benefit from clear logical thinking. To provide a solid foundation for your mastery of arguments and formal logic, we'll start by examining arguments and then move on to using formal logic in arguments.

14.1 What Is an Argument?

In its most basic form, an argument is simply a statement composed of two stated parts, the evidence and conclusion, and one or more unstated but implied parts, the assumption(s) or implication(s). Arguments as they appear on the MCAT have nothing to do with heated debates. Instead, they are simply conclusions the author makes (regardless of whether they are actually true or false), accompanied by the evidence the author uses to back up his or her conclusion. There are three levels of arguments that we call the **domains of discourse**: the basic difference between the three is very simply things *vs.* words *vs.* ideas. Though the domains can never be entirely separated from one another, each has distinctive parts and relationships that must not be confused.

DOMAINS OF DISCOURSE

- The **natural domain** corresponds to objects, events, and experiences—everything that can be found in the world around us.
- The **textual domain** corresponds to words, sentences, and paragraphs—everything that directly faces you in an MCAT passage.
- The **conceptual domain** corresponds to concepts, claims, and arguments—everything that underlies logic.

KEY CONCEPT

Logic is the formal study of arguments. It falls into the conceptual domain of discourse.

A **concept** is an idea that has a clear meaning or definition, but is not by itself true or false. A concept is distinct from the words that represent the concept, and from the objects or events that may exemplify a concept; rather a concept is the idea itself. Two or more concepts can be related in various ways, and often these relationships are indicated by **Relation keywords,** such as the very common Continuation and Contrast keywords, or the more rare Opposition, Sequence, and Comparison keywords.

KEY CONCEPT

Claims are the middlemen in the logical hierarchy, composed of concepts and their relationships and, in turn, composing arguments. Claims consist of at least a subject and a predicate. Claims have both meaning and truth value (the capacity to be true or false).

KEY CONCEPT

Unstated claims in arguments are known as inferences. Inferences are either assumptions (unstated evidence) or implications (unstated conclusions).

14.2 What Are the Elements of Arguments?

CONCEPTS

It might seem obvious, but the fundamental element of a logical argument is an idea, called a **concept.** Concepts have **meanings** but are not necessarily true or false. Note, though, that the CARS questions can employ synonyms and paraphrases of ideas in different wording than that used in the passage. In short, it will be essential on Test Day to look for concept-for-concept correspondences, not exact word-for-word matches.

CLAIMS

What distinguishes a **claim** from a mere concept is **truth value,** the capacity to be either true or false. Claims may be quite complex, potentially consisting of numerous concepts related together in diverse ways. However, having a truth value requires only a minimum of two parts: a **subject** and a **predicate,** such as "The yeti is ten feet tall."

- **Claims** can also be called assertions, statements, propositions, beliefs, or contentions.
- Claims are made up of combinations of concepts and relations of concepts.
- Claims possess truth value and can thus be true or false.
- Claims can also be related through various relationships.
  - If two claims are **consistent** (compatible or in agreement) with one another, then both can be true simultaneously.
  - If two claims are **inconsistent** (contradictory or conflicting) with one another, then it is impossible for both to be true simultaneously.
  - If one claim **supports** another, then this claim being true would make the other claim more likely to be true as well.
  - If one claim **challenges** (refutes or objects to) another, then this claim being true would make the other claim more likely to be false.

INFERENCES, ASSUMPTIONS, AND IMPLICATIONS

Although concepts and claims represent the stated parts of arguments, authors will often neglect to explicitly state parts of their arguments, due either to a lack of space, a desire to hide weak or irrelevant parts of their arguments, or a failure to recognize the missing parts. You will likely see an abundance of questions that require you to identify these missing parts, called inferences, which can be subdivided into assumptions and implications.

- **Inferences** are unstated parts of arguments. One way to recognize an inference is by the negative effect it would have on the argument if the inference was denied.
  - **Assumptions** are unstated pieces of evidence.
  - **Implications** are unstated conclusions.
- Inferences are claims that must be true or—at the very least—must be highly probable.

COUNTERARGUMENTS

A **counterargument** is an argument made against a conclusion. Some authors will offer only counterarguments, their purpose being to argue against some claim. Other authors raise counterarguments merely for the sake of refuting them, which is an indirect way for an author to support their own conclusion.

KEY CONCEPT

Counterarguments, also called refutations, objections, or challenges, are the opposite of evidence because they go against the conclusion.

14.3 How Will Arguments Be Tested?

INFERENCE AND ASSUMPTION QUESTIONS

Your skill in parsing arguments is most directly tested on the MCAT by implication and assumption questions, often asking what would weaken or strengthen them.

- There are three main ways of strengthening an argument:
  - One could provide a new piece of evidence that supports the conclusion.
  - One could support evidence that already exists, further supporting the conclusion.
  - One could challenge refutations against the conclusion.
- There are three main ways of weakening an argument:
  - One could provide a new refutation that goes against the conclusion.
  - One could support refutations that already exist.
  - One could challenge evidence for the conclusion.

ANALOGICAL REASONING QUESTIONS

The MCAT will also pose questions based on analogies, using the similarities between two things to argue for an additional commonality between them. The **known** entity is the one with characteristics that have already been established. The **unknown** entity is the one that is only partially understood. In some cases, the passage provides the known term, with its various characteristics, and the question gives the new context that establishes the unknown. In such questions, you are being asked to extrapolate, extend, or apply the ideas from the passage to a new situation. So you can take the information from the passage as a given.

MCAT EXPERTISE

Analogical Reasoning questions are a subtype of Apply questions. Apply questions involve applying passage information to new information provided in the question. In the case of Analogical Reasoning questions, application of passage information is done to identify which answer choice is most analogous (often sharing the same logical framework) to claims and concepts of the passage.

- An analogy can be strengthened by greater similarity between the known and unknown. The more points of similarity between the two, the stronger the analogy.
- The more relevant (structural as opposed to superficial) the similarities are between the two, the stronger the analogy. Alternatively, the fewer relevant differences there are between the two, the stronger the analogy.

14.4　**What Is Formal Logic?**

The most abstract application of logic, formal logic, examines patterns of reasoning to determine which ones necessarily result in valid conclusions. Formal logic consists of a conditional statement (e.g., if I am in Pennsylvania) and a necessary result (e.g., then I am in the United States). As you see, the conditional statement is sufficient to necessarily bring about the result. On the MCAT, arguments made using conditional claims, with conditional relationships, are featured in some form in every passage and play some role in most CARS questions.

14.5　**What Are the Elements of Formal Logic?**

CONDITIONALS

A **conditional** is a unidirectional relationship that exists between two terms.

- Conditionals can be represented with language (if **X**, then **Y**) or symbols (X → Y).
- The **antecedent** (**X**) can also be called a **sufficient condition**, **evidence** (in cases of justification), or a **cause** (in cases of causation).
- The **consequent** (**Y**) can also be called a **necessary condition**, a **conclusion** (in cases of justification), or an **effect** (in cases of causation).
- A **conditional claim** is true if it is impossible to have a true antecedent and a false consequent simultaneously.
- Operations of formal logic can be represented in a **truth table** (Table 14.1).

X	Y	X → Y
true	true	**true**
true	false	**false**
false	true	**true**
false	false	**true**

Table 14.1. Truth Table for Conditional Claims

APPLICATIONS FOR CONDITIONALS

Conditionals can function in several different ways in CARS passages and questions. Of the terms discussed in the following list, justification and causation are the most common ways that conditionals are used.

- **Justification** is the relationship of logical support between a piece of evidence and its conclusion.
- **Causation** is the one-way relationship of the antecedent leading to the consequent (cause and effect).
- **Correlation** is the relationship of two events accompanying one another.
- **Whole-parts relationship:**
  - One concept can be a part of another concept (the whole) in the conceptual domain.
  - One component or characteristic can be part of an object in the natural domain.

SUFFICIENT *VS.* NECESSARY

Sufficient and necessary refer to the one-way relationship between the antecedent (X) and the consequent (Y) and the impossibility of having an antecedent without its consequent. Revisiting the previous example, if you are in Pennsylvania (antecedent), then that is sufficient evidence to prove that you are in the United States (consequent). When put another way, the antecedent (X) is called a sufficient condition because if it is true, this is sufficient to say that the consequent (Y) is also true. On the other hand, if you are not in the United States at all, then you are *certainly* not in Pennsylvania. So being in the United States is necessary if you hope to have any chance of being in Pennsylvania specifically. For this reason, the consequent (Y) is called a necessary condition because in order for the antecedent (X) to be true, it is necessary that the consequent (Y) be true.

CONTRAPOSITIVE

Whenever an author makes any kind of conditional claim (if X, then Y), it is always possible to translate the conditional claim into other relationships, most notably the contrapositive. By definition, the contrapositive of "if X, then Y" is "if not Y, then not X." In the contrapositive, the X and Y terms switch positions, with the Y term now first. We've already seen one example: Our conditional claim was, "If you're in Pennsylvania, then you are in the United States." Turning this claim around into the contrapositive, "If you are not in the United States, then you are not in Pennsylvania." The contrapositive can be represented using a tilde (~) to stand for negation (~X thus means "not X" or "the negation of X"):

Conditional: $X \rightarrow Y$

Contrapositive: $\sim Y \rightarrow \sim X$

One of the most useful Test Day reasons for forming the contrapositive is that it's a guaranteed inference, a logical equivalent for any conditional claim made in a passage.

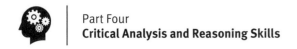
14.6 How Will Formal Logic Be Tested?

The MCAT will not provide you with a formal logic statement and require you to form the contrapositive. However, using formal logic will allow you to dig deeper into claims. If, for example, the condition is that all lions are mammals and you form the contrapositive that if it's not a mammal, it's not a lion, you have the information you need to answer a question about mammals and lions. Appreciating the general characteristics of formal logic will clarify your thinking and garner you many additional points.

14.7 Getting the Edge Using Arguments and Formal Logic

As we said in the beginning of this book, the MCAT is ultimately a test of critical thinking. That skill is manifest in your ability to recognize an argument, take it apart (sometimes using formal logic), and answer questions based on it. Although academic texts can be vague and subject to interpretation, every question you face in the CARS section will have only one defensible answer. The value of logic is precisely in its ability to clarify your thinking, allowing you to mirror the cognitive processes the test makers use to write the questions and to identify correct responses.

However, the abstract knowledge of arguments is not enough. The only way to be successful with the CARS questions is to practice questions and passages. Every question that you get wrong on a practice passage or question is an opportunity to review how you approached the question. Systematically reviewing questions to determine weaknesses in your critical-thinking skills will help you identify and address those weaknesses. If you find that you are stuck at a score plateau on practice tests, it is essential to take an honest look at your critical-thinking skills to break through that plateau.

CHAPTER 15

CARS Question Types

The MCAT is fundamentally a test of critical thinking, and this fact becomes very evident in the CARS section. Here you are not reading for the sake of reading but, instead, thinking about what you read to answer a range of question types. It's important to be able to identify each type because different question types are more efficiently answered with different approaches. As you go through the question types you'll see in this chapter, remember that there are no MCAT points to be had in reading a passage; all your points are in the questions. The more efficiently you can identify and attack a question, the greater your opportunity to answer the question correctly.

15.1 What Kinds of Questions Will You Be Asked?

Questions accompanying CARS passages range from ones that can be answered simply by referring to the passage text to those that require thinking about what is not stated but is implied in the text. Thus, question types require different approaches, involve different levels of difficulty, and ask you to think in different ways. You will have questions that require you simply to use the information in the text, called Foundations of Comprehension questions; questions that require deeper reasoning about the information in the text, called Reasoning Within the Text questions; and a third category that requires you to integrate new information, called Reasoning Beyond the Text questions. Regardless of the complexity of question type, all correct answers result in the same number of points. Think clearly and carefully about each question before you answer it.

15.2 Foundation of Comprehension Questions

Although there are a variety of Foundations of Comprehension question types, these questions have in common the fact that the answer can be found directly in the text or can be directly inferred from it. In this way, Foundations of Comprehension questions test your ability to identify basic components of a passage such as main ideas, examples, and arguments. From there, this question category requires inferring meaning from these components.

MAIN IDEA

MCAT EXPERTISE

According to our research of released AAMC material, Main Idea questions make up about 5 percent of the CARS section (about three questions).

Main Idea questions ask for the author's primary goal; why did the author write the passage? Less commonly, these questions can ask who the intended audience of the text is or what kind of publication would print this passage (e.g., magazine, journal, editorial).

Attacking Main Idea Questions

- **Type:** Main idea questions often contain words such as *central thesis*, *primary purpose*, or *main idea*. As these questions deal with the goal of the passage, they are best attacked *now*.
- **Rephrase:** Main idea questions are really asking, *Why did the author write this passage?*
- **Investigate:** Evaluate the major takeaway of each paragraph and consider how each paragraph builds to the overall goal of the passage. In addition, incorporate the author's tone in your prediction (positive versus negative, extreme versus moderate) as the author's tone can allow you to eliminate wrong answers quickly.
- **Match:** Match your prediction to an answer choice. If there is no clear match or if you cannot perform any of the earlier steps of the Kaplan Method for the CARS questions, use the process of elimination.
  - Wrong answer choices may be too narrow (Faulty Use of Detail) or too broad (Out of Scope). For example, a wrong answer may describe the purpose of a particular paragraph instead of the passage as a whole.
  - Wrong answer choices may have the wrong tone (positive, negative, ambivalent, or impartial) or wrong degree (too extreme or too moderate).

DETAIL

MCAT EXPERTISE

Scattered Detail questions can ask, which of the following did the author NOT state? As a result, these questions can demand testers to locate three separate passage references in order to eliminate the wrong answers. As a result, Scattered Detail questions can be inordinately time consuming. So triage these questions for later in the passage when you'll have greater familiarity with the passage.

Detail questions ask about details that are stated explicitly in the passage. Detail questions are the most likely to use the **Scattered** format, which uses Roman numeral options or words such as *EXCEPT*, *NOT*, or *LEAST*.

Attacking Detail Questions

- **Type:** Detail questions tend to use words and phrases such as *the author states* or *according to the passage*, with declarative language such as the words *is* and *are*. With the exception of Scattered detail questions, these questions are often best attacked *now*.
- **Rephrase:** Detail questions are really asking, *What did the author say?*
- **Investigate:** Before scanning the entirety of the passage hoping for the relevant portion of text to jump out at you, use content buzzwords in the question stem and the products of your Distill step (interrogative questions, passage outline, or highlighted terms) to determine where the relevant information is found. Reread the relevant sentence as well as the sentences before and after. Create your prediction by rephrasing the detail in your own words.
  - Make the prediction brief so you can repeat it to yourself between answer choices.
  - For Scattered Detail questions, locate all three of the wrong answers in the passage and eliminate them from the options.

MCAT EXPERTISE

According to our research of released AAMC material, Detail questions make up about 16 percent of the CARS section (about nine or ten questions).

- **Match:** Match your expectations to the right answer. If there is no clear match or if you cannot perform any of the earlier steps of the Kaplan Method for the CARS questions, use the process of elimination.

INFERENCE

Inference questions demand identifying the unstated parts of arguments. The answers must be true given what is claimed in the passage. Unstated parts of arguments include assumptions and implications. **Assumptions** are unstated evidence and **implications** are unstated conclusions. Whether the question demands identifying an assumption or implication, in both cases the correct answer is the choice that *must* be true based on the passage information.

Attacking Inference Questions

- **Type:** Inference questions often contain words such as *assume*, *because*, *conclude*, *imply*, *infer*, *justify*, *reasonable*, or *suggest*. These question stems can also be vague, often without any specific passage reference. Therefore it is advantageous to save inference questions for later.
- **Rephrase:** Inferences questions are really asking, *What must be true based on a passage argument or the passage as a whole?*
- **Investigate:** Determine whether you are looking for an assumption or an implication. Then determine which claim the answer is supposed to support (for assumption questions) or be supported by (for implication questions). Once you have identified the appropriate claim, consider the major arguments of the passage to make a general prediction.
  - For assumption questions, the answer is either similar to the evidence given or links the evidence to the conclusions.
  - For implication questions, the answer is either similar to the conclusions given or is another logical conclusion one could draw from the evidence.
- **Match:** If the question allows for a focused prediction, Match your prediction to an answer choice. If there is no clear match or if your prediction is more general, use a special form of the process of elimination called the Denial Test:
  - Negate each answer choice.
  - Whichever answer choice—when negated—has the most detrimental effect on the argument made in the passage is the correct answer choice.

MCAT EXPERTISE

Although the Denial Test always reveals the correct answer in an Inference question, it's very time-consuming. If you cannot set good expectations for the right answer during the Investigate step, triage the question and return to it later with the Denial Test.

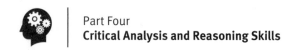

DEFINITION-IN-CONTEXT

Definition-in-Context questions ask you to define a word or phrase as it is used in the passage. These questions often call attention to the term to be defined using quotation marks or italics. To answer these questions, you have to consider *why* the author chose that particular word or phrase. In this way, Definition-in-Context questions require reading for purpose at the word/phrase/term level.

Definition-in-Context questions always reference a word, a phrase, or in rare cases, an entire claim from the passage.

Attacking Definition-in-Context Questions

- **Type:** Definition-in-Context questions can be quickly identified as they often have a passage reference and use language such as *in the context of passage, as used by the author,* or *most synonymous.* Because these questions point to specific parts of the passage, these questions are best attacked now.
- **Rephrase:** Definition-in-Context questions are really asking, *What does the author mean when using <phrase> in <paragraph>?*
- **Investigate:** Reread the sentence with the word or phrase and perhaps the surrounding context. Paraphrase the author's definition of the term in your own words as your prediction.
- **Match:** Match your prediction to an answer choice. If there is no clear match or if you cannot perform any of the earlier steps of the Kaplan Method for the CARS questions, then use the process of elimination.

KEY CONCEPT

Reading for Purpose

Both Main Idea and Definition-in-Context questions demand the reader to read for purpose. The Function question type in Reasoning Within the Text category of questions also demands this mode of reading. Simply put, each of these question types requires asking the question, *why did the author write/include this?* The difference between these question types is the scope of purpose.
- Main Idea: Why did the author write this passage?
- Function: Why did the author include this claim/paragraph?
- Definition-in-Context: Why did the author include this word/phrase?

15.3 **Reasoning Within the Text Questions**

KEY CONCEPT

Reading for Reasoning

This mode of reading aims to identify the connections that exist between different parts of a text. To facilitate reading for reasoning, practice asking yourself, *how* is this portion of the text different from what comes before it and *how* does this portion relate to what comes after it? Reading for reasoning is not done isolation. To read for reasoning effectively, you must also read for purpose by asking *why* the author wrote this portion of text.

Unlike Foundations of Comprehension questions, which demand that you identify components of a passage or infer their meaning, Reasoning Within the Text questions require that you see the connections between different components of a passage. In this way, these question types incorporate reasoning skills. The two most common question types in this category are Function questions and Strengthen–Weaken questions. *Reasoning Within the Text* questions account for 30 percent of the CARS questions you'll encounter on Test Day, according to the AAMC's official statements.

FUNCTION

Function questions ask about the author's purpose in writing a specific portion of the passage. These questions are similar to Main Idea questions. However, Function questions are narrower in scope as they focus on the purpose of only one portion of the passage (usually one sentence or one paragraph).

Attacking Function Questions

- **Type:** Function questions tend to use words such as *purpose*, *motive*, or *intention* or completions such as *in order to* or *because*. These questions are best attacked *now* since answering them will help deepen your understanding of the passage and therefore help you answer later questions.
- **Rephrase:** Function questions are really asking, *Why did the author include this portion of text?* or *What is the purpose of this portion of text?*
- **Investigate:** Use the products of your Distill approach (interrogative questions, passage outline, or highlighted terms) to locate the specific portion or portions of text referenced in the question stem. Reread those portions, and formulate a prediction about how they fit into the purpose of the paragraph and the overall passage.
- **Match:** Match your prediction to an answer choice. If there is no clear match or if you cannot perform any of the earlier steps of the Kaplan Method for the CARS questions, then use the process of elimination, removing any answer that conflicts with the author's main argument or the paragraph's purpose.
  - ○ Answer choices addressing the purpose of the passage, instead of the specified portion of text, are common traps in Function questions. Often, these answer choices are too broad and do not answer the question (Out of Scope/Faulty Use of Detail).
  - ○ Wrong answer choices may have the wrong tone (positive, negative, ambivalent, or impartial) or wrong degree (too extreme or too moderate).

MCAT EXPERTISE

Function questions, like Main Idea and Definition-in-Context questions, require *reading for purpose*. If you frequently miss questions in these three question types, that may indicate issues with understanding the author's purpose or identifying the organization and structure of the passage.

STRENGTHEN–WEAKEN (WITHIN)

Strengthen–Weaken questions concern the logical relationship between conclusions and the evidence that strengthens them or the refutations that weaken them. There are two subtypes: Strengthen–Weaken (Within) and Strengthen–Weaken (Beyond). Questions requiring information beyond the passage are discussed later in this chapter.

Attacking Strengthen–Weaken (Within) Questions

- **Type:** These questions often contain words such as *relate*, *support*, *challenge*, *relevance*, *significance*, or *impact*. These can be *now* or *later* questions depending on your passage familiarity when encountering the question.
- **Rephrase:** Strengthen–Weaken (Within) questions are really asking, *How do the concepts presented in the passage strengthen or weaken one another?*
- **Investigate:** Determine the two claims and the connection between them; you are usually given at least one of these elements and have to find the other(s).
  - ○ Identify where each piece of the argument can be found: in the question stem, in the passage, or in the answer choices.
  - ○ If no claims are given in the question stem, plan to triage and answer the question by the process of elimination later.
  - ○ If one claim is given in the question stem, determine whether it is a conclusion, a piece of evidence, or a refutation.
  - ○ If two claims are given in the question stem, identify the relationship between them.

  No matter the structure of the question, research the relevant text to determine the missing claim or the connection between them as your prediction. Use logic keywords to help assemble the argument.
- **Match:** Match your prediction to an answer choice. If there is no clear match or if you cannot perform any of the earlier steps of the Kaplan Method for the CARS questions, then use the process of elimination.

OTHER REASONING WITHIN THE TEXT QUESTIONS

Even though you will see mostly Function and Strengthen–Weaken questions representing the Reasoning Within the Text category, you should be able to identify three more types of questions that are also Reasoning Within the Text questions.

- **Clarification questions** ask for statements that are roughly synonymous. However, the clarifying statement tends to be supporting evidence for the conclusion because the statement is more specific or exact.
  - These questions often contain words such as *clarify*, *explain*, or *reflect*.
  - Approach these questions similarly to Strengthen–Weaken (Within) questions except that the meanings of the two claims are roughly synonymous.
- **Weakness questions** ask for implicit refutations to arguments discussed in the passage.
  - These questions often contain phrases such as *implicit weaknesses* or *reasonable objections*.
  - The correct answer to a Weakness question is the answer choice that is most detrimental to the argument made in the passage. Note that this strategy is similar to the use of the Denial Test for Inference questions, except that the answer choices in Weakness questions do not need to first be negated. Simply choose the answer that is the most detrimental as written.
- **Paradox questions** ask for the resolution of an apparent logical contradiction.
  - These questions often contain words such as *paradox*, *dilemma*, or *discrepancy*.
  - Approach these questions using the process of elimination, eliminating out any answer choice that is inconsistent with one or both of the claims of the paradox or with the passage as a whole.

KEY CONCEPT

Answering a Weakness question is just like using the Denial Test for Inference questions. The difference is that the correct answer choice is detrimental to the arguments in the passage without being negated.

KEY CONCEPT

A paradox is a set of two claims that appear to be inconsistent on the surface. The correct answer in a Paradox question is consistent with both of the claims and usually attempts to explain the surface inconsistencies between the two claims.

MCAT EXPERTISE

Intensive Kaplan study of released AAMC materials seems to indicate that Apply questions appear to be a bit more common than Strengthen–Weaken (Beyond) questions. Out of the approximately 24 Reasoning Beyond the Text questions you'll see in a CARS section, typically about 13 will be Apply questions and only about nine or ten will be Strengthen–Weaken (Beyond) questions, with perhaps one Reasoning Beyond the Text question that doesn't neatly fall into either type.

15.4 Reasoning Beyond the Text Questions

Questions that fall into the broad category of Reasoning Beyond the Text are easy to identify because they always involve novel information (in the question stem, the set of answer choices, or both) that is not stated or even suggested by the passage and that may not even seem to be related the the passage topic. There are two main categories of these questions: Apply questions and Strengthen–Weaken (Beyond) questions. The fundamental difference is one of direction. Apply questions go from passage to new information, whereas Strengthen–Weaken (Beyond) questions go from new information to passage. Despite these differences, both Reasoning Beyond the Text question types require reasoning through both the passage and novel information to resolve the connection between them.

APPLY

Apply questions require you to take the information given in the passage and extrapolate it to a new context. Apply questions may ask for one of three tasks.

- They may ask for the author's **response** to a situation, using words such as *response*, *reply*, *most likely to agree with*, or *least consistent with*.
- They may ask for the most probable **outcome** in a situation, using words such as *outcome, result, expectation,* or *consequence*.
- They may ask for an **analogy** or **example** of an idea discussed in the passage, using words such as *most similar, analogous,* or *example*.

Attacking Apply Questions

- **Type:** Apply questions often begin with words such as *suppose, consider,* or *imagine*, indicating the presence of new information. These questions can be attacked *now* or *later*, depending on your familiarity with the passage and its arguments.
- **Rephrase:** If the question stem is long, jump to the end to determine what it's asking. Read any information given in the question stem closely, looking for hints that connect it to the passage. Apply questions can be Rephrased as, *How does the passage information affect this new information?*
- **Investigate:** Most Apply questions reference an argument or claim from the passage. So start there by rereading the relevant text. If the question stem is more general, lacking specific passage references, consider how the major takeaway of the passage can be applied to the new information. These questions can apply passage concepts in several ways.
  - Response questions ask how the author would respond to the new information. Investigate by determining the author's key beliefs, which are generally reflected in the passage using Author keywords.
  - Outcome questions ask how passage information can predict the outcome of a novel situation. Investigate by paying attention to cause-effect relationships in the passage, which are generally reflected in the passage using Logic keywords.

○ Analogy questions require applying passage information to identify appropriate examples or analogies of passage information. Investigate by looking for text that provides definitions, explanations, or the author's own example, noting any necessary or sufficient conditions.

- **Match:** Match your prediction to an answer choice. If there is no clear match or if you cannot perform any of the earlier steps of the Kaplan Method for the CARS questions, use the process of elimination.
  ○ Eliminate any answer choices that are inconsistent with the author's views, especially for Response questions.
  ○ Eliminate any answer choice that does not contain necessary conditions (which must occur in all instances of a concept), especially for Analogy questions.

STRENGTHEN–WEAKEN (BEYOND)

Similar to Strengthen–Weaken (Within) questions, Strengthen–Weaken (Beyond) questions concern the logical relationship between conclusions and evidence that strengthens the conclusions or refutations that weaken them. However, in Strengthen–Weaken (Beyond) questions, at least one of the claims involved will not be from the passage but will be unique to the question stem or answer choices. Strengthen–Weaken (Beyond) questions are also distinct in that they treat the passage as flexible, subject to modification by outside forces.

Attacking Strengthen–Weaken (Beyond) Questions

- **Type:** These questions often contain words such as *relate*, *support*, *challenge*, *relevance*, *significance*, or *impact*. In contrast to Strengthen–Weaken (Within) questions, they often contain words such as *could* or *would*.
- **Rephrase:** Strength–Weaken (Beyond) questions are really asking, *How does this new information strengthen/weaken the argument from the passage?*
- **Investigate:** Start with the new information and Investigate its connection to passage information. The Investigate step generally proceeds as follows:
  ○ Identify the new information, it will be found in either the question stem or the answer choices.
  ○ Consider the new information's connection and relevance to the passage. Does it strength or weaken passage ideas?
  ○ Finally, consider how the new information impacts passage information; let this serve as your prediction.
- **Match:** Match your prediction to an answer choice. If there is no clear match or if you cannot perform any of the earlier steps of the Kaplan Method for the CARS questions, then use the process of elimination.

OTHER REASONING BEYOND THE TEXT QUESTIONS

MCAT EXPERTISE

Other question types, in both
the Reasoning Beyond the Text
and Reasoning Within the Text
categories of CARS questions,
are rare. On Test Day, expect
to see only a couple of these
other question types. Thus, it's
generally not worth memorizing
the specific steps to attack each
of these rare question types.
Instead, see how the Kaplan
Question Strategy can be used
to attack these questions.

Though not the most common type of Reasoning Beyond the Text questions, Probable
Hypothesis, Alternative Explanation, and Passage Alteration questions do occasionally
appear. They can be identified by the words in the questions themselves.

- **Probable Hypothesis questions** ask for causes of new situations presented in the
  question stem.
  - These questions often contain phrases such as *probable hypothesis*, *likely cause*, or
    most reasonable explanation.
  - Approach these questions similarly to the Apply questions, except that you are
    looking for analogous cause-effect relationships in the passage.
- **Alternative Explanation questions** ask for causes that differ from the ones given in
  the passage but that still provide an explanation for a phenomenon.
  - These questions often contain phrases such as *alternative explanation*, *other
    cause*, or *different reason*.
  - Approach these questions by eliminating any answer choice that would not lead to
    the effect in the question stem. If stuck between multiple answers, eliminate those
    that conflict most significantly with the passage.
- **Passage Alteration questions** ask for changes the author could make to the passage
  to make it consistent with new information.
  - These questions often contain words such as *alter*, *change*, or *update*.
  - Approach these questions by looking for the answer that produces the desired
    effect with the least amount of modification to the ideas in the passage.

15.5 How Will the CARS Question Types Appear on the Exam?

As you see in the review of all the question types, questions can be worded in different ways, ask for different types of answers, and require different types of thinking and reasoning. However, all of the CARS questions have one thing in common: they do not ask for any information outside the stated or implicit information in the passage, question, or answer choices. Everything you need to answer a question correctly can be extrapolated from one of these three parts, even when the question asks you to reason an implicit conclusion or apply information to a new situation. Bringing in outside information will set you on the wrong track, just as using an irrelevant formula in science will deflect you from the correct answer. You can be sure, then, that regardless of the question type or complexity, the MCAT test maker has given you everything you need to answer the question correctly.

15.6 Getting the Edge Using the CARS Question Types

One of the major turning points of any student preparing for the MCAT is learning to see the underlying structure and patterns of the test. Nowhere else is this advantage more pronounced than in the CARS section. Not only have you seen that the AAMC uses patterns in the passages, but in this chapter we focused on the patterns of the questions and answer choices themselves. To ensure you've developed the *edge* when attacking CARS questions, use this litmus test: from the question stem alone, can you plan how exactly how you'd attack that particular question? If so, that is a good indication that you're seeing the underlying question patterns in the CARS section.

Furthermore, as with all parts of the MCAT, the best way to improve your performance with the CARS questions is to practice and then effectively review. Systematic review of how you answer questions will help you determine weaknesses and formulate a study plan to ameliorate them. If you find that you are not improving steadily, take an honest look at your critical-thinking skills to determine what you need to do to improve your score. A helpful tool to self-diagnose the areas you need help with is *deconstruction*. For a missed question, try to identify the specific step of your Kaplan Method where you made a mistake. Did you miss the question behind the question? That's a *Type* and *Rephrase* issue! Did you return to the wrong part of the passage or not return at all? That's an *Investigate* (potentially a *Read and Distill*) issue! Did you fall for a wrong answer pathology? That's a *Match* issue! Once you have identified a specific step where your method needs improvement, spend time consciously working on it!

CHAPTER 16

Practicing with CARS Passages

This chapter of the CARS unit includes worked examples and practice passages. In the worked examples, you will witness the utilization of the Kaplan Method for passages, questions, and arguments in the context of two exceptionally challenging passages. After seeing the Kaplan Method in action, complete the practice passages on your own. Be sure to read the entire explanations to align your thinking with that of the test makers.

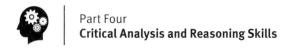

16.1   CARS Worked Example I

A PHILOSOPHY PASSAGE

Every student of the sciences is taught to be wary of mistaking correlation for causation, but few fully appreciate the difference. Among the first to give an account of this distinction was David Hume (1711–1776) in his early masterpiece *A Treatise of Human Nature*, the composition of which commenced at the prodigious age of 15 when Hume was himself but a student. Though often thought to be surpassed by his treatment of cause and effect in the more mature *An Enquiry Concerning Human Understanding*, the discussion in the *Treatise* is remarkable for situating causation squarely within the context of human psychology.

Hume's analysis began from a simple principle, "that all our ideas are copy'd from our impressions," by which he means that all knowledge ultimately derives from sense experience—an axiom he shared with fellow empiricists John Locke and George Berkeley. Causation is no different, and thus Hume set out to determine the original impressions (today more commonly called perceptions or sensations) whence this idea derives. According to his analysis, causation is nothing that is intrinsic to any particular object but rather emerges only in the relations between two objects, namely, cause and effect. Hume noted three specific relations that are essential to the idea of causation: contiguity (spatial proximity), temporal priority of cause before effect, and an additional "necessary connexion" between the two. This last is what distinguishes causation from mere coincidence, so Hume devoted several sections to uncovering what it is.

His conclusion may shock those unaccustomed to skeptical thinking. Hume argued that this necessary connection that makes one entity the cause of another is purely a creation of the mind: "Necessity is nothing but that determination of the thought to pass from causes to effects and from effects to causes, according to their experienc'd union." Such behavior is the product of custom, a mental habit established after we repeatedly perceive similar sequences of cause and effect, such as when a moving billiard ball transfers momentum to a resting one after they collide—one of parlor gamesman Hume's favorite examples. Logic does not dictate that momentum should be transferred in a collision, for we could easily imagine one ball colliding into another and producing any number of other results; only experience shows us it is so.

Hume's inquiries led him to formulate the following definition: "A cause is an object precedent and contiguous to another, and so united with it, that the idea of the one determines the mind to form the idea of the other, and the impression of the one to form a more lively idea of the other." He can remain confident that this determination of the mind is a customary connection, not a logical one, with his astute observation that all causal reasoning presupposes "that the future resembles the past," a claim that need not be true. In fact, such a claim could only ever be taken on faith—for how could it be proved? If one were to argue that, in the past, what would become the future at that point has always turned out to resemble the prior past, so we can expect the same in the future, one would be begging the question. How do we know the laws of nature won't change tomorrow?

If Hume was right, there is naught but the quirks of the psyche that properly distinguish causation from what he designated "constant conjunction" (correlation). Later thinkers would come to call this the "problem of induction," for it demonstrates how all inductive reasoning—which moves from particular pieces of evidence to a universal conclusion—is ultimately uncertain.

1. Which of the following statements is assumed without support in paragraph 3?

   A. Hume said that the necessary connection between cause and effect is simply a mental custom.

   B. Momentum is transferred if an object in motion collides with an object at rest.

   C. The mind infers a necessary connection after experiencing one instance of a cause and its effect.

   D. The truth of a claim is not logically determined if it can be imagined otherwise.

2. According to the discussion in the final paragraph, one example of inductive reasoning would be concluding that an automobile tire will never go flat on the basis of:

   A. repeated daily observations of the tire staying intact.

   B. the logical necessity of all tires being incapable of going flat.

   C. a customary habit of jumping to faulty conclusions.

   D. knowledge that the tire is made of an indestructible material.

3. Based on the passage, what best explains how "all causal reasoning presupposes 'that the future resembles the past'" (paragraph 4)?

   A. Reasoning about causality is ultimately founded on an assumption established by custom rather than by logic.

   B. The laws of nature must be unchanging from past to future.

   C. It is not necessarily the case that the past and the future resemble one another.

   D. Past conjunctions of cause and effect would yield no causal knowledge if the future operated by new laws of nature.

4. The claim "causation is nothing that is intrinsic to any particular object" most nearly means that objects:

   A. can never be adequately comprehended by the human mind.

   B. are by nature effects rather than causes.

   C. can be understood as causes only relative to other entities.

   D. cannot be the cause of other objects.

5. Which of the following, if true, would most undermine Hume's conclusions about cause and effect?

   A. There is no reason to believe that the laws of nature will change tomorrow.

   B. Some knowledge is attainable completely independent of experience.

   C. Most students of science fully appreciate the difference between correlation and causation.

   D. Claims about causal relations can always be doubted.

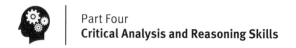

USING THE KAPLAN METHOD

Preview for difficulty: Spending 10 seconds or so to Preview the passage reveals the passage topic of philosophy, specifically Hume's philosophy. In addition, the first several words of each paragraph, specifically Hume's conclusions, reveal an argumentative passage.

Choose your approach: Argumentative passages require reasoning through arguments, connecting different portions of the passage to understand the passage's major takeaway. In addition, abstract topics such as a philosophy often require a deeper passage analysis to Distill effectively. As such, **Interrogation** is a viable choice for this passage.

Read and Distill:

P1: This paragraph can be chunked into two portions. The first chunk (sentences 1 and 2) introduces Hume and his first work *A Treatise of Human Nature*. The next chunk (sentence 3) compares *Treatise* to another work of Hume's. An interrogative question could be, *Why did the author make this comparison?* The author does this to emphasize the "remarkable" discussion connecting causation and human psychology in *Treatise*. This is the major takeaway of the paragraph.

P2: This paragraph can be chunked into two portions. The first chunk (sentences 1 and 2) describes the first principle of Hume's theory, that all of our ideas come from our experiences. An Interrogative question connecting this chunk to the previous can be, *How do causation and impressions from P2 relate to causation and human psychology?* Perceptions and sensations are part of human psychology.

The second chunk (the remainder of the paragraph) describes Hume's findings. Causation does not come from any individual object but, rather, emerges from the relation between different objects. This is the major takeaway of the paragraph. The author repeats this idea in the final two sentences terming it the "necessary connexion". An Interrogative question could be, *How does this chunk help you anticipate what's coming up next?* The passage will dive deeper into this concept.

P3: As expected, paragraph 3 expands on the "necessary connexion" and does so in two ways, which is also how this paragraph can be chunked. The first chunk states that the necessary connection is a creation of the mind, while the second chunk provides a more concrete example. The boundary between the chunks can be placed at the phrase "such as."

An Interrogative question that leverages the example would be, *How does the collision and momentum transfer example relate to the necessary connection being a creation of the mind?* There is no logical reason why momentum should be transferred in a collision; we know this to be true only because of our experience (experiments). From here we can even connect the collision example back to P2, as it is an example of an idea that comes from our experiences.

P4: This paragraph begins with Hume's definition of causation, which may come as no surprise if the earlier paragraphs were successfully interrogated. Put briefly, Hume believes that causation is a relationship between two (or more) objects and emerges from our experience of the past. This explanation continues until the end of the chunk, which ends at "for how could it be proved?" The second chunk, beginning with "If one were," states an implication of Hume's definition. In order for cause and effect to continue to have meaning, the future must have the same rules of nature as the past. Interrogate: *How do these two chunks relate to previous paragraphs and chunks?* This paragraph is the conclusion of Hume's thoughts and principles.

P5: This last paragraph is a single chunk that presents an implication of Hume's philosophy, that causation is an example of inductive reasoning and is ultimately uncertain.

---

1. Which of the following statements is assumed without support in paragraph 3?
   A. Hume said that the necessary connection between cause and effect is simply a mental custom.
   B. Momentum is transferred if an object in motion collides with an object at rest.
   C. The mind infers a necessary connection after experiencing one instance of a cause and its effect.
   D. The truth of a claim is not logically determined if it can be imagined otherwise.

KEY CONCEPT

Reasoning Within the Text: Inference (Assumption)

---

① Type the question

In addition to the reference to the third paragraph, the most important words in the question stem are "assumed without support." The phrasing suggests an Inference question, most likely an Assumption. The correct choice is a statement that must be true, given what is said in that paragraph, but is not backed up with its own reasoning. Given that the scope is limited to only one paragraph, a question such as this is probably worth doing as soon as it is encountered.

② Rephrase the question stem

Based on the question type and phrasing of the stem, this can be Rephrased as, *Which answer is stated in P3 as a standalone fact, without support or evidence?*

③ Investigate potential solutions

The question stem does not specify what part of paragraph 3 to look at, so it may be worth doing a quick reread of the paragraph or considering your interrogations of the paragraph. Inference question stems are often vague. So let your general understanding of paragraph 3 be your prediction. After this preparation, the process of elimination is the way to go. Read each choice, and then find the relevant text in paragraph 3. If a choice is not assumed by the author, it can be eliminated. That's not all. The wording in the stem suggests another way an answer can be ruled out: if a choice is a claim that the author would endorse but is supported elsewhere in paragraph 3.

④ Match your prediction to an answer choice

Start with (**A**). The relevant text is the following:

"Hume argued that this necessary connection that makes one entity the cause of another is purely a creation of the mind: 'Necessity is nothing but that determination of the thought to pass from causes to effects and from effects to causes, according to their experienc'd union.' Such behavior is the product of custom, a mental habit established after we repeatedly perceive similar sequences of cause and effect . . ."

Clearly the language in this choice is cobbled together from the sentence that surrounds the quotation, so it must be something the author would endorse. However, this is ultimately a claim about what Hume said. The best way to strengthen claims that offer interpretations of a writer is to quote the writer directly. Because the author does quote Hume directly, this is not "assumed without support," so (**A**) can be eliminated.

For (**B**), look to this part of the paragraph:

"Logic does not dictate that momentum should be transferred in a collision, for we could easily imagine one ball colliding into another and producing any number of other results; only experience shows us it is so."

TAKEAWAYS

When a question asks for a statement "assumed without support," the correct answer may be directly stated or only implied in the passage. Regardless, if a statement is "assumed without support," then the author writes nothing else about why to believe that statement.

Although the first part of this sentence states that the claim cannot be supported logically, the clause following the semicolon notes that this claim is demonstrated by experience. That reference to support rules out (**B**) as well.

With (**C**), there is actually an inconsistency with the passage. This inconsistency is found when the author noted that custom is "a mental habit established after we *repeatedly* perceive similar sequences of cause and effect" (emphasis added). There's no reason to believe that the mind does this after only one experience, so cross off (**C**) as well.

At this point, the process of elimination shows that the correct response is (**D**).

Considering the general prediction while evaluating the answer choices leads to the elimination of (A), (B), and (C), indicating that (D) is correct. This choice is confirmed with the first part of the last sentence in the third paragraph: "Logic does not dictate that momentum should be transferred in a collision, for we could easily imagine one ball colliding into another and producing any number of other results." The Evidence keyword *for* suggests the author takes the ability to imagine something to be otherwise as evidence that it is not dictated, or determined, by logic. But why should the imagination be any guide about what is logically determined? The author offers no reasons, so this assumption is unsupported.

THINGS TO WATCH OUT FOR

Watch out for when a question stem presents multiple ways of eliminating incorrect responses.

> **2.** According to the discussion in the final paragraph, one example of inductive reasoning would be concluding that an automobile tire will never go flat on the basis of:
>
>   **A.** repeated daily observations of the tire staying intact.
>   **B.** the logical necessity of all tires being incapable of going flat.
>   **C.** a customary habit of jumping to faulty conclusions.
>   **D.** knowledge that the tire is made of an indestructible material.

KEY CONCEPT

Reasoning Beyond the Text: Apply (Analogy/Example)

① Type the question

The paragraph reference, quotation, and use of the term *example* help identify this question as a subtype of Apply question. The stem provides a lot of clues, so this one is worth attempting now.

② Rephrase the question stem

The question asks for an application of inductive reasoning as explained in the last paragraph. To answer this question, it is essential to have a clear understanding of inductive reasoning; be sure to incorporate this into your task. The question can be Rephrased as, *What evidence would be needed to reason inductively that an automobile tire will never go flat?*

③ Investigate potential solutions

To furnish an example of a concept from a passage, it is essential to be clear on the meaning of that concept. Go back to the passage and learn as much as possible about the cited term: "All inductive reasoning—which moves from particular pieces of evidence to a universal conclusion—is ultimately uncertain." The dashes set apart a definition for the term, recognizing two key components that make up induction. The question stem provides half of this, the "conclu[sion] that an automobile tire will never go flat." This is a universal claim (one that applies in every case), as suggested by the word *never*, which admits no exceptions. The words *on the basis of* confirm that the correct answer is the evidence that supports this conclusion.

TAKEAWAYS

Anything that appears in a question stem should be taken for granted, regardless of how peculiar it may seem. The claim that a tire will never go flat is clearly false; the physical world provides ample evidence that everything eventually succumbs to entropy. However, what matters for this question is the reasoning behind the conclusion, not its truth value.

The correct choice must exemplify particular pieces of evidence, but what does this really mean? The final paragraph notes how the problem that Hume identified with causation was later called the "problem of induction," suggesting that causal reasoning and inductive reasoning are closely related (although the author does not specify precisely what this relation is). Because of this connection, it is possible to use the examples that the passage provides of causal reasoning as a basis for predicting what will count as inductive reasoning.

The third paragraph offers a crucial hint, with its reference to the formation of customary casual associations "after we repeatedly perceive similar sequences of cause and effect." These repeated perceptions are the particular pieces of evidence mentioned in the fifth paragraph. Put it all together now; the correct answer should make reference to multiple cases in which the tire does not go flat.

THINGS TO WATCH OUT FOR

Although every choice provides some basis for making that conclusion, the most tempting is (C), which echoes a lot of the language from the passage. The problem with it, though, is that there is no indication in the passage that inductive conclusions must be faulty or wrong, only that they are uncertain, which is far less negative.

④ Match your prediction to an answer choice

(**A**) presents an immediate match for these expectations. The general conclusion, "that an automobile tire will never go flat," could be inductively supported by *repeated daily observations of the tire staying intact*.

---

3. Based on the passage, what best explains how "all causal reasoning presupposes 'that the future resembles the past'" (paragraph 4)?

    A. Reasoning about causality is ultimately founded on an assumption established by custom rather than by logic.
    B. The laws of nature must be unchanging from past to future.
    C. It is not necessarily the case that the past and the future resemble one another.
    D. Past conjunctions of cause and effect would yield no causal knowledge if the future operated by new laws of nature.

KEY CONCEPT

Reasoning Within the Text: Other

① Type the question

Questions that ask for explanations often fall into one of the two Other types. Because no new situation is suggested, this is Other Reasoning Within the Text, rather than Other Reasoning Beyond the Text. Because Other questions often are difficult, this may be worth saving for the last question of the passage, though the direct quotation does make doing research a bit easier.

② Rephrase the question stem

Rephrasing this question stem requires understanding the context of the quoted phrase. Consider the in-depth Interrogation; we may recall that P4 was aimed at summarizing Hume's argument. Thus we can Rephrase this question stem as, *What best explains Hume's view on causation and its requirement that the future resembles the past?*

③ Investigate potential solutions

To answer this question, we must first recall from the Interrogation or Investigate the passage anew to ensure a clear understanding of Hume's views. Let that understanding serve as a general prediction, and Match it to an answer choice.

P4:

"[Hume] can remain confident that this determination of the mind is a customary connection, not a logical one, with his astute observation that all causal reasoning presupposes 'that the future resembles the past,' a claim that need not be true. In fact, such a claim could only ever be taken on faith—for how could it be proved? If one were to argue that, in the past, what would become the future at that point has always turned out to resemble the prior past, so we can expect the same in the future, one would be begging the question. How do we know the laws of nature won't change tomorrow?"

This is the most intricate idea in the entire passage, though it's given a relatively brief formulation. The author (echoing Hume) is saying that the claim "the future resembles the past" is an assumption in any argument made with a conclusion about cause and effect. Rely on an example the passage itself furnishes. Throughout human history, there have been repeated observations that a collision causes momentum to be transferred from a moving object to a static (but not immobile) one, such as seen with a rolling ball hitting a standing ball in games such as billiards or croquet. In physics, a change in momentum is known as an impulse, so abbreviate this idea as "a collision causes an impulse," or $C \rightarrow I$.

Past observations have always confirmed $C \rightarrow I$. To be able to claim that this statement is universally or generally true, though, one also must say that $C \rightarrow I$ is equally true for the future. Because the future is something that, by definition, has not yet been observed, there can be no experience to draw on to support $C \rightarrow I$. To argue that $C \rightarrow I$ is true, one must assume that what has not been experienced (the future) will produce the same results (more examples of $C \rightarrow I$) as what has been experienced (the past).

Let this unpacking of Hume's argument serve as the prediction. Then work through the answer choices for the Match.

④ Match your prediction to an answer choice

Begin with (**A**). The last part is simply a reference to the claim that the future resembles the past, which means that altogether this choice is simply a restatement of the quoted line from the question stem. This provides at most a minimal explanation. So it is unlikely to be the correct answer, particularly given that the question asks for *what best explains*.

The statement in (**B**) is, as was noted in the Plan step, simply another way of saying the future resembles the past. This is another restatement, this time of only part of the quotation in the question stem. So it's even less helpful than (**A**). It can safely be ruled out.

Although (**C**), does not rehash the quoted claim, it is effectively a reiteration of something said in the fourth paragraph, that the claim that the future resembles the past "need not be true." This is another way of saying the claim is not logically or necessarily true, but it does not explain how the claim is presupposed in causal reasoning. Thus, (**C**) can also be eliminated.

The process of elimination suggests the answer must be (**D**). Be sure to evaluate it first to ensure that it is superior to the minimal explanation given by (**A**).

Upon examination, (**D**) provides by far the best explanation, going beyond the mere repetition of claims to some of the underlying ideas in the text. Causal knowledge must be referring to the knowledge gained from causal reasoning, that is, conclusions that are backed by observation. Now, these observations (*past conjunctions of cause and effect*) would be worthless if the future stopped resembling the past because that past knowledge would no longer apply. The author's rhetorical question at the end of the fourth paragraph ("How do we know the laws of nature won't change tomorrow?") is hinting at this same idea, but this choice spells it out explicitly.

TAKEAWAYS

When asked to provide an explanation for a claim, the correct answer will do more than just make the same assertion in slightly different language. It will offer an account of why or how the claim is true.

THINGS TO WATCH OUT FOR

Question stems that use superlative language (*most*, *best*, and other -est words) occasionally feature choices that seem to provide minimal answers to the question but pale in comparison to the correct response.

KEY CONCEPT

Foundations of Comprehension: Definition-in-Context

---

4. The claim "causation is nothing that is intrinsic to any particular object" most nearly means that objects:

   A. can never be adequately comprehended by the human mind.
   B. are by nature effects rather than causes.
   C. can be understood as causes only relative to other entities.
   D. cannot be the cause of other objects.

① Type the question

Phrases such as *most nearly means* almost always indicate a Definition-in-Context question, which carries the task of identifying the meaning of a term, statement, or other segment of the text. Because of the specific passage reference, these questions can be attacked immediately.

2 Rephrase the question stem

Definition-in-Context questions require reading for purpose. As such this question can be Rephrased as, *What did the author mean when using this phrase? Why did the author include it?*

3 Investigate potential solutions

From our in-depth Interrogation, causation emerges from a relationship between two objects and therefore is not a property of an object itself. The question stem claim was included to support this view of causation. If unable to recall the context of the passage claim, seek it out during the Investigate step. An understanding of the author's view of causation can serve as a focused prediction for your Match step.

4 Match your prediction to an answer choice

(C) presents a match for the latter prediction, saying that objects *can be understood as causes only relative to other entities.*

TAKEAWAYS

Having a broader range of expectations, such as recognizing two equivalent ways of making the same prediction, can lead to homing in on the correct choice more quickly.

THINGS TO WATCH OUT FOR

Answers similar to **(A)** can be tempting because they might seem to have a similar tone as language in the passage, such as "ultimately uncertain" in the fifth paragraph. However, **(A)** excludes the essential element of causality, so it cannot capture the meaning of the quoted phrase.

KEY CONCEPT

Reasoning Beyond the Text: Strength–Weaken (Weaken)

---

5. Which of the following, if true, would most undermine Hume's conclusions about cause and effect?

    A. There is no reason to believe that the laws of nature will change tomorrow.

    B. Some knowledge is attainable completely independent of experience.

    C. Most students of science fully appreciate the difference between correlation and causation.

    D. Claims about causal relations can always be doubted.

---

1 Type the question

The phrase *if true* typically indicates a Strengthen–Weaken (Beyond) question, and *undermine* is just a synonym of weaken. The vaguely worded *Hume's conclusions about cause and effect* could refer to just about any part of the passage. This question likely requires some process of elimination (especially given the word *most*) and may also require research in multiple paragraphs. So it's one best reserved for later, after several other questions have been successfully tackled and the passage is more familiar.

2 Rephrase the question stem

Most simply, this question can be Rephrased as, *What would weaken Hume's view on causation?*

③ Investigate potential solutions

Before evaluating answer choices, it is essential to understand Hume's views on causation. Once done, let that understanding serve as your prediction. The Interrogation provided a fairly deep understanding of Hume's concept of causation, specifically that *causation is a relationship between two objects, ultimately based on our perceptions and thus our experiences.*

Once armed with this understanding, evaluate the impact that each choice's truth would have on arguments made in the passage. How strong the language is or how implausible the situation described may be do not matter—the question stem asks only for the most powerful negative effect on Hume's ideas in particular.

④ Answer by matching, eliminating, or guessing

For (**A**), the laws of nature changing tomorrow does relate to Hume's argument that causation is based on experiences. Specifically, if causation is based on experiences, it must be based on the past. Thus, we need to assume that the future will operate in the same manner as the past in order for causation to hold. So (**A**) is on topic. However, it states that there is *no reason to believe that the laws of nature will change tomorrow.* If anything, this would support Hume's views.

(**B**) directly pertains to the discussion at the start of the second paragraph: "Hume's analysis began from a simple principle, 'that all our ideas are copy'd from our impressions,' by which he means that all knowledge ultimately derives from sense experience—an axiom he shares with fellow empiricists John Locke and George Berkeley."

TAKEAWAYS

It's always possible to revise a Plan as it is being Executed if the answer choices lead in such a direction. Just because you begin the process of elimination does not mean that you have to finish it when you come across a choice that perfectly answers the question. Save the time reading the remaining wrong options for working on another question.

THINGS TO WATCH OUT FOR

In passages with multiple viewpoints, such as the author and another writer who the author discusses, watch out for choices in all question types that reflect the wrong views.

Again, (**B**) refers to the connection between causation and experience. Hume holds that causation is ultimately based on experience, but (**B**) states that some knowledge can be attained without experience. Choice (**B**) is correct.

Although (**C**) directly conflicts with the opening sentence, "Every student of the sciences is taught to be wary of mistaking correlation for causation, but few fully appreciate the difference," this claim constitutes the author's lead-in to the discussion of Hume. It undermines the author's framing of the issue, but it is not relevant to any idea tied to Hume himself.

As expected, (**D**) also fails to have a negative impact. In fact, the statement *claims about causal relations can always be doubted* is completely consistent with the author's concluding thought in the fifth paragraph that "all inductive reasoning . . . is ultimately uncertain." Because it supports the author and the author is never critical of Hume, there is no way this choice could undermine Hume.

After checking the other answers, it's clear that only (**B**) has a significantly negative impact on anything that can be connected immediately to Hume. In fact, its impact is so detrimental (analogous to demolishing a house's foundation) that such an answer can safely be taken as correct without consulting the remaining options.

This chapter continues on the next page. ▶ ▶ ▶

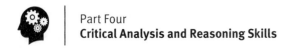

16.2   CARS Worked Example II

A SOCIAL SCIENCE PASSAGE

According to a 2014 report by Oxfam International, the world's richest 85 people possess as much as the poorest 3.5 billion, and nearly half of all wealth is owned by just 1 percent of the global populace. Many measures of inequality, when plotted annually, adopt a potentially disconcerting U-shape: declining after the reforms implemented by many industrialized populations in the wake of the Great Depression, inequality is now returning to levels not seen since the 1920s—and is on the verge of surpassing them. With statistics such as these, elite figures, from the president of the United States to the pope of the Catholic Church, have had to admit that inequality has become a prominent issue.

The truly interesting question concerns neither the existence of economic inequality nor the fact of its continuing growth but its origin. What has caused—and even more crucially, what is perpetuating—this polarization in wealth? After weighing the evidence, my contention is that this development is ultimately a political outcome, not an economic one. By this I mean it is the product of deliberate decisions by political leaders (elected, appointed, or otherwise) and other influential socioeconomic elites, not the natural result of market forces, as many other scholars have suggested.

At issue are the differing political fortunes of two factions, the centrality of which have been recognized by economists from Karl Marx to Thomas Piketty, laborers, capitalists, and the class of workers and the owners who employ them. When labor was politically ascendant (for instance, in the aftermath of Franklin D. Roosevelt's New Deal), inequality decreased. However, with the rise of the political ideology of neoliberalism (embraced by leaders on both ends of the accepted political spectrum, such as the United Kingdom's Margaret Thatcher and Tony Blair and the United States's Ronald Reagan and Bill Clinton), inequality began to rebound.

Neoliberalism purports to promote free markets, but perhaps a better characterization of it is the promotion of the free movement of capital. Capital tends to have its own law of gravity, except that it seems to fall upward, accumulating in floating paradises known as tax havens that contain the coffers of the planet's wealthiest. Few people would vote explicitly for this program, yet most governments in democratic nations throughout the world are filled with officials who act in ways that further the polarization of wealth, whether knowingly or unwittingly.

Much of the ascendance of neoliberal ideology stems from a discrepancy in organization. The United States presents a clear-cut example of one side of this phenomenon. From 1940 to 1980, between about one-fifth and one-fourth of all employed workers in the United States were members of labor unions. According to Piketty and associates 1940–1980 also is the bottom of the inequality U-curve. Subsequently, there was a precipitous decline in union participation in the 1980s, followed by continuing erosion, so that now only about one-ninth of all US workers are union members—all the while, inequality has steadily climbed upward.

On the other side, the capitalists have become better organized. In fact, their mobilization—not coincidentally—shortly precedes the extensive disempowerment of unions in and around the 1980s. For example, the infamous yet influential Powell Memorandum (written in 1971 by a man who would become a US Supreme Court Associate Justice) explicitly advocated coordinated action among capitalists: "Strength lies in organization, in careful long-range planning and implementation, in consistency of action over an indefinite period of years, in the scale of financing available only through joint effort, and in the political power available only through united action and national organizations." That careful long-range planning has paid serious dividends.

1. Which of the following would specifically bolster the author's primary line of argumentation?

    I. Evidence that coordination among capitalists in the 1970s directly contributed to the decline of labor unions in the 1980s

    II. Findings demonstrating that current levels of inequality have eclipsed the historical records set in the 1920s

    III. A study showing that the rate of polarization of wealth has increased since the global financial crisis of 2007–2008

    A. I only

    B. I and II only

    C. II and III only

    D. I, II, and III

2. Based on the passage, what is the author's most likely reason for regarding a U-shaped curve as "potentially disconcerting" (paragraph 1)?

    A. Inequality has returned to a level not seen since before the Great Depression.

    B. Deliberate choices by political leaders have led to an increase in inequality.

    C. The extreme polarization of wealth has detrimental consequences for society.

    D. The growth in inequality shows how capitalists are motivated solely by greed.

3. Which of the following, when taken in conjunction with the information presented by the passage, would best explain the author's use of "not coincidentally" (paragraph 6)?

    A. The ascendance of neoliberalism in democratic politics is largely responsible for the rise in inequality.

    B. The capitalists began coordinating their efforts immediately after recognizing unions were losing their power.

    C. A majority of citizens decided to relinquish membership in the working class and become capitalists instead.

    D. The democratically elected politicians financed by neoliberal organizations enacted antilabor policies.

4. The author suggests a correlation between each of the following pairs of phenomena EXCEPT:

    A. more coordination among capitalists and less coordination among laborers.

    B. higher participation in labor unions and lower levels of equality.

    C. strength of organization and political success in democratic nations.

    D. the rise of neoliberalism and a widening of the gap between rich and poor.

5. In Citizens United *v*. Federal Election Commission (2010), the US Supreme Court ruled that restrictions on political advocacy spending by capitalist corporations, labor unions, and other associations were prohibited by the First Amendment. Assuming that such spending is effective, the most reasonable expectation based on the passage about inequality in the United States is that inequality will:

    A. stop increasing because the ruling eliminates regulations that promoted the polarization of wealth.

    B. continue increasing because corporations will be able to outspend unions, resulting in more pro-capitalist policies.

    C. begin decreasing because unions will be able to outspend corporations, resulting in more pro-labor policies.

    D. remain at its present level because corporations and labor unions are treated equally under the ruling.

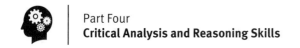
USING THE KAPLAN METHOD

Preview the passage: A quick ten-second glance through the passage shows that it is a social sciences passage, more specifically, an economics-focused passage. The passage is fairly long and detailed but with evenly sized paragraphs. Many would decide this passage to be relatively medium or ambiguous in difficulty.

Choose your approach: A detail-heavy passage with evenly spaced paragraphs is best suited for the Outlining method.

Read and Distill:

P1: The first sentence introduces the topic of wealth inequality with some statistics. The next few sentences talk about historic precedence showing that measures to redistribute the wealth work for a short period of time but that wealth goes back to being unequal after time. We end the paragraph with acknowledgement that this is a problem.
Outline: Wealth inequality; historic redistribution not lasting

P2: The next paragraph starts with, "The truly interesting question . . . ," indicating that a key idea is going to be discussed in this paragraph. The author focuses not on how to fix the inequality but on how it originates. There's a rhetorical question in the second sentence, which further highlights the emphasis. The usage of personal pronouns ("my contention" and "I mean") indicates that this is the author's opinion, so we need to pay attention. The author thinks that the cause of the inequality is due to purposeful actions on the part of political leaders.
Outline: Author → inequality caused deliberately by political leaders

P3: The first half of the first sentence tell us more about the politics, specifically calling out two factions. It might be tempting to think that the people and groups in the second part of sentence 1 are parts of these factions. However, the statement is just saying that many recognize that there are two factions. The first group is labor. We're told that when the labor faction is in power, the inequality drops. The second faction, triggered by the word "however," is neoliberalism, which causes the rise of inequality.
Outline: Two factions: labor → inequality decrease; neoliberalism → inequality increase

P4: The first word of this paragraph is "neoliberalism," so we're focusing on the second of two factions. The "better characterization" of neoliberalism is the movement of capital upward as tax havens, which is pushed in that direction by political officials.
Outline: Neoliberalism → free movement capital in tax havens

P5: Again, this paragraph has a clear topic sentence right at the beginning that talks about how neoliberalism came to rise. We're told it's an issue with organization. The author uses an example to illustrate this. When a large proportion of labor workers were unionized, it correlated to the lowest amount of wealth inequality.
Outline: Labor unionized → lowest wealth inequality

P6: The phrase "on the other hand" tells us we're pivoting in topic, probably talking about how labor is contrasted with neoliberalism. When capitalists had better organization, unions couldn't have as much power. The rest of the paragraph is an example supporting this idea.

Outline: Capitalist organization → unions less power

---

1. Which of the following would specifically bolster the author's primary line of argumentation?

   I. Evidence that coordination among capitalists in the 1970s directly contributed to the decline of labor unions in the 1980s
   II. Findings demonstrating that current levels of inequality have eclipsed the historical records set in the 1920s
   III. A study showing that the rate of polarization of wealth has increased since the global financial crisis of 2007–2008

   A. I only
   B. I and II only
   C. II and III only
   D. I, II, and III

KEY CONCEPT

Make sure that on Test Day, you create an outline that makes sense to you. Your outline should use symbols, abbreviations, shorthand, and other notation methods to ensure you spend as little time writing as possible. Practice with creating outlines to identify the most effective ways to write quickly and clearly.

KEY CONCEPT

Reasoning Beyond the Text: Strength-Weaken (Strengthen), Roman numeral

1 Type the question

The word *bolster* indicates a Strengthen question of some kind, with the subjunctive *would* suggesting Reasoning Beyond the Text. The fact that the stem is looking specifically for an effect on the author's primary line of argumentation suggests that the Roman numeral options may include evidence that bolsters related arguments that are only incidental to the author's real concerns. Given the lack of references to particular parts of the text and the fact that there are multiple pieces of evidence to consider, this question might be better saved for later.

2 Rephrase the question stem

Which of the following Roman numerals support the author's argument?

3 Investigate potential solutions

One key preparation is essential before beginning the attack: clarifying the author's primary argument. We hear the author's voice mostly clearly in paragraph 2, which states that the wealth inequality was due to the deliberate decisions on the part of political leaders. Moreover, the suggestion that "neither the existence of economic inequality nor the fact of its continuing growth" are interesting is worth noting because this can help set expectations for the wrong kind of support.

With a Roman numeral question, a divide-and-conquer strategy is the best approach. Before doing a close reading of the Roman numerals, look at the answer choices to see if any of them appear in exactly two of the four options. This is the answer choice you'll want to test first. If it's true, you can eliminate the two choices in which it does not appear. If it's false, you can eliminate the two choices in which it does appear. Then, with the two remaining options, you'll have to evaluate only one numeral that differs between them. (If more than one numeral appears twice, then start with whichever one seems easier for you. If no numeral appears twice, you may have to test all of them; so just begin with the easiest.)

④ Answer by matching, eliminating, or guessing

Following the Investigate steps outlined previously, start with numeral III. Although such evidence would support the claim that inequality is continuing to grow, this is precisely what the author suggests is uninteresting, definitely not the author's primary line of argument. To support the main argument, this item would need to offer some indication that decisions by socioeconomic elites caused this accelerating growth. However, the mere mention of the financial crisis is insufficient to establish that.

Given that numeral III is false, both **(C)** and **(D)** are ruled out, and it can be inferred that I is true. Looking at II, it is readily apparent that this is more support for inequality's existence and growth, not for the cause proposed by the author. Numeral II is thus false for roughly the same reason that III is, so **(B)** also can be eliminated.

The divide-and-conquer approach reveals that **(A)** is correct after evaluating only two of the numerals. Though you would want to select **(A)** on Test Day without further delay, we can confirm that only I is true by considering the impact of the sentence *evidence that coordination among capitalists in the 1970s directly contributed to the decline of labor unions in the 1980s*. This points to another paragraph, the sixth paragraph, where the author states that capitalist "mobilization—not coincidentally—shortly precedes the extensive disempowerment of unions in and around the 1980s" and cites the Powell Memorandum. Numeral I would definitely help to support the author's account of how inequality was caused to increase in the 1980s and would thus bolster the primary argument.

2. Based on the passage, what is the author's most likely reason for regarding a U-shaped curve as "potentially disconcerting" (paragraph 1)?

   A. Inequality has returned to a level not seen since before the Great Depression.
   B. Deliberate choices by political leaders have led to an increase in inequality.
   C. The extreme polarization of wealth has detrimental consequences for society.
   D. The growth in inequality shows how capitalists are motivated solely by greed.

1 Type the question

The question stem asks for the most likely reason behind a judgment the author makes, which is another way of asking for an assumption. So this question type is an Inference. There's a direct reference to paragraph 1. This might make this question a bit more workable and worth trying now, when you first encounter it, even though it concerns implicit parts of an argument.

2 Rephrase the question stem

Why does the author think the U-shaped curve is possibly disturbing?

3 Investigate potential solutions

Start by returning to the context of the quoted words: "Many measures of inequality, when plotted annually, adopt a potentially disconcerting U-shape: declining after the reforms implemented by many industrialized populations in the wake of the Great Depression, inequality is now returning to levels not seen since the 1920s—and on the verge of surpassing them." The clauses following the colon explain the U-shape but do not really get at the reason for it being potentially disconcerting, that is, why it might be alarming or troubling. The correct answer has to do more; it has to explain *why* the return to high levels of inequality is a negative outcome. Evaluate each answer choice to assess whether it accomplishes this goal.

4 Match your prediction to an answer choice

(**A**) may seem tempting because it mentions the Great Depression. However, it simply restates the author's description of the U-curve without explaining why it's a negative, which is a typical Faulty Use of Detail trap.

The issue with (**B**) is different: it offers an explanation, albeit the wrong one. It may be true that the author's primary argument concerns the causes of this increase in inequality, but this question asks specifically about the evaluation the author makes of this increase. Asking for the reason *why* an outcome is good or bad is conceptually distinct from asking for the cause of that outcome. (**B**) is incorrect.

Although (**C**) does not employ the word *inequality* as do the other options, it does use a synonymous phrase: *extreme polarization of wealth*. Moreover, unlike the previous choices, this answer actually gives a reason for why this trend could be disturbing: it carries negative social consequences. The author does suggest that the wealth inequality of the 1920s was responsible for an event so negative that it came to be known as the Great Depression. So this is precisely what we are looking for. (**C**) matches the prediction made in the Plan step.

(**C**) can be confirmed as the correct option by briefly considering the final contender, (**D**). Although greed may not be an emotion that most people applaud, (**D**) is similar to (**B**) insofar as it addresses the cause of the outcome rather than an appraisal of its value. Thus, we can be confident that (**C**) is right.

TAKEAWAYS

Sometimes Inference questions ask for very specific assumptions or implications, such as pieces of information that explain a normative (value) judgment.

THINGS TO WATCH OUT FOR

A valid inference from the passage could still be an incorrect answer if it fails to meet the requirements of the question stem. Use the clues the stem provides to make a more thorough prediction, and such traps will be much less tempting.

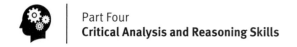

3. Which of the following, when taken in conjunction with the information presented by the passage, would best explain the author's use of "not coincidentally" (paragraph 6)?

   A. The ascendance of neoliberalism in democratic politics is largely responsible for the rise in inequality.
   B. The capitalists began coordinating their efforts immediately after recognizing unions were losing their power.
   C. A majority of citizens decided to relinquish membership in the working class and become capitalists instead.
   D. The democratically elected politicians financed by neoliberal organizations enacted antilabor policies.

❶ Type the question

The line *in conjunction with the information presented by the passage* suggests the answer choices present new ideas, meaning that this is Reasoning Beyond the Text. Because the question asks for an explanation of the author's use of a term, this does not exactly fall into either the Apply or Strengthen-Weaken (Beyond) types. There's a specific reference to the text, which may make this question more manageable. However, Other questions often can be challenging, so you may want to triage this one.

❷ Rephrase the question stem

Along with passage information, what will help explain "not coincidentally"?

❸ Investigate potential solutions

A question that asks for the best explanation, especially one that seems likely to bring in new information, is one that likely requires examining every answer choice. A good explanation makes the author's intention with the phrase clear. So begin your preparation by returning to the relevant part of the text. After establishing in the fifth paragraph that labor has become less organized, the author writes the following in the sixth paragraph:

"On the other side, the capitalists have become better organized. In fact, their mobilization—not coincidentally—shortly precedes the extensive disempowerment of unions in and around the 1980s. For example, the infamous yet influential Powell Memorandum (written in 1971 by a man who would become a US Supreme Court Associate Justice) explicitly advocated coordinated action among capitalists . . ."

The suggestion is that the improved organization of the capitalists is directly connected (is not a coincidence) to the diminution of organized labor. Given that the author stresses that the one event shortly precedes the other, there is a hint that the two are causally connected (because a cause typically comes immediately before its effect). Thus, the correct response should account for how better organization among capitalists could lead to worse organization among laborers.

4 Answer by matching, eliminating, or guessing

Although **(A)** mimics the language of the passage, even echoing the author's thesis, it fails to account for the use of this particular phrase. It is too general to account for the specific phenomenon referenced in the sixth paragraph. Eliminate it.

(B) seems a bit more promising because it connects the activities of the two classes. However, *the capitalists began coordinating their efforts immediately after recognizing unions were losing their power* gets the timing backward. The author says that the capitalist coordination came first, followed by the decline of the unions. So **(B)** is also wrong.

It may seem as if **(C)** provides a possible explanation, but it fails for a number of reasons. The first line of the passage notes the huge discrepancy in numbers between the wealthy class of owners and the poor class of laborers. Although the author mentions that deliberate decisions are important in the second paragraph, these are the decisions of political leaders and other elites, not the decisions of the majority of people. It's not clear from the passage that laborers have the power simply to switch roles from employee to employer. Even if some employees could become employers (for instance, entrepreneurs and the self-employed), it seems highly unlikely that a majority of citizens could do so. Finally, this choice does not take care to distinguish between membership in organized labor unions and membership in the class of laborers (employees). The previous paragraph discusses a decline in union membership, not a decline in membership in the working class. Thus, **(C)** clashes with the passage too much to be a plausible answer.

The Plan was to check all four answers, so **(D)** should also be evaluated although we now expect it is correct. The statement *the democratically elected politicians financed by neoliberal organizations enacted antilabor policies* would indeed provide the necessary explanation, one that is consistent with the discussion in the passage. The quote from the Powell Memorandum even mentions financing as a means of attaining political power, a number of neoliberal politicians are noted in the third paragraph, and the fourth paragraph cites the actions of democratic officials who promote the polarization of wealth (in other words, antilabor policies). So the agreement between this choice and the passage is resounding.

Executing the Plan led to the elimination of the wrong options, revealing **(D)** as the correct answer.

TAKEAWAYS

Questions that ask for possible explanations can often be tricky. Be clear on exactly what must be explained.

THINGS TO WATCH OUT FOR

Answer choices in Reasoning Beyond the Text questions can present entirely new situations completely unaddressed by the passage without such choices automatically being wrong. However, watch out for situations that directly conflict with the passage; these are most likely incorrect.

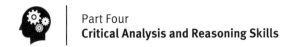

KEY CONCEPT

Foundation of Comprehension:
Inference (Implication, Scattered)

> **4.** The author suggests a correlation between each of the following pairs of phenomena EXCEPT:
>
> **A.** more coordination among capitalists and less coordination among laborers.
> **B.** higher participation in labor unions and lower levels of equality.
> **C.** strength of organization and political success in democratic nations.
> **D.** the rise of neoliberalism and a widening of the gap between rich and poor.

❶ Type the question

The prominent *EXCEPT* calls attention to the fact this is a Scattered variant of either a Detail question or an Inference question—the word *suggests* is regularly used in both types. However, because it asks for something as complex as a correlation, this question most likely requires deducing some implications from the text. Given the amount of time that is potentially involved in answering a Scattered Implication question (a lot of searching through the passage for ideas that might not be explicitly stated, only implied), this would best be saved for later in a question set.

❷ Rephrase the question stem

Which of the following pairs of occurrences have a relationship? Eliminate those that follow this statement.

❸ Investigate potential solutions

Scattered questions (featuring words such as *EXCEPT*, *NOT*, and *LEAST*) typically require the process of elimination to answer. However, it's still worthwhile to set some expectations. The correct answer will be either something that the text fails to mention or—more likely—a twisted version of information contained in the passage. Any choice that contradicts the passage or otherwise distorts its content would have to be right and could potentially be selected without testing the remaining options.

On the other hand, wrong answer choices are pairs of phenomena for which the author states or implies a correlation. Keep in mind that cause-and-effect relationships always entail a correlation between the cause and the effect. So any indication by the author of causation would thereby be a suggestion of correlation as well.

❹ Match your prediction to an answer choice

For (**A**) the relevant text is at the start of the sixth paragraph: "On the other side, the capitalists have become only better organized. In fact, their mobilization—not coincidentally—shortly precedes the extensive disempowerment of unions in and around the 1980s." The fact that the author stresses that this is not a coincidence reinforces that the relationship is intended to be more significant, potentially cause and effect. That there is at least a correlation is clear, so **(A)** should be ruled out.

With **(B)**, however, there is an issue when returning to the relevant text, this time from the fifth paragraph: "From 1940 to 1980, between about one-fifth and one-fourth of all employed workers in the United States were members of labor unions. According to Piketty and associates, 1940–1980 also is the bottom of the inequality U-curve." There's definitely a correlation being highlighted, but it's between high union participation and low inequality, not low equality. If inequality is low, then equality must be relatively high. So this choice is the opposite of what the passage suggests. Thus, without further ado, it's safe to conclude that **(B)** is correct.

This can be double-checked by finding the other choices in the text. The correlation in **(C)** is implied in the discussion beginning with "much of the ascendance of neoliberal ideology stems from a discrepancy in organization," and continuing throughout the final two paragraphs. For **(D)**, the relevant text is from the third paragraph: "with the rise of the political ideology of neoliberalism . . . inequality began to rebound." An increase in inequality entails a widening of the gap between rich and poor.

TAKEAWAYS

On occasion, Scattered questions can be answered without actually hunting down information for every choice. If you find a direct contradiction (or another obvious distortion), you've likely found your answer.

THINGS TO WATCH OUT FOR

When you find an answer choice that perfectly answers the question, don't waste any more time reading wrong answers. Get the point and use that extra time where it could gain you even more!

KEY CONCEPT

Reasoning Beyond the Text: Apply (Outcome)

5. In Citizens United *v.* Federal Election Commission (2010), the US Supreme Court ruled that restrictions on political advocacy spending by capitalist corporations, labor unions, and other associations were prohibited by the First Amendment. Assuming that such spending is effective, the most reasonable expectation based on the passage about inequality in the United States is that inequality will:

   A. stop increasing because the ruling eliminates regulations that promoted the polarization of wealth.
   B. continue increasing because corporations will be able to outspend unions, resulting in more pro-capitalist policies.
   C. begin decreasing because unions will be able to outspend corporations, resulting in more pro-labor policies.
   D. remain at its present level because corporations and labor unions are treated equally under the ruling.

❶ Type the question

The lengthy question stem, chock full of new information, tells us this is a Reasoning Beyond the Text question. The language of *most reasonable expectation* tells us that this is an Apply question, specifically one that asks for an Outcome. These kinds of questions can take a while (especially with long answer choices), so consider saving them for later.

❷ Rephrase the question stem

What will the US do if there are no restrictions on political advocacy by groups?

❸ Investigate potential solutions

With a new scenario, the key is finding the points of connection (or analogy) with the passage. The stem says that *restrictions on political advocacy spending were judged to be prohibited* and that this affected corporations, unions, and other groups. In short, that means these organizations gained additional freedom to spend money on political issues at their discretion. The question stem goes on to say explicitly *assuming that such spending is effective,* which tells you to take it for granted that this spending can have an impact on who gets elected and what policies get enacted. The actual question amounts to the following, *Given the new freedom of these groups to spend money and assuming it works, what will likely happen to inequality in the United States?* Answering this is the task presented.

Before tackling these wordy answer choices, it's worthwhile to make a prediction for the correct one. Start by clarifying the nature of the trend in inequality leading up to the Supreme Court ruling. The first paragraph mentions the more recent date of 2014, within only a few years of the date from the question stem, so it offers a good reference point. There, we're told that "inequality is now returning to levels not seen since the 1920s—and is on the verge of surpassing them." This is hardly an isolated statement. The idea that inequality is increasing is noted throughout the passage, which largely seeks to answer the question of why this occurs.

Now the question becomes, *How will this upward trend be affected?* The third paragraph offers some guidance on this question: "When labor was politically ascendant . . . inequality decreased. However, with the rise of the political ideology of neoliberalism . . . inequality began to rebound." Thus, if the ruling benefits labor more, we should expect to see inequality decrease or at least see the rate of its increase slow or stop. However, if the ruling benefits the capitalists more, inequality should continue its rise or even accelerate.

So, who benefits more? Even though the ruling applies to both capitalist corporations and labor unions, the discussion in the last two paragraphs suggests that capitalists are in a much stronger position to take advantage of the ruling. In the fifth paragraph, the author notes that about half as many US workers belong to unions as once did (one-ninth versus one-fourth or one-fifth). The sixth paragraph is explicit about the success of capitalists in working together, even hinting that their coordinated efforts may have caused the decline in organization among laborers. Because capitalists have the advantage, the ruling will likely only exacerbate the discrepancy between rich and poor, leading to even greater inequality.

④ Match your prediction to an answer choice

More thorough preparation means a quicker match when you finally look at the answer choices. Only (**B**) is consistent with the prediction made.

(**A**) and (**C**) can both immediately be discounted because they indicate a downward trend. Moreover, there's no reason to suppose that the restrictions prohibited by the ruling promoted the polarization of wealth nor to suspect that unions would have the ability to outspend corporations.

(**D**) comes closer to the truth but fails to take into account the realities described in the passage. If corporations and unions began on equal footing, it would be true that this ruling would help neither because it grants the same freedom to both. However, the passage makes it abundantly clear that the two groups are not at all on equal footing; the capitalists were ascendant when this ruling was handed down. To suggest that inequality remains at its present levels would also ignore the fact that it continues to increase. If the ruling truly had no effect on the status quo, then presumably inequality would just keep following the upward trend described in the passage.

TAKEAWAYS

Although a lengthy question stem takes longer to read, it also gives you more material to work with. Be sure to use that to your advantage and formulate a more thorough prediction for the correct answer.

THINGS TO WATCH OUT FOR

Some wrong answer choices may be completely consistent logically but be incorrect because they neglect vital information from the passage.

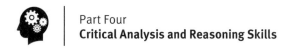
16.3   CARS Practice Passage I

PRACTICE PASSAGE I: A HUMANITIES PASSAGE

Using the Kaplan Method

(QUESTIONS 1–6)

Hope and fear are the quintessential political emotions, for both take as their object an unknown future, rife with possibilities for cultural flourishing or social dissolution. One always accompanies the other, for we inevitably dread that our aspirations might remain unrealized, and we cannot but yearn for our anxieties to prove unwarranted. An era may come to be dominated by one or the other pole, but its opposite can be repressed only temporarily—witness the opportunistic ascendance of the theme of "hope" in US politics subsequent to the unabashed fear-mongering of the "War on Terror."

Given the centrality of hope and fear in politics, there can thus be no question that the most authentically political of all works of fiction are novels of utopia and dystopia. The former term, a hybrid of "good place" (the ancient Greek *eutopos*) and "no place" (*outopos*), is a coinage of Sir Thomas More, whose 1516 *Utopia* is regarded as the urtext of both genres, notwithstanding that the literary construction of ideal societies is found as early as Plato's *Republic* nearly two millennia prior. Utopian fiction celebrates human potential, particularly the power of reason, which is supposedly capable of engineering a more perfect world than the one that the arbitrary forces of nature and tradition have yielded.

The first great dystopian novel was not published until 1921, more than four centuries after More's original *Utopia*. Yevgeny Zamyatin's *We* depicts the dark side of human reason, what has come to be known as "instrumental rationality," a robotic logic in which efficiency is valued for its own sake, and citizens are mere means for the advancement of political ends, which must remain unexamined. Zamyatin's literary personae are granted numbers rather than names and treated accordingly. Instrumental rationality is readily apparent in other icons of dystopia: Aldous Huxley's *Brave New World*, George Orwell's *Nineteen Eighty-Four*, Margaret Atwood's *The Handmaid's Tale*, and (more recently) Suzanne Collins's *The Hunger Games*. Although each novel uniquely paints a dire tomorrow, all portray humans as cogs in a vast social contraption, the overarching illogic of which belies the tidy sensibility of its everyday operations.

As with their emotional antecedents, utopia and dystopia are inextricably intertwined, evident in their deep structural commonalities. Each in its distinctive way emphasizes the fate of the transgressor, the individual who would privilege personal desires over the ironclad imperatives of state. Such free spirits cannot be tolerated within the body politic any more than a cancerous cell within the body physical. The analogy is imperfect, of course, because a tumor does not feel. From the transgressor's perspective, a vantage taken up far more commonly in novels of dystopia, the well-oiled social machine becomes a torture apparatus. Indeed, a tremendous amount of toil and violence are required for the proper maintenance of a device that runs so contrary to nature; the most effective social lubricants are blood, sweat, and tears.

Ironically, utopias and dystopias are intended to be immutable and self-perpetuating, which would preclude the very possibility of politics; a certain future will bring either despair or confidence but not the restless blend of hope and fear that accompanies uncertainty. In other words, both genres represent human coexistence as a problem and the state as its solution. The utopian novel seeks to answer the political question, whereas its counterpart calls into question an emerging answer. The most profound works of speculative political fiction reject this dynamic entirely—which, in its crudest form, merely recapitulates instrumental rationality—suggesting perhaps that the real problem is envisioning human life as a problem to be solved.

1. Which of the following statements, if true, would most strengthen the author's claim that "utopia and dystopia are inextricably intertwined" (paragraph 4)?

   A. A dystopian society always seems like an ideal political order to the members of its ruling class.

   B. Most utopian societies allow for the questioning of overarching political objectives.

   C. Dystopias do not actually require significant amounts of violent force to be maintained.

   D. Many works of speculative fiction can be classified as neither utopian nor dystopian.

2. Which of the following does the author consider to be a point of difference between utopian and dystopian literature?

   I. The depiction of violence as necessary for maintaining social order

   II. An emphasis on the role that reason plays in shaping society

   III. The likelihood of considering the point of view of a social deviant

   A. I only

   B. III only

   C. II and III only

   D. I, II, and III

3. By stating that "the analogy is imperfect" in the fourth paragraph, the author most likely intends to suggest that:

   A. people in a society should be regarded as more than just parts making up a whole.

   B. human societies are far more complex than the cells that constitute a single human body.

   C. comparisons between any two ideas can only ever be imprecise.

   D. transgressors are not treated identically under utopian and dystopian social orders.

4. The author refers to *The Handmaid's Tale* in paragraph 3 in order to:

   A. argue that women are just as talented as men at writing speculative fiction.

   B. challenge the idea that society should be organized rationally.

   C. give an example of utopian literature that explores the concept of instrumental rationality.

   D. offer an instance of a novel in which humans are treated as means rather than ends.

5. Based on the discussion in paragraph 4, which of the following would be LEAST likely to be regarded as a transgressor?

   A. A citizen of a dystopia who tries to lead a rebellion against the powers that be

   B. A citizen of a utopia who neglects political duties to spend more time with loved ones

   C. An official in a dystopian society who uses torture to reprogram disobedient citizens

   D. A criminal in a utopian society who is punished for questioning the state's legitimacy

6. The author's primary concern in the passage is to:

   A. advocate for the superiority of dystopian over utopian fiction.

   B. discuss the characteristics of utopian and dystopian literature.

   C. challenge the notion that human life is a problem to be solved.

   D. argue that the most politically relevant emotions are hope and fear.

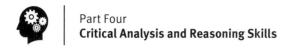

16.4 CARS Practice Passage II

PRACTICE PASSAGE II: A HISTORY PASSAGE

Using the Kaplan Method

(QUESTIONS 7–11)

In the late 18th century, citizens throughout rural Massachusetts shut down courthouses in an attempt to conduct debt collection hearings, farmers in western Pennsylvania and other parts of the western frontier refused to pay an excise on whiskey, and members of the Pennsylvania Dutch community harassed officials attempting to assess a direct tax on houses. In each case, the government's initial response to protests of "taxation without representation" led to an exacerbation of tensions: radicalized citizens banded together, creating armed militias in open rebellion against the ruling regime.

These popular uprisings against taxation and economic hardship were not—as many Americans would now assume when hearing such descriptions—revolts against the British monarchy in prelude to the American Revolution (1775–1783). Rather, Shays' Rebellion (1786–1787), the Whiskey Rebellion (1791–1794), and Fries's Rebellion (1798–1800) occurred after the British had been vanquished. Although each episode has distinctive historical significance, it is particularly instructive to examine the evolving reaction to popular protests by the incipient U.S. government.

In the case of the uprisings throughout western and central Massachusetts that would come collectively to be known as Shays' Rebellion, the federal government existed in a much attenuated form, enfeebled as a result of the considerable amount of sovereignty ceded to the 13 original states under the Articles of Confederation. After subsistence farmers, veterans of the Continental Army, and other rural citizens found themselves hard-pressed in 1786 by debts incurred during hard times and taxes newly levied by the Massachusetts government, they began to revolt, at first closing down courts but soon organizing armed militias, culminating in an attempt led by veteran Daniel Shays to seize a federal armory in Springfield, Massachusetts. The federal government lacked the funds to assemble its own militia and counter the uprising, so it was left to the governor of Massachusetts, James Bowdoin, to handle—and he had to turn to assistance from more than 100 wealthy merchants to bankroll mercenaries, who quashed the rebels.

The moneyed and propertied interests—creditors to whom many debts were owed—had been unnerved by the events in Massachusetts, and they were instrumental in creating and ratifying the new Constitution, which greatly concentrated power in a more robust central government. When many western farmers refused to pay a 1791 excise tax on whiskey, the newly empowered federal government was able to muster a formidable response after resistance grew more organized. In 1794, President Washington himself led a massive federalized militia of nearly 13,000 troops that would effortlessly scatter the resistance forces. The reaction by President Adams to the smaller rebellion led by John Fries years later would be similarly heavy-handed.

This tendency toward increased centralization of power has only worsened since the 18th century. As the federal government has accumulated strength, state and municipal governments—and, ultimately, the people—have lost their sovereignty. And although the moneyed had to foot the bill directly to protect their property (and continue collecting their rents) in quelling Shays' Rebellion, since the adoption of the new Constitution in 1789, the federal government has been able to make the people pay directly for their own repression—a fact recently highlighted in the assault, covertly orchestrated across several cities by the Federal Bureau of Investigation and the Department of Homeland Security, on the 2011 Occupy movement. In the end, the people have traded one master for another: the feudal relic of British monarchy has been usurped by a modern bureaucratic behemoth, ultimately in thrall to the nouveau aristocracy of corporate persons and the rapacious class of executives that constitute the homunculi within.

7. The author writes in paragraph 5 that "the federal government has been able to make the people pay directly for their own repression." Based on the rest of the passage, this is most likely intended to signify that:

   A. popular uprisings no longer occur in the United States because of the more successful control of citizens.

   B. imprisoned protestors are sent a bill for the expenses accrued while they are behind bars.

   C. protesting ultimately incurs worse consequences for individuals today than it did in the 18th century.

   D. the government requires citizens to pay taxes, which are partly used to fund police and military responses to protests.

8. The author's attitude toward "moneyed and propertied interests" (paragraph 4) can best be characterized as:

   A. indifferent.

   B. positive.

   C. negative.

   D. ambivalent.

9. The author most likely omits specific details of the events in the first paragraph in order to:

   A. set an expectation that is reversed in the following paragraph.

   B. express the primary thesis of the passage more concisely.

   C. downplay the significance of the events being addressed.

   D. conceal a general lack of knowledge on the subject matter.

10. Which of the following is assumed by the author in the second paragraph?

    A. The response to Fries's Rebellion was more heavy-handed than the response to Shays' Rebellion.

    B. The British monarchy is entirely unlike the U.S. federal government that eventually replaced it.

    C. A significant number of Americans today are unfamiliar with the rebellions that occurred after the American Revolution.

    D. The British played a covert role in the rebellions that took place after their defeat in the American Revolution.

11. Some scholars have argued that in response to the 2007–2008 financial crisis, the U.S. federal government did less to protect citizens whose homes were taken away in fraudulent foreclosures than to defend the banks that engaged in this criminal behavior. If true, what impact does this have on the passage?

    A. It challenges the author's central argument.

    B. It supports the author's central argument.

    C. It weakens the assertion that the U.S. people have exchanged one master for another.

    D. It strengthens the claim that the wealthy shaped the creation of the U.S. Constitution.

Practice Passage I Explanations

PRACTICE PASSAGE I: A HUMANITIES PASSAGE

1. (A)

Look at the line in context to get a better sense of what to expect: "As with their emotional antecedents, utopia and dystopia are inextricably intertwined, evident in their deep structural commonalities." The "emotional antecedents" refers to the discussion of hope and fear in the first paragraph, which noted how "one always accompanies the other," even though one might come to dominate for a time. **(A)**, which suggests that a dystopian society always looks like a utopian one from the perspective of the rulers, would definitely support this point, showing how utopia is inseparable from dystopia.

(B) Opposite. In the third paragraph, the author notes that "instrumental rationality," featured regularly in dystopian fiction, creates a society in which "citizens are mere means for the advancement of political ends, which must remain unexamined." If utopias allowed the examination of political ends, this would constitute a point of difference rather than a similarity.

(C) Opposite. Violence is addressed predominately in the fourth paragraph where the author discusses commonalities between utopia and dystopia. Because utopias are suggested to be violent, this choice would create another point of difference if true.

(D) Faulty Use of Detail. Although this choice does not weaken the claim, as the other wrong answer choices do, it is largely irrelevant. Just because utopia and dystopia are both absent sometimes does not mean they must always occur together, as "inextricably intertwined" suggests.

2. (B)

Roman numeral I appears twice, so begin with it. Violence is discussed in the fourth paragraph as a commonality between utopian and dystopian literature, so this is not a point of difference. Because I is false, **(A)** and **(D)** can be eliminated. Numeral III must be true because it appears in the two remaining options (confirmed by a line from the fourth paragraph: "From the transgressor's perspective, a vantage taken up far more commonly in novels of dystopia . . ."). So only II needs to be evaluated. At the end of the second paragraph, the author asserts, "Utopian fiction celebrates human potential, particularly the power of reason . . ." So utopian literature does emphasize reason. In the third paragraph, the author discusses the crucial role that "instrumental rationality" ("the dark side of human reason") plays in *We* and a number of other dystopian novels. As another point of similarity, II is thus false, so **(C)** is wrong. Because only III is true, **(B)** is correct.

3. (A)

Return to the line in context: "Such free spirits cannot be tolerated within the body politic any more than a cancerous cell within the body physical. The analogy is imperfect, of course, because a tumor does not feel." The suggestion is that humans are different from cells. They deserve to be considered as more than just expendable parts of a larger whole because they (unlike tumors and other cells) *can* feel. **(A)** matches most closely with this reasoning.

(B) In the analogy, cells (parts of the larger whole that is the body) are being likened to people (parts of the larger whole that is society). This choice mischaracterizes the analogy because it compares the whole on one side (society) to the parts on the other (cells).

(C) Distortion. The author is not suggesting that every analogy is imperfect, only that the particular analogy being discussed is.

(D) Although this might pose a different kind of problem for the analogy, it does not make sense in context. The author cites "a tumor does not feel" as a reason for the breakdown, which has nothing to do with the differences between utopia and dystopia.

4. (D)

In the third paragraph, the author lays out the various characteristics of dystopian fiction, emphasizing especially the idea of "instrumental rationality," which is described as "a robotic logic in which efficiency is valued for its own sake, and citizens are mere means for the advancement of political ends, which must remain unexamined." The author mentions "Margaret Atwood's *The Handmaid's Tale*" as part of a list of icons of dystopia and so is giving an example of a novel that explores the concept of instrumental rationality. Thus, **(D)** is correct.

(A) Out of Scope. The author never discusses gender explicitly and never compares authors of different genders.

(B) Although the author seems to be critical of instrumental reason in this paragraph, the idea is not significantly challenged until the fifth paragraph.

(C) Opposite. *The Handmaid's Tale* is said to be one of the icons of dystopia. So it would not be utopian fiction, as suggested by this choice.

5. (C)

To determine the least likely example, first clarify what the author means by a transgressor in the fourth paragraph: "the individual who would privilege personal desires over the ironclad imperatives of state." Someone would not be a transgressor if he or she acted on behalf of the state, such as an official who was trying to reprogram actual transgressors in a dystopian society, as in **(C)**.

(A) Opposite. This would be a textbook case of transgression because the citizen is fighting against the state (*the powers that be*).

(B) Opposite. Although this might not seem so bad, this would count as privileging some other value over the state. So the individual would be a transgressor.

(D) Opposite. Questioning the society's legitimacy would clearly be acting against the imperatives of state, so this criminal would count as a transgressor.

6. (B)

Although the author begins with a discussion of hope and fear in the first paragraph, the primary focus of every other paragraph is on the qualities of utopian and dystopian fiction, as in **(B)**.

(A) Out of Scope. The author primarily emphasizes the similarities between the two genres and never really suggests that one is better than the other.

(C) Faulty Use of Detail. This is raised only in the final paragraph, so it does not address the passage as a whole.

(D) Faulty Use of Detail. The argument concerning hope and fear is almost entirely limited to the first paragraph. It serves as an introduction to utopia (which represents hope) and dystopia (which represents fear) but is not the primary concern of the entire passage.

Practice Passage II Explanations

PRACTICE PASSAGE II: A HISTORY PASSAGE

7. (D)

Read the quote from the question stem in context to get a sense of what to look for: "And although the moneyed had to foot the bill directly . . . in quelling Shays' Rebellion, since the adoption of the new Constitution in 1789, the federal government has been able to make the people pay directly for their own repression." The contrast with Shays' Rebellion is instructive. The author notes in the third paragraph that "the federal government lacked the funds to assemble its own militia and counter the uprising." However, this is not a problem in the fourth paragraph with the federal response to the Whiskey Rebellion. The inference to be drawn is that the new government can levy taxes, which it can then use to respond to a popular uprising—even if that uprising is itself a reaction to the taxes levied, as was the case with the Whiskey Rebellion. The only answer that reflects this line of thinking is (D).

(A) Opposite. The author cites a recent example (the 2011 Occupy movement) of a kind of popular uprising immediately after raising this point, so this choice is contradicted by the passage.

(B) Out of Scope. Although this offers a possible explanation, the passage never discusses anything of this sort.

(C) Out of Scope. No comparison is ever made between the kinds of consequences dissenters face today versus the 18th century, so this choice could not reflect the passage.

8. (C)

Although the language used to describe the "moneyed and propertied interests" tends to be relatively neutral in the fourth paragraph, the author's negative attitude toward the wealthy comes through in the fifth paragraph. This is particularly true in the closing sentence, with the mention of a "rapacious class of executives." Thus, (C) is correct.

(A) Although the author is relatively neutral in the fourth paragraph, the language used in the fifth paragraph suggests that the author is far from indifferent.

(B) Opposite. The author never says anything positive about the moneyed.

(D) Because the author says nothing to praise the wealthy but uses only negative language in describing them, this indicates that the author's attitude is not one of ambivalence (a mix of positive and negative feelings).

9. (A)

Although this is ostensibly a question about the first paragraph, properly answering it requires understanding how the first paragraph connects to the rest of the passage. A key hint comes in the transition into the second paragraph: "These popular uprisings against taxation and economic hardship were not—as many Americans would now assume when hearing such descriptions—revolts against the British monarchy . . ." The author has made the descriptions in the first paragraph deliberately ambiguous to create an expectation (these tax protests are against unfair British taxes) that is almost immediately overturned (the protests are actually against taxes imposed by American authorities). This serves to highlight the fact that the American officials were acting just as unfairly as the British. This corresponds most closely to (A).

(B) Although concise expression would be a reason to omit details, the primary thesis does not really emerge until later in the passage, particularly in the final paragraph.

(C) Opposite. This choice is contradicted by the discussion in the second paragraph, where the author notes that "each episode has distinctive historical significance" and goes on to state how "particularly instructive" their contrast is.

(D) Opposite. Plenty of details are provided in the third and fourth paragraphs. So it's clear that the author does not generally lack knowledge about the subject.

10. (C)

Be sure to stick to the discussion in the second paragraph because the question stem specifically references it. The author suggests that "many Americans would now assume" that the rebellions described in the first paragraph were against British authorities when the rebellions were actually against American authorities. In suggesting that many Americans will make that assumption, the author is actually assuming these individuals are unfamiliar with the events described and would not be able to recognize the events from their descriptions. This matches with **(C)**.

(A) Although the end of the fourth paragraph suggests that the reactions to the Whiskey Rebellion and Fries' Rebellion were both heavy-handed, this is not an assumption made in the second paragraph.

(B) Opposite. The author deliberately compares the American Revolution against the British monarchy to these rebellions against American authorities to highlight similarities, not differences.

(D) Out of Scope. The passage does not suggest that the British played any role in these rebellions. The British are merely raised as a point of comparison.

11. (B)

The situation described in the question stem seems to echo the idea from the last sentence, that the U.S. federal government is "ultimately in thrall to the nouveau aristocracy of corporate persons and the rapacious class of executives that constitute the homunculi within." This is an aspect of the author's central argument, that the people have been disempowered as more power has been accumulated in the federal government and that this government represents the interests of the wealthy first and foremost. Thus, **(B)** is right.

(A) Opposite. As explained previously, the author's argument is actually bolstered by the new information.

(C) Opposite. If anything, this claim would be strengthened because the evidence in the question stem makes it clear that the people are not in charge.

(D) Although the new situation makes it clear that the wealthy have influence in the 21st century, this in itself proves nothing about what happened in the 18th century, when the new Constitution was created and ratified (explained in the fourth paragraph).